Progress and pathology

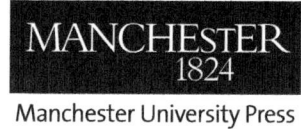
Manchester University Press

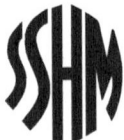

SOCIAL HISTORIES OF MEDICINE

Series editors: David Cantor and Keir Waddington

Social Histories of Medicine is concerned with all aspects of health, illness and medicine, from prehistory to the present, in every part of the world. The series covers the circumstances that promote health or illness, the ways in which people experience and explain such conditions, and what, practically, they do about them. Practitioners of all approaches to health and healing come within its scope, as do their ideas, beliefs, and practices, and the social, economic and cultural contexts in which they operate. Methodologically, the series welcomes relevant studies in social, economic, cultural, and intellectual history, as well as approaches derived from other disciplines in the arts, sciences, social sciences and humanities. The series is a collaboration between Manchester University Press and the Society for the Social History of Medicine.

Previously published

The metamorphosis of autism *Bonnie Evans*

Payment and philanthropy in British healthcare, 1918–48 *George Campbell Gosling*

The politics of vaccination *Edited by Christine Holmberg, Stuart Blume and Paul Greenough*

Leprosy and colonialism *Stephen Snelders*

Medical misadventure in an age of professionalization, 1780–1890 *Alannah Tomkins*

Conserving health in early modern culture *Edited by Sandra Cavallo and Tessa Storey*

Migrant architects of the NHS *Julian M. Simpson*

Mediterranean quarantines, 1750–1914 *Edited by John Chircop and Francisco Javier Martínez*

Sickness, medical welfare and the English poor, 1750–1834 *Steven King*

Medical societies and scientific culture in nineteenth-century Belgium *Joris Vandendriessche*

Managing diabetes, managing medicine *Martin D. Moore*

Vaccinating Britain *Gareth Millward*

Madness on trial *James E. Moran*

Early Modern Ireland and the world of medicine *Edited by John Cunningham*

Feeling the strain *Jill Kirby*

Rhinoplasty and the nose in early modern British medicine and culture *Emily Cock*

Communicating the history of medicine *Edited by Solveig Jülich and Sven Widmalm*

Progress and pathology

Medicine and culture in the nineteenth century

Edited by
Melissa Dickson, Emilie Taylor-Brown,
and Sally Shuttleworth

Manchester University Press

Copyright © Manchester University Press 2020

While copyright in the volume as a whole is vested in Manchester University Press, copyright in individual chapters belongs to their respective authors, and no chapter may be reproduced wholly or in part without the express permission in writing of both author and publisher.

An electronic version of this book is also available under a Creative Commons (CC-BY-NC-ND) licence which permits non-commercial use, distribution and reproduction provided the editors, chapter authors and Manchester University Press are fully cited and no modifications or adaptations are made. Details of the licence can be viewed at https://creativecommons.org/licenses/by-nc-nd/4.0/legalcode

Published by Manchester University Press
Altrincham Street, Manchester M1 7JA

www.manchesteruniversitypress.co.uk

British Library Cataloguing-in-Publication Data
A catalogue record for this book is available from the British Library

ISBN   978 1 5261 3368 7   hardback

ISBN   978 1 5261 4754 7   open access

First published 2020

The publisher has no responsibility for the persistence or accuracy of URLs for any external or third-party internet websites referred to in this book, and does not guarantee that any content on such websites is, or will remain, accurate or appropriate.

Typeset
by Toppan Best-set Premedia Limited
Printed in Great Britain
by TJ International Ltd, Padstow

Contents

List of figures and tables	*page* vii
List of contributors	ix
Acknowledgements	xiii
Introduction *Melissa Dickson, Emilie Taylor-Brown, and Sally Shuttleworth*	1
Part I: Constructing the modern self	25
1. Revolutionary shocks: the French human sciences and the crafting of modern subjectivity, 1794–1816 *Laurens Schlicht*	27
2. Medical negligence in nineteenth-century Germany *Torsten Riotte*	56
3. Imperfect bodies: the 'pathology' of childhood in late nineteenth-century London *Steven Taylor*	78
4. Phrenology as neurodiversity: the Fowlers and modern brain disorder *Kristine Swenson*	99
Part II: Paradoxes of modern living	125
5. A disease-free world: the hygienic utopia in Jules Verne, Camille Flammarion, and William Morris *Manon Mathias*	127

6. 'Drooping with the century': fatigue and the *fin de siècle* 153
   Steffan Blayney
7. 'A rebellion of the cells': cancer, modernity, and decline in *fin-de-siècle* Britain 173
   Agnes Arnold-Forster
8. The curse and the gift of modernity in late nineteenth-century suicide discourse in Finland 194
   Mikko Myllykangas

Part III: Negotiating global modernities 215
9. From physiograms to cosmograms: Daktar Binodbihari Ray Kabiraj and the metaphorics of the nineteenth-century Ayurvedic body 217
   Projit Bihari Mukharji
10. From Schenectady to Shanghai: Dr Williams' Pink Pills for Pale People and the hybrid pathways of Chinese modernity 247
    Alice Tsay
11. Poisonous arrows and unsound minds: hysterical tetanus in the Victorian South Pacific 269
    Daniel Simpson

Part IV: Reflections and provocation 293
12. What is your *complaint*? Health as moral economy in the long nineteenth century 295
    Christopher Hamlin

Bibliography 328
Index 364

Figures and tables

Figures

4.1	'Numbering and Definition of the Organs', O. S. Fowler and L. N. Fowler, *The Illustrated Self-Instructor in Phrenology and Physiology with over One Hundred Engravings* (New York: Fowler and Wells, 1859), p. vi.	page 106
4.2	'Parental Love', O. S. Fowler and L. N. Fowler, *The Illustrated Self-Instructor in Phrenology and Physiology with over One Hundred Engravings* (New York: Fowler and Wells, 1859), p. 81.	107
9.1	Nagendranath Sengupta, *Sachitra Susruta Samhita*. Author's personal collection.	234
9.2	Gopalchandra Sengupta, *Ayurveda Samgraha* (Calcutta, 1871). Author's personal collection.	235
9.3	Lecture on the Nervous System from 1860. Wellcome Images.	236
10.1	Dr Williams' Pink Pills for Pale People. Wellcome Images.	250
10.2	1915 *Shenbao* advertisement for Dr Williams' Pink Pills featuring testimonies from Mr Cui Xiwu (top) and Mr Zhao Shaoqin (bottom). The advertisement,	

published on 3 April 1915, is now in the public
domain. Original copy used for this scan belongs
to the University of Michigan.   259
10.3 Dr Williams' yuefenpai poster designed by Hang
Zhiying, 1922. Museum of Applied Arts and Sciences.
Photo Credit: Penelope Clay.   262

Tables

8.1	Suicide per 1 million inhabitants in Finland, 1841–90	*page* 206
10.1	Contents of Dr Williams' Pink Pills for Pale People	252

Contributors

Agnes Arnold-Forster is a Wellcome Trust funded Postdoctoral Researcher at the University of Roehampton. She received her PhD on the history of cancer in nineteenth-century Britain from King's College London in 2017 and now works on the emotional landscape of the NHS from 1948 to the present. She has been published by *Social History of Medicine*, *Gender & History*, and the *British Medical Journal*.

Steffan Blayney is a Research Fellow in the Department of History at the University of Sheffield. His research focuses on the relations between health, the body, and society, and on histories of political activism in modern and contemporary Britain.

Melissa Dickson is a Lecturer in Victorian Literature at the University of Birmingham. She has a PhD from King's College, London, and an MPhil, BA, and University Medal from the University of Queensland, Australia. She is the author of *Cultural Encounters with the Arabian Nights in Nineteenth-Century Britain* (2019) and co-author of *Anxious Times: Medicine and Modernity in the Nineteenth Century* (2019).

Christopher Hamlin is a historian of science, technology, and medicine, Professor in the Department of History and the Program in the History and Philosophy of Science at the University of Notre Dame, and Honorary Professor at the London School of Hygiene and Tropical

Medicine. His research focuses broadly on the application of knowledge to public needs, mainly in areas relating to health. In nearly six dozen articles and several books, he has examined concepts of disease and disease causation, forensic science and expert disagreement, the assessment of water and air, the regulation of environmental nuisances, social epidemiology (focusing on issues of hunger and exposure), alternative agricultures, and cultural and religious concepts of nature. He is author of *A Science of Impurity* (1990), *Public Health and Social Justice in the Age of Chadwick: Britain, 1800–1854* (1998), *Cholera: The Biography* (2009), *More than HOT: A Short History of Fever* (2014), and most recently co-editor of *Global Forensic Cultures* (2019).

Manon Mathias is a Lecturer in French at the University of Glasgow. She has published several book chapters and journal articles on the nineteenth-century novel, particularly the works of George Sand. Her monograph, *Vision in the Novels of George Sand*, was published in 2016. Her current research project focuses on the digestive system in nineteenth-century French medicine and culture. She is the co-editor of *Gut Feeling and Digestive Health in Nineteenth-Century Literature, History and Culture* (2018).

Projit Bihari Mukharji is an Associate Professor at the University of Pennsylvania. He was educated in India and the UK and researches the histories of science and medicine in modern South Asia. Mukharji is particularly interested in how different traditions of knowledge making interact. He is the author of two monographs, *Nationalizing the Body: The Medical Market, Print and Daktari Medicine* (2009) and *Doctoring Traditions: Ayurveda, Small Technologies and Braided Sciences* (2016).

Mikko Myllykangas is a Postdoctoral Researcher in the History of Sciences and Ideas at the University of Oulu, Finland. In 2014, he defended his doctoral dissertation, in which he studied the medicalisation of suicide and the history of medical suicide research in Finland in the nineteenth and twentieth centuries. Since then, he has done research on the history of social psychiatry and psychiatric epidemiology of suicide, on the history of child suicide, and on the history of suicide prevention during the modern era. Currently, he is working on the history of stress and the proliferation of the concept of stress in the discourses of psychiatric and somatic medicine.

Torsten Riotte is currently Acting Professor for Modern European History at the University of Tübingen. Educated at Cologne and Cambridge, he has worked at the German Historical Institute, London, and the Goethe University Frankfurt. He has published widely on nineteenth-century European history with a special focus on Germany, Britain, and France. His latest research project deals with medical malpractice and professional liability insurance in nineteenth-century Germany as part of a broader study on the transformation of individual and collective responsibility in Modern Europe.

Laurens Schlicht is a historian of science and a Research Associate on the 'Mind Reading as Cultural Practice' project based at Humboldt University in Berlin. He has a PhD from Frankfurt University and is author of *Tabula Rasa: Beobachtung von Sprache und Geist am Menschen in der Société des observateurs de l'homme 1789–1830* (forthcoming), and co-editor of *Mind Reading as Cultural Practice* (forthcoming).

Sally Shuttleworth is a Professor of English Literature at the University of Oxford. She has published extensively on the inter-relations of science and culture, including *George Eliot and Nineteenth-Century Science* (1984), *Charlotte Brontë and Victorian Psychology* (1996), and *The Mind of the Child: Child Development in Literature, Science and Medicine, 1840–1900* (2010). Between 2014 and 2019 she directed two large research projects, 'Constructing Scientific Communities: Citizen Science in the 19th and 21st centuries', www.conscicom.org (AHRC funded) and 'Diseases of Modern Life: Nineteenth-Century Perspectives', www.diseasesofmodernlife.org (ERC funded).

Daniel Simpson is a Caird Fellow at the National Maritime Museum. His research interests include the history of ethnographic collecting by the Royal Navy in Australia in the late eighteenth and nineteenth centuries, and the circulation of museum objects through British ports. He is currently writing a book, provisionally titled *The Royal Navy in Indigenous Australia, 1795–1855: Maritime Encounters and Museum Collections*.

Kristine Swenson is a Professor and Department Chair in English and Technical Communication at Missouri University of Science and Technology in Rolla, MO. Her research areas are Victorian literature and culture, literature and medicine, and women's cultural history. Swenson's publications include *Medical Women in Victorian Fiction* (2005); 'Mindblindness: Metaphor and Neuroaesthetics in the Works of Silas Weir Mitchell and Simon Baron-Cohen', *Literature, Neurology and Neuroscience: Historical and Literary Connections*, Progress in Brain Research, 205 (2013); and 'Scholarship in Victorian women and medicine: a critical overview', *Literature Compass*, 10:5 (May 2013), 461–72. Her most recent scholarly projects concern heterodox medical practices, particularly as they were employed by women practitioners.

Steven J. Taylor is a historian of childhood and medicine. His research explores ideas and constructions of childhood health, lay and professional diagnoses, ability and disability, and institutional care. His first monograph, *Beyond the Asylum: Child Insanity in England, 1845–1907*, was published in 2017. He is currently researching the experience of special schools in the early twentieth century as a Wellcome Trust ISSF Fellow at the University of Leicester.

Emilie Taylor-Brown is a Postdoctoral Researcher on the ERC-funded 'Diseases of Modern Life: Nineteenth-Century Perspectives' project based at the University of Oxford. She is currently writing two monographs: one on Victorian understandings of gut health, the other on parasitology and the British literary imagination in the nineteenth century. Her research interests include history of medicine, health humanities, nineteenth-century fiction, and literature and science studies.

Alice Tsay earned her PhD in English Language and Literature as well as a Graduate Certificate in Museum Studies from the University of Michigan. She works in the Office of the President at The Huntington Library, Art Collections, and Botanical Gardens and previously held the role of Director for Library Programming and Public Affairs at Pepperdine University in Malibu, California.

Acknowledgements

Progress and pathology is the product of a large European Research Council project, 'Diseases of Modern Life: Nineteenth-Century Perspectives', led by Sally Shuttleworth and funded from the European Research Council (ERC) under the European Union's Seventh Framework Programme ERC Grant Agreement number 340121. We are extremely grateful to the ERC for making this research possible, and for giving us the freedom and the time to develop our ideas over the past five and a half years. The project has involved a large team of researchers and we have benefitted immensely from years of interdisciplinary research and collaboration, as well as from the lively programme of seminars, workshops, and conferences run by the project. The chapters in this volume are the outcome of a two day interdisciplinary conference on medicine and modernity which took place at St Anne's College, Oxford in 2016, and we are grateful to all our interlocutors at this early stage, and team members Amelia Bonea and Jennifer Wallis who helped organise the conference. Profuse thanks are also owed to St Anne's College, Oxford, who have housed the project since its inception, and been an endless source of practical and intellectual support.

Introduction
Melissa Dickson, Emilie Taylor-Brown, and Sally Shuttleworth

Nervous exhaustion, wrote the New York physician and early neurologist George Miller Beard in 1881, is 'a result and accompaniment and barometer of civilisation'.[1] Throughout his study, *American Nervousness*, Beard was very explicit in drawing out the relationship between the new technologies, work, and education patterns of a modernising, industrialising society, and the nervous exhaustion, or what he called neurasthenia, of its subjects. The human nervous system had been held culpable for a range of diseases since at least the late seventeenth century, and anxieties about nervous diseases and other mental ailments arising from the general pressures of modern life were not unique to America in the nineteenth century. Nonetheless, Beard insisted upon the distinct status of neurasthenia not simply as a general condition of modern life, but as a culturally specific, new disease with characteristic symptoms that were induced by that life.[2] In support of this claim, he drew together medical hypotheses with cultural critique and social observation, constructing the figure of the neurasthenic as one who both produces, and is produced by, the practices and structures of industrial modernity. Only the nineteenth century, Beard insisted, was capable of suffering from neurasthenia because, while other civilisations had undoubtedly experienced weak nerves and fatigue, it was this period alone that had produced the five elements which he believed inculcated such severe nervous exhaustion: 'Steam power, the periodical press, the telegraph, the sciences, and the mental activity of women.'[3]

Held in a continual state of socio-cultural, economic, and technological flux, the nineteenth-century American citizen was supposedly living in an almost permanent state of nervousness. Furthermore, Beard noted, because America, a 'young and rapidly growing nation, with civil, religious, and social liberty', was more advanced in each of these categories than any other nation, it was only natural that nervous exhaustion was more pronounced in the United States than it was anywhere else in the world.[4]

Beard's insistence upon the profound connection between the social and economic factors of modern living, and the state of the nerves, was distinctly nationalistic in its avowal of neurasthenia as a malady of what he deemed to be the most evolved, 'civilised' societies. This may, in part, account for the fact that the term neurasthenia was not widely used to refer to conditions relating to overwork and fatigue outside the United States. Beard's nationalism is, moreover, increasingly problematic throughout his analysis, as it is deployed to establish national and racial hierarchies in the context of modernity and modernisation, and to affirm the superior status of American social and economic institutions globally. Beard's descriptions of the disease were, as David Schuster has noted, 'rife with religious, racial, and regional assumptions'.[5] Those peoples Beard regarded as content to live in ignorance, indifferent to science or the mysteries of life, or who lived robust, 'primitive' lives without overexerting their mental faculties, were supposedly spared the sufferings of the neurasthenic. Thus, Schuster notes, 'by explaining who was not susceptible to neurasthenia – Catholics, southerners, Indians, blacks – Beard was framing neurasthenia as a primarily white, Anglo-Saxon, Protestant, Yankee condition'.[6] Implicit in Beard's claims is a form of social change whereby 'civilisation', figured here as an external and rather violent force, '*invades* any nation' in the form of specific social and technological innovations, and individuals react by feeling overworked, overstimulated, fatigued, and generally anxious.[7] He assumes a global history of discontinuous, asynchronous cultures on an imperial scale, against which societies might measure and define themselves as more or less neurotic, and therefore as more or less 'modern'. Disease itself becomes for Beard a marker of industrial and technological modernity, the privilege of the overcultured and the affluent, and a critical component of the national identity.[8] Neurasthenia, or 'Americanitis' as it was sometimes dubbed, was, as one New

York doctor reflected in 1904, one of the nation's 'most distinctive and precious pathological possessions', and an 'important stimulus to patriotism and racial solidarity'.[9] The pathological conditions seeming to emanate from specific changes in the social and physical environment were, at least for some, a matter of national pride.[10]

The present volume, which examines the correlations that were being drawn between notions of progress and pathology across a diverse range of socio-economic cultures in the long nineteenth century beginning with the French Revolution, interrogates such notions of exceptionalism. Our purview is deliberately transnational, drawing on case studies from Britain, America, France, Germany, Finland, Bengal, China, and the South Pacific, in order to provide rich comparative perspectives on medical responses to, and constructions of, modernity, while demonstrating that anxieties about mental and physical ailments arising from the general pressures of modern life were not unique to America, or to Britain, in the nineteenth century, but engendered concern across national boundaries and cultures. Central to this study is the question of how self-referential concepts of 'the modern' worked to structure perceptions of health, disease, and medical treatment in the long nineteenth century. Neurasthenia was not the only disease constituted in relation to problems of modernity or to national character. Similar claims were, as our volume demonstrates, made around the world for other conditions such as fatigue, cancer, suicide, and general cultural or intellectual degeneration. Analogous concerns about the interaction between the environment and individual and social well-being also emerged in movements for self-improvement and self-care, public health and sanitation, and the 'rescue' and reform of the poor and disabled. These preoccupations influenced public policies, with numerous commissions and scientific inquiries into, for example, incidences of suicide and other causes of death amongst expanding urban populations, and instances of medical negligence and professional accountability. Through such activities, new connections were established between environmental conditions, social pressures, and bodily and mental pathologies. By highlighting such intricate interactions across the history of literature, psychiatry, and social and public health and reform in the nineteenth century, the chapters in this volume seek to understand more broadly how societies and discourses construct and formulate health and disease.

Nineteenth-century advances in the fields of technology, science, and medicine, while clearly constituting 'progress' for some, nonetheless prompted deep concern about the problems and pathologies that would potentially be induced by modern life. An increasing number of references to the problems of 'modern times' and to the 'wear and tear' of modern life can be traced throughout the nineteenth-century medical and general press across national boundaries and cultures. In Italy in 1891, for example, the physiologist Angelo Mosso's La Fatica famously proffered his formulation of the laws pertaining to exhaustion, while in Russia in 1879, the psychologist I. A. Sikorskii studied various conditions of mental fatigue in young people over the course of the school day.[11] In Germany the shocking number of suicides occurring among secondary school students was attributed to the extreme mental and physical overburdening of school children, and such a mass of German literature emerged on the subject of mental overpressure that the politician August Reichensperger observed that simply staying abreast of the proliferating number of pamphlets and articles addressing the issue could overburden the mind.[12] The poet Victor Laprade similarly decried what he called the *'L'Éducation homicide'* of French lycées and colleges, describing theirs as a 'regimen entirely contrary to nature, which lowers the vital force and enervates the constitution of both the individual and the race subjected to it for too long'.[13] The physician Aimé Riant in his study, *Le surmènage intellectuel*, in 1889, and Alfred Binet and Victor Henri in their work, *La Fatigue intellectuelle*, in 1898, equally registered their alarm at what they considered to be the chronic overwork and exhaustion of young French citizens.[14] At times, as Anson Rabinbach has shown in his study of *The Human Motor* (1992), the scientific and cultural frameworks through which notions of progress and industry were deployed drew on remarkably similar metaphors pertaining to work, energy, and exhaustion. In nations with distinctive politics, practices, and body imaginaries, stress, fatigue, and nervous exhaustion were generally deemed to be the inevitable corollaries of the pressures and pace of modern civilisation.

'Life at high pressure' was, according to the eminent London-based physician Thomas Stretch Dowse, 'the prominent feature of the nineteenth century', and tracing this concept across nineteenth-century cultures affords new insights into both popular and medical understandings of the body and mind. Dowse declared in his 1880 study of brain and nerve exhaustion that 'we cannot be surprised when we find that the so-called nervous diseases and exhaustions, dipsomania and insanity, are increasing beyond all proportion to the rapid increase of the population'.[15] People were suffering as never before, he believed, from varying states of physical and mental exhaustion, which were themselves symptoms of a much broader national deterioration. Here again, it seems, a nation's pride was at stake, as Dowse draws a direct correlation between a general decline in the country's health, and its future standing in a competitive industrial economy.[16] In his 1875 address to the Royal Institution, published in an enlarged form in the *Contemporary Review* with the title 'Life at High Pressure', the manufacturer and journalist W. R. Greg similarly argued that the disconcertingly hurried pace of the 'high-pressure style of life' was the result of both technological and social factors.[17] First, the 'rapidity of railway travelling', which, Greg noted, 'produces a kind of chronic disturbance in the nervous system of those who use it much', had forever accelerated the individual's rate of movement.[18] Secondly, he argued, the incessant demands placed upon professional and public figures such as lawyers, physicians, ministers, and politicians – 'even', he noted, 'the literary workman or the eager man of science' – required 'a greater strain upon both bodily and mental powers, a sterner concentration of effort and of aim, and a more harsh and rigid sacrifice of the relaxations and amenities which time offers to the easy-going and unambitious'.[19] Excess physical and mental exertion, Greg makes clear, could disrupt or even deplete an exhausted nervous system, rendering it incapable of further function and highly susceptible to a range of diseases. A defining feature of the modern civilised subject, heightened nervousness was paradoxically rendering the human race less fit for survival.

It is a central aim of this volume to explore changing perceptions of health and disease in the context of burgeoning global modernities of the long nineteenth century. The concept of 'modernity', often defined exclusively by its Western or European model, is of course a relative term, often predicated on a break with the past across social, cultural, political, and economic institutions, and conferred by historians as a means of determining major shifts in orientation.[20] L. S. Jacyna, in his recent work on medicine and modernism, contends that historians have typically employed this term in such a manner, to 'refer to the interrelated series of economic, social, and political transformations that occurred in Western societies during the period of the long nineteenth century.'[21] However, 'modernity' is also a self-referential concept, an actors' category, employed and applied within any given social and cultural moment by those seeking to express what they regard as new conditions in the social, political, and economic order. In this view, as Shmuel N. Eisenstadt has argued, modernity is inherently multiple and contingent, with different groups of social actors 'holding very different views on what makes societies modern'.[22] Differences of perception are particularly marked once the question of modernity is placed in a global frame. It is these varying perceptions of modernity which we are concerned with here, as set within a distinctly medical framework, since understandings of the human mind and body were increasingly challenged, modified, and reframed by the politics and structures of 'modern life' in the long nineteenth century. Rather than seeking to determine what was precisely 'modern' about this historical moment, or indeed to label the period itself, or any specific geographical or cultural location as 'modern', we are interested in tracking a range of anxieties and varieties of experience, as they were expressed and explored in the literature, science, and medicine of the time in terms of their impact upon social, cultural, and medical formations of the mind and body. Our principal concern is how the structures of industrial, commercial, and technological modernity came to be deeply embedded within understandings of physiological and psychological identity. As a whole, therefore, this volume offers a series of explorations of the ways in which modernity was constructed and performed within a range of medical discourses across the nineteenth century. Together, these chapters demonstrate the complexity and relativity of the term 'modernity' itself, and its fundamental instability as a category of analysis in the history of medical practice.

As Charles E. Rosenberg suggested in his influential article, 'Pathologies of progress: the idea of civilization as risk', the 'use of disease incidence and theories of causation and pathology as vehicles for the articulation and legitimation of cultural criticism' have persisted for centuries, as 'disease has always been construed as both indicator and product of less than ideal social conditions'.[23] This 'progress-and-pathology narrative', to use Rosenberg's terminology, is an oft-recurring, yet extremely fluid narrative that 'can be used in a variety of contexts with a variety of social motives'.[24] As such, as this volume demonstrates, it has been appropriated for and implicated in a range of social, cultural, and psychological formations, providing a useful rhetorical framework for, but also affording insight into, the cultural and ideological characters of its users. By interrogating the deployment of this narrative across diverse modes of expression, we ultimately seek to establish the ways in which medical, political, and cultural discourses have interacted in defining concepts of health and disease as peculiarly 'modern'.[25]

Our concern to situate medical knowledge in relation to specific sites of social and cultural experience responds to recent currents in history of medicine scholarship which explore nineteenth-century anxieties about health and modernity. It has often been noted, for example, that the jarring effects of new modes of transport, machinery, communications technologies, and the expansion of print culture fundamentally altered human perceptions of space and time, and prompted concerns about the equivalent velocity necessary in human thought and action in order to keep pace.[26] The emergence in mid-Victorian Britain of the condition known as 'Railway Spine', a physical disorder often said to be caused by the excessive vibrations passing through the human body during railway travel, and the British *fin-de-siècle* condition known as 'Bicycle Face', in reference to the wild, staring eyes, strained expression, and projecting jaw of the avid female cyclist, were discrete complaints that have been explicitly connected to contemporary anxieties surrounding the effects on public health of modern technologies and the shocks and strains they imposed.[27] Similarly, concerns were being raised by British and French doctors in the 1860s surrounding the sexual excitement supposedly being induced in female users of the sewing machine.[28] In such diagnoses, it is clear that definitions and perceptions of disease actively inform and are informed by their broader social contexts in terms of class, race, gender, and sexual politics. In more general terms, also, however, conditions such as 'nervous shock' and 'traumatic hysteria', emergent in the nineteenth century, have been noted as medicalised expressions of the new and apparently shocking conditions of modern life in various contexts.[29] Socially and culturally inflected experiences of neurasthenia have also been located within a multiplicity of medical practices and across a range of modernising discourses, for example in imperial Germany, nineteenth-century Russia, modern China, and Victorian England.[30] In Japan, as Sabine Frühstück has argued, neurasthenia was closely connected to concerns about masculinity, masturbation, and homosexuality.[31] Contrastingly, debates about neurasthenia in nineteenth-century Argentina were, as Kristin Ruggiero's work on modern diseases in the national Argentinian identity demonstrates, deeply informed by historical, politicised disputes about national honour and social responsibility.[32] This particular disease of modern life carried different meanings in different social, cultural, and political contexts.

Part of the function of this collection, then, is to register both the disciplinary convergences that give rise to such diagnoses, and the varying and culturally specific conditions of what constituted medical modernity around the world. Nineteenth-century anxieties about health and modernity have attracted a good deal of attention in recent scholarship, much of this focusing upon discrete disease entities or conditions. The field of public and environmental health, for example, tends to be treated in isolation from consideration of nervous diseases, whilst work on nervous diseases has tended to look at single aspects within this category, such as neurasthenia, shock, or agoraphobia.[33] It is alongside such works that we situate *Progress and pathology*. However, rather than focusing on a specific condition or concern as symptomatic of the nineteenth-century psyche, we seek to address the broad range of ways in which anxieties about health and disease manifested themselves in the period. In its ambition and multidisciplinary scope, our project follows the path set by the Victorians themselves in the ways in which they traced the relationships between physiological, psychological, and social health, or disease. This kind of holistic approach was taken by a number of contemporary writers, most notably Benjamin Ward Richardson in his 1876 work, *Diseases of Modern Life*. In this volume, we intend to disrupt the frequent compartmentalisation of psychiatric, environmental, and literary histories in present practice, in order to re-contextualise the problems of modernity.[34] Taking our cue from Richardson's work, we thus address anxieties about physical debility, hygiene and sanitation, nervous illness and exhaustion, psychology and mental health, and commodity culture. Each of the following chapters represents a specific avenue of concern as it was expressed and explored by nineteenth-century commentators, and each case study shows how medicine, broadly and culturally conceived, is intricately embedded in, and responsive to, the larger worlds in which it operates. The emphasis of this work is deliberately interdisciplinary, as we strive to tease out the range of public and private practices in which the supposed ill effects of modern life were being mobilised, from developments in psychiatric and public health, to new forms of cancer and suicide research, to speculations as to what was being lost in the movement from subjectivity to biomedical objectivity. This diverse range of source material highlights the often close dialogue that took place between medical professionals and the general public via the pages of popular newspapers and magazines, and the circulation of medico-scientific knowledge. In analysing these interactions, we demonstrate that debates concerning the impact of modern life on mental and physical well-being were being voiced across disciplines, in discussions that dovetailed with constructions of modern selfhood in medical, psychological, political, and literary spheres.

Medicine serves a crucial intermediary role in the processes of negotiation between the self and its environment, between pathologies of the body and the broader dynamics of social, cultural, and economic exchange. In a condition such as neurasthenia, those dynamics are explicitly drawn upon to structure new and evolving identity formations. For this reason, Roger Cooter has identified neurasthenia alongside degeneration in his study of 'medicine and modernity', as one of those 'new-fangled theories' that 'were themselves signs of modernity in medicine', as they 'cut new social paths in medical thinking at the same time as they established new medicalized ways of thinking about society and identity'.[35] Medical theories and treatments of the diseases of modern life were not only deeply embedded in social and cultural operations; modernity itself was actively constructed and deployed from within nineteenth-century medical discourses.

This volume is framed by questions of epistemology and revolves around a tightly focused series of medical and cultural responses to the general pressures of modern life. We begin by asking what role medicine played in the formation of new and evolving definitions of the modern self during the French Revolution, and end by raising this question again with reference to medicine more generally when it is set alongside the historical record of the long nineteenth century. Our intention is not to provide a comprehensive account of the medical and cultural transformations of this dynamic period; rather, we ask how medical theories, practices, and technologies both structured and were constituted in relation to problems of modernity across literature, science, and medicine. The authors gathered here illustrate how changing social, political, and economic dynamics were drawn upon across multiple emergent disciplines to support new conceptions of the healthy or unhealthy mind and body. Such conceptions are read within and across evolving practices in psychiatry, psychology, psychopathology, physiology, marketing, and education. Drawing on current scholarship on the history of medicine, science, and technology, disability studies, childhood, and consumer culture, we explore how emotional and physical ailments in this period were often understood as uniquely 'modern'. By interrogating the practices and ideologies that underpin these understandings, we offer new ways of thinking about how the mind and body were situated in relation to rapidly changing external environments.

Laurens Schlicht, in the first chapter, opens our discussion at the moment of the European age of revolutions, which inculcated not only a wave of physical displacement, but also a profound sense of moral and political shock. In France, contemporary writers within medicine, politics, and the developing human sciences maintained that it had been necessary to inflict this kind of shock in order to dismantle the rigid structures of French society and make way for a radically new regime. Sustained metaphors of the medicalised human body, the social body, and the body politic commingled in the critical questions that were raised about the nature of the relationship between individuals and their wider social collective, and about the ways in which the passions of France's citizens might be either stirred into action or carefully regulated by external influences. Manifestations of this conscious interaction between medical and political spheres, Schlicht shows, included the emergent psychiatric practice of intentionally shocking patients as a form of therapy, and the evolving instruction of deaf-mute pupils, as schools and asylums provided experimental spaces for controlling and adjusting the human passions. In addition to an overt politicisation of the body and its responses to shock and strain, these discussions carried sustained analyses of the medicalised human body, and informed an evolving scientific practice directed towards an essentialised sphere of individuality.

In the second chapter, Torsten Riotte takes up the interaction between medical and political spheres in the context of nineteenth-century Germany, and poses questions about accountability, medical negligence, and the nature of individual and collective responsibility in relation to accidents. Beginning with the first recorded court case in 1811, when a doctor at the Berlin Charité hospital sued a colleague over the death of a female patient, Riotte draws upon the files of the so-called medical commissions (medical advisory boards to ministries of the interior in the German states) in order to analyse the professional and public debate that ensued and to engage in a discussion of medical negligence as an aspect of professional accountability. The emergence of medical courts of honour from the mid-1870s onwards, and the complementary development of liability insurance for doctors, illuminate the shifting moral, economic, and social structures in which medical practices were embedded.

The interaction of medical and political spheres regarding questions of public health also actively informed notions of individual and collective responsibility regarding the figure of the child, who became a primary focus for concerns about the moral powers of education and the corrupting effects of urban life. Notions of a youthful, 'natural' state of innocence and purity stem, it has often been noted, from Jean-Jacques Rousseau's *Émile, ou de l'éducation* (1762), in which he declared that 'childhood has its own ways of seeing, thinking, and feeling', and that the child mind 'should be left undisturbed until its faculties have developed'.[36] Educational treatises of the late eighteenth and early nineteenth centuries generally advised parents to maintain a child's 'natural' state of innocence and purity through vigilant protection and preferably physical removal from cities and society in general, and from dangerous reading materials or formal training in particular. In the next chapter, Steven Taylor traces this now very familiar model of childhood through to nineteenth-century concerns surrounding the protection and, where necessary, the rescue, of children of the urban poor. During this period of rapid industrialisation and urbanisation in England, Taylor argues, there was increased political and evangelical attention directed towards children as members of a distinct and vulnerable population in a morally dangerous and increasingly adult urban society. The romantic desire to 'protect' children from the ill effects of modern urban life was, in the context of the child rescue efforts of 1870 to 1914, underpinned by a desire to produce useful, morally upright, and productive citizens of future generations. Those children who were deemed physically or mentally incapable of rendering themselves 'useful' to society were, therefore, thought to be beyond the scope of state improvement and educational intervention. Taylor focuses specifically on the Church of England-sponsored Waifs and Strays Society, and examines the manner in which discourses drawn on by health and educational professionals pathologised disabled children as 'imperfect', and even as a potential source of violence. Viewed through a lens of pathological difference, children living with impairment represented physiological and psychological deviations from a socially and politically accepted model of childhood and its patterns of development.

Kristine Swenson further interrogates this model of the pathologisation of physiological and psychological variation in the following chapter, by turning to popular reform movements which arose in response to what mainstream medicine considered largely innate and unchangeable conditions, and actively pursued alternative methods of constructing such difference. Drawing on the emergence of the American Fowler family – led by the brothers Orson and Lorenzo, their sister, Charlotte, and her husband Samuel Wells – as her central case study, Swenson considers the Fowlers' empire of phrenological lecture tours, publishing, and therapeutics as a practice that not only kept phrenology in the public eye long after its dismissal from scientific practice, but that responded to the perceived ills of industrialised capitalism by touting progressive self-improvement and self-care. The Fowlers, Swenson shows, exploited the potential of phrenology as a form of practical self-help (or 'self-culture') allied to hydropathy, dietetics, vegetarianism, dress reform, and temperance. The concept of self-help, largely associated in Victorian studies with the work of Scottish writer and government reformer Samuel Smiles (1812–1904) whose *Self Help*, published in 1859, sold a quarter of a million copies in his lifetime, permeated British and American cultures well beyond Smiles's works.[37] As cultural fears of degeneration and race suicide became widespread, and the middle classes were increasingly seen as subject to the 'modern illnesses' of neurasthenia and dyspepsia, the Fowlers sought means of facilitating social and personal adjustment to the demands of a newly industrialised society. Their reform-oriented late-century phrenology promised personal improvement through proper living habits and the 'exercising' of the faculties, and seemed to mitigate the harsh physiological and psychological consequences of Darwinian evolution and hereditary conditions, which fuelled degenerationist discourse.

Moving from the first section of this volume, which explores varying constructions of modernity and the modern subject in relation to medical practice, Chapters 5 to 8, collectively titled 'Paradoxes of Modern Living', are devoted to 'diseases' and conditions that seemingly emerged from a dialectical relationship between notions of progress and pathology. Degenerationist discourses across the medical, biological, and psychiatric sciences of the *fin de siècle* illuminated the 'dark side of progress', as the supposed advancement of the human race was understood to be constantly threatened with potential reversals through collapse, physical and psychological deviancy, or decay.[38] Late nineteenth-century society appeared to many commentators increasingly to manifest degenerate symptoms of nervous exhaustion, neurosis, psychosis, and general debility derived from prolonged exposure to the speed, noise, and constant stimuli of the urban environment. Such noxious influences as hysteria, neurasthenia, insanity, criminality, and even homosexuality, induced fears concerning the possible corruption of the species through the determinism of heredity. As Max Nordau explained in his study, *Degeneration* (1892), when an organism becomes debilitated, its successors will not resemble the healthy, normal type of the species with its capacities for development, but will form a new subspecies.[39] Images of reversion to lower animal or protoplasmic states proliferated in the art and literature of the period, and were frequently employed, as William Greenslade and Daniel Pick have shown, in order to demonstrate the risks of this kind of atavistic decline, while also paranoically creating and enforcing political boundaries between races, genders, and nationalities.[40] Despite, or indeed, because of its progress, the modern, civilised Western subject was continually confronted with its own fear of a backwards slide and the loss of control.

Manon Mathias opens this section by analysing new attitudes towards disease and hygiene in the nineteenth century in the context of the unprecedented growth of cities in this period, which provoked a parallel rise in diseases from human excrement (such as typhus, typhoid fever, and cholera). This analysis is placed in the context of new scientific understandings of bacteria that began to develop in the late nineteenth century, as the realisation that germs spread through human contact led to an acute fear of dirt and an increased obsession with cleanliness. As human excrement came to dominate discussions of public health and disease, fictions of the period provoked and explored imaginative extensions of these concerns. Jules Verne's *Cinq cents millions de la Bégum* (1880), Camille Flammarion's *Uranie* (1889), and William Morris's *News from Nowhere* (1890) each created compelling fantasies of alternative, faeces-free societies in which bodily waste and dirt have been eradicated. These somewhat anodyne and sterile hygienic utopias, however, also reveal the potential unintended consequences of extreme cleanliness. Implicated in the rational rejection of disease and infection, Mathias argues, is a rejection of human physicality, intimacy, and passion.

In Chapter 6, Steffan Blayney pursues this concept of the human being who is at odds with their environment by tracing an ongoing tension between the overwhelmingly fast pace of industrial modernity, and the natural rhythms and pulses of the finite energies of the human body. Demands for increased velocity of thought and action inculcated a variety of concerns about modernity and its limits, and about social, political, and cultural decline. Fatigue, rarely mentioned in scientific or medical textbooks before the 1860s, emerged in the latter decades of the century as a particularly disturbing symptom of modernity, representing both its degrading effects and its immanent limits. Blayney examines constructions of fatigue at the end of the nineteenth century, as both scientific object and cultural metaphor, situating this condition alongside other such *fin-de-siècle* signifiers as decadence and degeneration. In this context, Blayney approaches fatigue as the bodily manifestation of the second law of thermodynamics, as well as a critical part of the new medical terminology that proliferated in order to designate the exhausting effects of modern life. It was expressive of the inevitable dissipation of energy that accompanied the performance of work in this period. Paradoxically, an epidemic of fatigue appeared both as the main obstacle to the progressive development of industrial civilisation, and as the most indubitable evidence of its ascendancy.

The aetiology of nineteenth-century fatigue as a kind of built-in counter to the dangers of excess was deeply embedded in social, economic, and political realities, and it relied upon a new scientific understanding of the material world and of the body, grounded in the concepts of 'energy' and 'work'. In her seminal text, *Illness as Metaphor* (1991), Susan Sontag traced similar anxieties about the expenditure of energy to the social and cultural perceptions that accrued around more specific diseases such as syphilis, tuberculosis, and cancer, which consumed or stored energy at varying rates. 'The Victorian idea of TB as a disease of low energy (and heightened sensitivity)', Sontag argues, 'echo[ed] the attitudes of early capitalist accumulation' in that the sufferer was understood to have a limited amount of energy, which may be depleted, or wasted away, without appropriate regulation. In contrast, cancer 'evokes a different economic catastrophe: that of the unregulated, abnormal, incoherent growth'.[41] As a disease with a monstrous capacity for growth and expansion, cancer thus typically conjures notions of invasion, attack, and unrestraint. In Chapter 7, Agnes Arnold-Forster takes up this ongoing interplay between medical understandings of cancer and broader social and economic shifts, which, she notes, has given rise to cancer's fluid metaphoric identity. Arnold-Forster situates the 'new cancer epidemic' of the *fin de siècle* within a climate of widespread anxiety about the vitality of the British Empire and concerns about imperial over-reaching, as well as fears of the revolt of an apparently unruly, ungovernable, and newly enfranchised urban population. The metaphoric associations of the cancerous growth resonated in many colonial contexts, as doctors who reflected on medicine in non-European contexts became particularly engaged with the conceptualisation of certain races as more or less prone to the disease, and therefore as more or less 'modern'. Commentators on the domestic 'cancer epidemic' perceived its presence as an unintended consequence of the public health successes of industrial modernity, such as lower infant mortality, increasing hospitalisation, and sanitary reforms. In these parallel, but conflicting, constructions of cancer as a pathology of progress, the disease itself emerged as a symptom of modern life that nonetheless manifested a national deterioration in health.

Another phenomenon discursively connected both to the conditions of modern life and to social degeneration and decline at the *fin de siècle* was suicide. The rise of the new science of social statistics in the early decades of the nineteenth century had enabled researchers to collect new forms of data on suicide incidence and causes of death amongst expanding urban populations and to reinforce their suspicions about the disruptive, even fatal, consequences of urbanisation and industrialisation. Like cancer, suicide was constructed both as a by-product of progress, and as a source of social and cultural decline. In 1879, the Italian professor of psychological medicine, Enrico Morselli, drew on the language of Darwin and Spencer to argue that suicide was 'an effect of the struggle for existence, and of human selection', and that urban societies therefore had higher rates of suicide than rural societies because the struggle for existence was intensified by city living.[42] The pioneering social scientist, Émile Durkheim, also drew explicit parallels between individual and social maladies in his definitive study, *Le Suicide* in 1897. In Finland, too, the principal case study of Mikko Myllykangas's chapter, the psychiatrist Thiodolf Saelan explicitly attributed the slowly increasing suicide rates in Finland to modern urban lifestyles, in an effort to accentuate the cultural differences between so-called 'modernised' Western nations, and other cultures. Myllykangas interrogates such claims in the context of Finnish society, which, he notes, was at a very different stage of industrial transition than many of its Western European counterparts. In this specific social and political context, counterarguments to the widespread conception of suicide in Europe were put forward by figures such as the physician and anthropologist F. W. Westerlund, who argued that it was in fact the lack of progress and modernisation in Finland that constituted its main causes of suicide. Likewise, Hannes Gebhard, a member of the Finnish Parliament, criticised what he considered the excessively deterministic view of human nature that had been put forward by other commentators. These divergent constructions of the role of modernity in relation to suicide ultimately illustrate the ways in which physiological and psychological problems of the period were being constituted in relation to their social contexts and to the changing dynamics of urbanisation and industrialisation. It also points to the multiplicity of modernities being organised around different and evolving definitions of the subjective and/or suicidal self. The notion of modernity here, and throughout this volume, is clearly far from static. It is a constantly changing accretion of history, social context, and material conditions.

The third part of the book investigates the fluctuating boundaries between medical theory, social change, and cultural representation in this era within non-European contexts. Drawing on Johannes Fabian's work on the conceptual geography of anthropology, which, Fabian contends, regards different cultures as living in different moments of historical development, Projit Bihari Mukharji points to a similar denial of coevalness in the history of medicine.[43] The distinctions drawn between 'Western' (later 'bio') medicine and various so-called 'traditional medicines', Mukharji argues, have consistently relegated the latter to the practices of a bygone era. Nonetheless, 'Western' medicine is not the only tradition to have engaged with constructions of modernity. During the nineteenth century, so-called 'traditional' medicines around the globe were also forced to confront the notion of modernity in all its diversity. The Ayurveda tradition of South Asia was one such medical practice, and at the core of Mukharji's chapter is a demonstration of the modernity of Ayurveda. The interplay between Ayurvedic practice and social, cultural, and economic change in nineteenth-century South Asia was, he shows, twofold. Ayurvedic physicians such as Daktar Binodbihari Ray Kabiraj not only developed a self-conscious discourse about modernity and its effects upon the body and mind, but they explicitly drew upon the language of modernity in order to radically reconfigure the Ayurvedic body. Metaphors, as Laura Otis points out, are not, after all, about producing 'objective knowledge' but about 'creating productive thought'.[44] Railways and telegraphs, for these physicians, were not simply new material realities; they were also a rich ideational resource that encouraged and inspired them to think in new ways about the human body and its operations.

In the following chapter, Alice Tsay tracks the global history of a patent medicine known as Dr Williams' Pink Pills for Pale People, from its invention in Canada in 1866 to promotional spreads dedicated to these greatly popular pills in Chinese-language publications in Shanghai in the early twentieth century. Dr Williams' Pink Pills were only one instance of the plethora of treatments which were being patented, marketed, and experimented with as a means of countering nervous exhaustion in the latter decades of the nineteenth century. By the time they made their appearance in Shanghai in the early decades of the twentieth century, however, Dr Williams' pills were widely derided in England and North America as an archetypal example of quackery, with commentators identifying the pills' continued ubiquity as a sign of the public's refusal to recognise scientific progress. Like the 'traditional' medicines evoked by Mukharji in the previous chapter, patent medicines were now associated with notions of backwardness and regression, particularly when they were encountered abroad. Foreign advertisements for Dr Williams' pills, however, engaged with notions of modernity from within their own social and cultural framework. Resisting the claims of scholars such as Erik Elinder and Theodore Levitt, who argue that worldwide advertising is a form of standardisation and gradual homogenisation across the globe, Tsay's comparative study reveals a more nuanced, localised form of engagement with the product in question.[45] Rather than simply translating their Anglo-American counterparts, Shanghai advertisements for the pills came to articulate a distinctly Chinese vision of twentieth-century society in their depiction of new gender roles, their absorption of non-Western medical discourse, and their use of *baihua*, the emerging vernacular. The discourse of the modern, at least in the case of this consumer product, was carefully tailored to its audience, while also responding to that audience, and was part of an ongoing dialogue between producers and consumers.

In Chapter 11, Daniel Simpson delineates a complex model of imperial and cultural entanglement in the context of a controversial medical debate surrounding poison arrows in the Victorian South Pacific. The death of the naval captain James Graham Goodenough under a hail of poisonous arrows on the Santa Cruz Islands in 1875 was, Simpson argues, a moment in which previously vague British fears of the poisons of Santa Cruz – supposedly a place of primitivism and a source of mysterious and dangerous knowledge unknown to the West – were seemingly confirmed. Amidst evangelical formulations of Goodenough's death as a kind of Christian martyrdom which he had suffered while heroically spreading Western 'civilisation' to the region, research into Pacific poisons by the ship's surgeon, Adam Brunton Messer, pointed to certain medical, cultural, and environmental factors that countered the popular hysteria. The prevailing superstitious dread of the reputed poisons of the region, Messer argued, had predisposed British sailors to a nervous irritability, which either mimicked or encouraged the onset of tetanus. Furthermore, he insisted, endemic neurosis amongst sailors was responsible for the increasing prevalence of tetanus in the wounds of those struck by ostensibly poisonous arrows. The suffering of many naval men, then, was in fact symptomatic of the mental strain associated with working in the Pacific during a period of increasingly violent encounters. In drawing upon new scientific, psychopathological understandings of the relations between mind and body, Messer effectively collapsed the distinctions between the 'civilised' and the 'uncivilised' peoples clashing in the South Pacific by imagining that modern medical education might work in both cases to supplant antiquated superstitions and anecdotal evidence. His medical practices and hypotheses, deployed at a juncture of intense intercultural contact, served both to characterise and to realise a form of medical modernity.

'The modern' was a widely deployed nineteenth-century signifier without a clearly corresponding signified, and the question of what constituted the diseases of modern life was partly the work of social perception and consensus, and partly the work of medical analysis and hypothesis. In the final section of this volume, 'Reflections and provocation', Christopher Hamlin takes up this unstable and often polarised relationship between cultural experience and interpretation on the one hand, and biomedical objectivity on the other, in order to draw our attention to a phenomenon which is so frequently missing from current scholarship: embodied subjectivity. In so doing, Hamlin does not offer us a single case study, like those of the preceding chapters. Rather, he ranges widely from public health archives to literary texts in a highly individual style and form, interrogating E. P. Thompson's seminal concept of the 'moral economy' through the social history of health, and questioning how we might meaningfully register the experiences of those whose words, emotions, and details of everyday lives are lost to history, and indeed were scarcely registered in their own times. Questioning the very voices and vocabularies through which the social history of health has been constructed, Hamlin warns us against complacency by recognising both the usefulness and the limitations of our approaches to illness and the history of medicine, while adopting an integrative and holistic approach to notions of disease. In a provocative paralleling of the historical figure of the nuisance inspector with the gamekeeper (or lover) in D. H. Lawrence's *Lady Chatterley's Lover*, and the tales of patients of Hardwicke Hospital, Dublin, in 1840–41 and 1844, with the complaints of Agnes Fleming in Charles Dickens's *Oliver Twist*, he opens up the possibilities of work which crosses literary and medical histories as a context in which the formation of an embodied subjectivity might be considered.

Although our work focuses on the range of ways in which anxieties about health and disease manifested themselves in medical and cultural discourses of the long nineteenth century, the authors in this volume frequently draw parallels to the present, positing Victorian perceptions of the diseases of modern life as close precursors to early twenty-first-century worries about the psychological and physiological strains of our own 'modern', technology-saturated lives. While we do not wish to draw a direct line of comparison between nineteenth-century attitudes to such technologies as the telegraph, train, telephone, and expanding print culture, and our own responses as a culture to the advent of the internet, the mobile phone, and associated complaints of 'fake news' and information overload, the longer historical context of such concerns, and their resonances across multiple fields of operation, is made evident throughout this volume. What emerges from such analysis is an increased alertness, not only to the anxieties induced by new developments and 'modern' technologies in and of themselves, but to the broader, and deeply intertwined, social, cultural, economic, and political contexts from which they have developed.

Notes

1 George M. Beard, *American Nervousness: Its Causes and Consequences* (New York: G. P. Putnam's, 1881), 186.
2 The nerves were central to the work of, for example, the English physician Thomas Willis (1621–75) and, subsequently, the Scottish Enlightenment physician George Cheyne (1671–1743), and the French physiologist Xavier Bichat (1771–1802). A detailed outline of this nervous history is provided in Roy Porter, 'Nervousness, Eighteenth and Nineteenth Century Style: From Luxury to Labour', in M. Gijswijt-Hofstra and R. Porter (eds), *Cultures of Neurasthenia from Beard to the First World War* (Amsterdam: Rodopi, 2001), 31–49.
3 Beard, *American Nervousness*, p. iv.
4 *Ibid.*, 176. Charles E. Rosenberg, in 'The place of George M. Beard in nineteenth-century psychiatry', *Bulletin of the History of Medicine*, 36 (January 1962), 245–59 (pp. 255–7), explores the 'long and familiar' tradition of nationalism underpinning Beard's aetiology of neurasthenia.
5 David Schuster, *Neurasthenic Nation: America's Search for Health, Happiness, and Comfort, 1869–1920* (New Brunswick: Rutgers University Press, 2011), 22.
6 Schuster, *Neurasthenic Nation*, 22.
7 Beard, *American Nervousness*, 186. Our emphasis.
8 For a detailed examination of the relationship between neurasthenia and the era's politics of race, nationalism, and citizenship, see Brad Campbell, 'The making of "American": race and nation in neurasthenic discourse', *History of Psychiatry*, 18:2 (2007), 131–56.
9 Charles L. Dana, 'The partial passing of neurasthenia', *Boston Medical and Surgical Journal*, 150:13 (1904), 339–44 (p. 341).

10 For a discussion of peculiarly British views on the concept of neurasthenia, and its advent as a useful addition to the British medical lexicon, see Janet Oppenheim, 'Shattered Nerves': Doctors, Patients, and Depression in Victorian England (Oxford: Oxford University Press, 1991), 79–109.
11 On the history of education in Russia and the late nineteenth-century concerns surrounding overpressure, see Patrick L. Alston, Education and the State in Tsarist Russia (Stanford, CA: Stanford University Press, 1969).
12 James C. Albisetti, Secondary School Reform in Imperial Germany (Princeton, NJ: Princeton University Press, 1983), 123.
13 Victor Laprade, L'Éducation homicide. Plaidoyer pour l'enfance (Paris: Didier, 1868), 30.
14 Aimé Riant, Le Surménage intellectuel et les exercices physiques (Paris: J. B. Baillère, 1889); Alfred Binet and Victor Henri, La Fatigue intellectuelle (Paris: C. Reinwald, 1898).
15 Thomas Stretch Dowse, On Brain and Nerve Exhaustion: 'Neurasthenia', Its Nature and Curative Treatment (London: Ballière, Tindall, and Cox, 1880), 40.
16 These claims were reflective of more general cultural perceptions of the dissipation of mechanical, mental, and physical energy under the strain of modernity. As Anson Rabinbach has shown, a decline in nervous energy was understood to create a corresponding decline in labour and productivity and was, therefore, in many ways an important indicator of a nation's longevity. See Anson Rabinbach, The Human Motor: Energy, Fatigue, and the Origins of Modernity (New York: Basic Books, 1990).
17 W. R. Greg, 'Life at High Pressure', Contemporary Review (December 1874), 623–38 (p. 627).
18 Ibid., 627. Greg adds to this form of chronic disruption, the anxiety to be on time and the hurrying pace to catch trains which further the daily wear and tear of the nervous system.
19 Ibid., 629.
20 Marshall Berman, for example, identifies three distinct transitional periods in his investigation of modernism and its complexities: 1500 to c. 1800, the nineteenth century, and the twentieth century. Crane Brinton and Richard Tarnas argue that a distinctly 'modern' world view emerged in the Enlightenment period. According to Richard Tarnas, it is science that dictates these shifts in orientation, while according to Warren W. Wagar, it is the process of secularisation. See Marshall Berman, All That is Solid Melts into Air: The Experience of Modernity (London: Verso, 1983); Crane Brinton, The Shaping of Modern Thought (Englewood Cliffs, NJ: Prentice-Hall, 1963); Richard Tarnas, The Passion of the Western Mind: Understanding the Ideas that have Shaped our World View (London: Pimlico, 1996);

Warren W. Wagar (ed.), *The Idea of Progress Since the Renaissance* (New York: John Wiley, 1964).
21 L. S. Jacyna, *Medicine and Modernism: A Biography of Sir Henry Head* (London: Pickering and Chatto, 2008), 4.
22 S. N. Eisenstadt, 'Multiple modernities', *Daedalus* 1:129 (2000), 1–29 (p. 2). See also Dominic Sachsenmaier, S. N. Eisenstadt, and Jens Riedel (eds), *Reflections on Multiple Modernities: European, Chinese, and Other Interpretations* (Leiden: Brill, 2002). For further exploration of the notion of multiple modernities, see Alberto Martinelli, *Global Modernization: Rethinking the Project of Modernity* (London: SAGE, 2005).
23 C. E. Rosenberg, 'Pathologies of progress: the idea of civilization as risk', *Bulletin of the History of Medicine*, 72:4 (1998), 714–30 (p. 716).
24 *Ibid.*, 730.
25 The emphasis throughout this study on the interrelations of modernity and the human mind and body has resonances with Michael Sappol's recent book, *Body Modern: Fritz Kahn, Scientific Illustration, and the Homuncular Subject* (Minneapolis: University of Minnesota Press, 2017), which locates modernity within the human body in the context of art and design, and considers the ways in which 'the surfaces of modernity' are 'brought into the depths of the body, and the depths of the body' are brought out 'onto modernity's industrial, urban, and domestic surfaces' (165).
26 The jarring effect of new modes of transport, machinery, or technological advances have been explored by Rabinbach in *The Human Motor*, Andreas Killen in his *Berlin Electropolis: Shock, Nerves, and German Modernity* (Berkeley: University of California Press, 2006), and in the more recent edited collection by Laura Salisbury and Andrew Shail, *Neurology and Modernity: A Cultural History of Nervous Systems, 1800–1950* (Basingstoke: Palgrave Macmillan, 2010). Now 'classic' texts in the field, such as Wolfgang Schivelbusch's *The Railway Journey: The Industrialization of Time and Space in the 19th Century* (Berkeley: University of California Press, 1986) are also instructive in considering how contemporary technological and scientific developments could alter perceptions both of the world and of the individual's place within it.
27 On railway spine, see Jane F. Thraikill, 'Railway Spine, Nervous Excess and the Forensic Self', in Salisbury and Shail (eds), *Neurology and Modernity*, 96–112. A detailed medical-historical analysis is provided by Michael R. Trimble, *Post-Traumatic Neuroses: From Railway Spine to Whiplash* (Chichester: John Riley, 1981). On Bicycle Face, see Patricia Anne Vertinsky, *The Eternally Wounded Woman: Women, Doctors, and Exercise in the Late Nineteenth Century* (Manchester: Manchester University Press, 1990), 75–81.

28 On the influence of the sewing machine on female sexual health, see Judith Coffin, 'Credit, consumption, and images of women's desires: selling the sewing machine in late nineteenth-century France', *French Historical Studies*, 18 (1994), 749–83, and Shelley Trower, *Senses of Vibration: A History of the Pleasure and Pain of Sound* (London: Continuum, 2012), 132–8.
29 See, for example, Mark S. Micale and Paul Lerner (eds), *Traumatic Pasts: History, Psychiatry and Trauma in the Modern Age, 1870–1930* (Cambridge: Cambridge University Press, 2001), which offers a variety of perspectives on shock in technological, industrial, and medical modernity, and Tim Armstrong, 'Two types of shock in modernity', *Critical Quarterly*, 42 (2000), 61–73.
30 See Joachim Radkau, 'The Neurasthenic Experience in Imperial Germany: Expeditions into Patient Records and Side-Looks upon General History', in M. Gijswijt-Hofstra and R. Porter (eds), *Cultures of Neurasthenia from Beard to the First World War* (Amsterdam: Rodopi, 2001), 199–217; Laura Goering, 'Russian nervousness: neurasthenia and national identity in nineteenth-century Russia', *Medical History*, 47:1 (2003), 23–46; Arthur Kleinman, *Social Origins of Distress and Disease: Depression, Neurasthenia, and Pain in Modern China* (New Haven, CT: Yale University Press, 1990); Janet Oppenheim, *'Shattered Nerves': Doctors, Patients, and Depression in Victorian England* (Oxford: Oxford University Press, 1991), 79–109.
31 Sabine Frühstück, 'Male anxieties: nerve force, nation, and the power of sexual knowledge', *Journal of the Royal Asiatic Society*, 15 (2005), 71–88.
32 Kristin Ruggiero, *Modernity in the Flesh: Medicine, Law, and Society in Turn-of-the-Century Argentina* (Stanford, CA: Stanford University Press, 2004), 139–43.
33 For work in the field of public and environmental health, see Christopher Hamlin, *Public Health and Social Justice in the Age of Chadwick: Britain, 1800–1854* (Cambridge: Cambridge University Press, 1998), Pamela Gilbert, *Cholera and Nation: Doctoring the Social Body in Victorian England* (Albany: State University of New York Press, 2008), and Mary Poovey, *Making a Social Body: British Cultural Formation, 1830–1864* (Chicago: University of Chicago Press, 1995). Previous work focusing on nervous diseases includes Janet Oppenheim, *'Shattered Nerves': Doctors, Patients, and Depression in Victorian England* (Oxford: Oxford University Press, 1991), and Mark Micale, *The Mind of Modernism: Medicine, Psychology, and the Cultural Arts in Europe and America, 1880–1940* (Stanford, CA: Stanford University Press, 2004), and *Hysterical Man: The Hidden History of Male Nervous Illness* (Cambridge, MA: Harvard University Press, 2008). Work on the history of neurasthenia includes Frederick Gosling, *Before*

Freud: Neurasthenia and the American Medical Community (Chicago: University of Illinois Press, 1987), Gijswijt-Hofstra and Porter (eds), *Cultures of Neurasthenia*, and Schuster, *Neurasthenic Nation*. On shock, see Jill Matus, *Shock, Memory and the Unconscious in Victorian Fiction* (Cambridge: Cambridge University Press, 2009), and on agoraphobia David Trotter, *The Uses of Phobia: Essays on Literature and Film* (Oxford: Wiley Blackwell, 2010).

34 Benjamin Ward Richardson, *Diseases of Modern Life* (London: Macmillan, 1876).

35 Roger Cooter, 'Medicine and Modernity', in Mark Jackson (ed.), *The Oxford Handbook of the History of Medicine* (Oxford: Oxford University Press, 2015), 100–16 (p. 103).

36 Jean-Jacques Rousseau, *Emile*, trans. Barbara Foxley (London: Everyman's Library, 1992), 54.

37 For more on the rise of Victorian self-help culture, see J. F. C. Harrison, 'The Victorian gospel of success', *Victorian Studies*, 1:2 (1957), 155–64, and Kenneth Fielden, 'Samuel Smiles and self-help', *Victorian Studies*, 12:2 (1968), 155–76. Boyd Hilton discusses self-help in a religious context in *The Age of Atonement: The Influence of Evangelicism on Social and Economic Thought, 1795–1865* (Oxford: Clarendon Press, 1988).

38 J. Edward Chamberlin and Sander L. Gilman, *Degeneration: The Dark Side of Progress* (New York: Columbia University Press, 1985).

39 Max Nordau, *Degeneration* (London: William Heinemann, 1896 [1892]).

40 William Greenslade, *Degeneration, Culture, and the Novel, 1880–1940* (Cambridge: Cambridge University Press, 2010) and Daniel Pick, *Faces of Degeneration: A European Disorder c. 1848–c. 1918* (Cambridge: Cambridge University Press, 1989).

41 Susan Sontag, *Illness as Metaphor and AIDS and its Metaphors* (London: Penguin, 1991 [1968]), 64.

42 Enrico Morselli, *Suicide: An Essay on Comparative Moral Statistics* (New York: D. Appleton, 1882), 354.

43 Johannes Fabian, *Time and the Other: How Anthropology Makes its Object* (New York: Columbia University Press, 2014).

44 Laura Otis, *Networking: Communicating with Bodies and Machines in the Nineteenth Century* (Ann Arbor: University of Michigan Press, 2001), 12.

45 Theodore Levitt, 'The globalization of markets', *Harvard Business Review*, 83:3 (1983), 92–102 and Erik Elinder, 'How international can European advertising be?' *Journal of Marketing*, 29 (1965), 7–11.

I
Constructing the modern self

1

Revolutionary shocks: the French human sciences and the crafting of modern subjectivity, 1794–1816

Laurens Schlicht

Between 9 August and 9 October 1793, the French city of Lyon was besieged by military forces of the central authority in Paris. Earlier that year, the Jacobin municipality at Lyon had been overthrown by a counter-revolutionary insurrection. Subsequently, the *ville rebelle* was besieged by the National Convention in Paris and ultimately defeated. The Hôtel-Dieu hospital at Lyon was reduced to ruins in the battle. Three years later, in 1796, Antoine Petit, a surgeon who was present during the siege, gave an account of that disturbing episode in the inaugural lecture of his anatomy course at the rebuilt Hôtel-Dieu on the 'Influence of the French Revolution on public health'. Petit believed in the healing effects of the Revolution: rather than emphasising his mental or physical suffering at the hands of the revolutionary forces, he used his medical training to highlight what he regarded as the positive political and therapeutic aspects of fear and terror. The first and most necessary function of political revolution, according to Petit, was radically to change the existing social and political habits of the populace in order to clear the way for new and better ones:

> Revolutions are, for the political body they shake, what medicines are for the impaired human body whose harmony they must restore. In both cases, the first effect is a disorder, the first sensation pain.[1]

Petit thereby claimed that the 'shock of all passions' which had been inflicted by the Revolution had revealed hitherto unknown powers of the mind.² It was, he argued, the reign of malicious customs among the enslaved peoples in particular – causing a 'moral fever' – that had led to the outbreak of Revolution.³ He believed that women, especially, offered proof that 'moral affections' contributed to healing, providing the example of a case of dropsy stemming from puffiness in the legs.⁴ As Nina Gelbart has shown, doctors during the Revolution were increasingly expected to understand and cure not only individual but also social diseases and the Revolution thus was seen as a 'medical event'.⁵ The French and American Revolutions thereby created spaces within which this new expertise could be practised and which provided material for reflecting on the behaviour of people during what George Rosen has termed 'social stress'.⁶ As a part or result of these reflections, a new way of thinking about the human mind was formed, whose empirical study became a task for the emerging human sciences. According to Robert Wokler, they replaced the speculative anthropology and conjectural history of the eighteenth century.⁷ One part of this project of creating an empirical knowledge system was a rearrangement of philosophical reflections about the human mind through the lens of medical and pedagogical expertise. When most administrative and pedagogical systems of the *ancien régime* for organising people were abolished or deeply transformed during the French Revolution, this necessitated at the same time a new way of thinking about the human mind, of new systems of control, of disciplining and organising people: the 'citizen' of a 'republic' was a different kind of subject, a subject at the same time demanding 'equality', 'liberty', and individuality.⁸ As Jan Goldstein has shown, after 1800 one new version of subjectivity consisted of a separation of the enigmatic inner world and the phenomenal appearance of the soul, which I will refer to as one version of 'modern subjectivity'.⁹ By focusing on interpretations of the shock of the Revolution I want to show how in the beginning the positive potential of the collective shock was a discursive option, while after 1800 shock as a medical intervention became an instrument of experts in controlled spaces.

Petit's short text is only one example from a series of interpretations of the political shocks inflicted on the French population, from the outset of the French Revolution in 1789 until the rise of Napoleon Bonaparte (1769–1821) to power in 1799. In 1789, for example, the well-known physician Philippe Pinel (1745–1826) observed in the *Journal de Paris* that, from the viewpoint of a 'physician observer', it was impossible to ignore the 'salutary effects of the progress of liberty', which had injected 'vigour' and 'energy' into the 'animal economy'. Like Petit, Pinel discussed this topic through the lens of gender, expressing his belief that 'moral causes' like the Revolution especially affected the 'weaker sex', that is, women.[10] Pinel also did more than any other physician in France to disseminate the concept of 'moral treatment', which was based on the assumption that 'moral causes', in contrast to 'physical' ones, could cure mental diseases.[11] In 1805, his student Jean-Étienne Esquirol (1772–1840) introduced the concept of the 'moral shock' (*sécousse morale*), which relied upon the notion of moral treatment and made further suggestions on how to strategically use moral shocks to cure types of insanity.[12]

This chapter argues that the therapeutic, educational, and scientific approach to the moral shock that arose after 1800 was only possible in a new framework for treating the human mind within spaces of expert knowledge and control such as the asylum and the school. Furthermore, this framework depended on a specific assessment of the history of the French Revolution. At various stages of the Revolution, optimistic interpretations of the shock were discarded. In the beginning, the universal concepts of equality and liberty had opened up the possibility of conceiving of a comprehensive shock as an equalising force that would create something like a *tabula rasa*.[13] After the fall of Robespierre in 1794, however, this essentially positive image of the 'people' became questionable, since it was precisely the 'people' who had been seduced by leaders of the Terror into committing appalling crimes, as the now ascendant Thermidorians believed. While these leaders still used a medical vocabulary to interpret the shock of the Revolution and to suggest a means of pacifying France, they no longer believed in the universal goodness of human beings and suggested avoiding immoderate affects.[14] After Napoleon's *coup d'état* the idea of the shock was again transformed.[15] Within the new interpretative scheme, which redefined the 'mind' and subjects' relation to it, a relegitimation of moral shock became possible in the form of the intervention of medical or educational experts within spaces of control, or of research strategies for finding something out about the enigmatic content of the mind. This chapter aims to show that this version of modern subjectivity was defined, on the one hand, as a semi-autonomous unit that came to be called the ego, the *Moi*. It was understood to be visible through careful introspection only and had an inexhaustible content. On the other hand this modern version of what Jan Goldstein has called the 'mental stuff' allowed for a sphere of scientific and administrative expertise, dealing with observing, experimenting on, and controlling the modern self and its deviations.[16] Unlike, for example, 'the citizen' at the beginning of the Revolution who, in Sieyès's eyes, could deal with 'good shocks', this kind of modern self was vulnerable, irritable, and principally unstable.[17] While the shock as a conscious intervention therefore had to be controlled by medical experts, the regime of inwardness was a prerogative of bourgeois subjects, and administrative professionals took over the control of spaces in which passions arose as threatening forces. What I call the 'modern subject' here, has to be understood as a result of these three agencies of acting on an inner zone.

Advocates of the evolving human sciences believed that the mind was characterised by some specifically human essence, some core, that was at least partially invisible.[18] The moral shock was thereby confined to spaces where it was used to encourage the development of individual human beings or groups of human beings and to find out something about their specific potential. From the perspective of moral shock, it is thus possible to show how, in the treatment of the human mind, a specific relationship between experts and subjects evolved on the basis of modern subjectivity and contributed to its production.

The first two sections of the chapter describe the first phase of revolutionary shock after the Terror, while the following three sections analyse the interventions of experts during the Consulate (1799–1804) on the basis of whether they rejected or adopted the technique of moral shock for the treatment of *sourds-muets* (deaf or hard-of-hearing persons),[19] the 'wild boy' Victor, and the insane. The moral shock and political disruption of the French Revolution led ultimately, the chapter concludes, to a new consciousness of the passions and the harmonies or disharmonies of the inner self, and to an evolving scientific practice directed towards an essentialised sphere of individuality. In the concluding section, I focus on the question of how these examples might help elucidate our understanding of a version of modern subjectivity.

The shock of the Revolution after the terror, 1794–99

The idea of moral shock was, from the onset, a political one that also had therapeutic, educational, and institutional corollaries. Its basic argumentative premise can be summed up as follows: despotic regimes, such as the *ancien régime*, have the tendency to keep the general populace in ignorance in order to keep it subordinate. This ignorance prevents people from reasoning well enough, for example, to identify their natural rights and interests. Therefore, some kind of shock has to break down these rigid structures and open up the possibility of creating new ones. Fundamental to this notion of the political shock of the Revolution was the belief that the nation's individuals could become alienated from their inner, rational, and universal mind that nevertheless remained intact even under very unfavourable external and internal conditions.[20] As the views of Pinel show above, the idea of insanity as a kind of obstruction of the principally undamaged rational mind also inspired a medical analysis of the early history of the Revolution.

At the beginning of the French Revolution, the inner self corresponded in many ways to the classical sensationalist theory of mind, especially as it was expressed by Étienne Bonnot de Condillac (1714–80) and, based on his theories, Antoine Louis Claude Destutt de Tracy (1754–1836).[21] In his essay on the origin of human knowledge (*Essai sur l'origine des connoissances humaines* (1749)), for example, Condillac provided an explanation of the mind that relied solely on the faculty of sense perception and the mind's basic capacity for 'attention'. Within this framework, the mind was continually affected by three possible causes: impairment of the sense organs, different ways of processing sense perceptions, and types of storage and connection of these perceptions in the form of ideas.[22] His basic hope, and that of Destutt de Tracy as well, was to discover laws governing the workings of the human mind that were analogous to the laws of physics. The intervention of the expert on the human mind should one day be based on the knowledge of these laws of, for example, 'morals', that is for Destutt de Tracy, the 'knowledge of the effects of our inclinations and our sentiments on our happiness.'[23] In Destutt de Tracy's eyes then, these experts would, on the basis of such 'human laws', help to create the optimal conditions for human social life.[24] While Destutt de Tracy wrote this after the fall of Robespierre, when he had embraced a moderate stance highlighting the dangerous potential of any kind of disturbance, before 1794 the positive effects of shock had been more pervasive in both political and scientific discourses.

The idea that shocks could heal was not without precedent, especially in medical circles, where the practice of curing patients by inducing a state of terror in them had existed since at least the beginning of the eighteenth century. A professor of medicine at Leiden University, for instance, Johannes Oosterdyk Schacht (1704–92) had supposed, with reference to Stoic philosophy, that even if terror (*terrore*) were a rather devastating disturbance of the soul (*perturbatio animi*), submerging an ill person in cold water could induce a shock that might cure rabies.[25] This kind of shock was adopted by the evolving psychiatric discourse at the end of the eighteenth century, as Philippe Pinel popularised the idea of the 'moral treatment' through his work at the Bicêtre hospital, claiming that dopted interventions – that is, those not involving direct physical contact – could cure insanity. In Pinel's case, as Goldstein argues, these moral interventions were understood to be effective because the faculty of imagination seemingly had an organising effect on the mind and could be affected by every external stimulus (including pictures, theatre plays, and sounds).[26] It was not absurd to transfer this idea of the effects of the imagination to the interpretation of the shock of the Revolution, which, for the advocates of the Revolution, could be interpreted as salutary, while in the eyes of its critics it was detrimental.[27]

The Thermidorians' stance

As Bronisław Baczko has demonstrated through sustained analysis of political debates after the Terror, providing a plausible explanation as to how a freed people could have succumbed to the seductive voices of the discourse of the Terror, and especially to that of Robespierre, became a central task of the post-Terror period.[28] The figure of a people easily seduced gained in prominence during this period, and the idea of the gentle and uniform progress of reason was delegitimated. Instead, the discourse of the Thermidorian Convention (1794–99), which had replaced the regime of the Terror, betrayed a deep-seated anxiety that the people might again be seduced by 'tyrants' (referring mainly to

Robespierre and Louis XVI). One of the central figures of this Thermidorian reaction, Jean-Lambert Tallien (1767–1820), made this stance very clear in his speech soon after the fall of Robespierre, on 28 August 1794.[29] While speaking about the concrete system of Terror that was, in his eyes, instituted primarily by Robespierre and Saint-Just, he drew attention at the same time to the medical concept of terror:

> the terror is a general and regular shock, an exterior shock that affects the most hidden fibres, which degrades man and reduces him to a beast. It is the shock of all physical forces, the concussion of all moral faculties, the disturbance of all ideas, the reversal of all feelings (*affections*). It is a genuine disorganisation of the soul, which, because it leaves the soul only the ability to suffer, robs it of both the sweetness of hope and of the resources of despair.[30]

Several texts published soon after the end of the Terror presented narratives similar to Tallien's, which utilised vocabulary of the human sciences in order to demonstrate how the people had been either deceived or driven mad by the abuse of passions or of words (the so-called *abus des mots*).[31] In 1798, for example, Destutt de Tracy published a series of articles in the *Mercure de France* in response to a prize question posed by the Class of Moral and Political Sciences at the National Institute, one of the first institutionalisations of the 'human', 'moral', 'political', or 'social' sciences.[32] The question read: 'What means should be considered to establish morality among a people?' (the question was later modified, so Destutt's essay did not enter the competition). Referring to the disturbing experiences of the Terror, de Tracy sharply criticised faith in the gentle progress of reason and instead put forward the thesis that the basic social and political operations of humanity are defined by the conflict of interests. To mitigate these conflicts one had, in his eyes, not to convince people by the force of arguments, but rather to 'indoctrinate' them, to 'use every indirect means to influence the dispositions of its [the people's] members'.[33] Morality, Destutt contended, is not something 'out there', it must be produced through a knowledge-based process aimed at changing people's customs (*habitudes*) by instituting good laws, promptly executing these laws, and furnishing the requisite material resources. For Destutt, the transition from one system to the other always generates a 'crisis where one experiences all the problems of both systems', which could, if prolonged, lead to 'irremediable disorders'.[34]

One of the major figures of the Thermidorian reaction was Benjamin Constant (1767–1830), a staunch defender of the ideals of moderation and harmony. Constant considered the idea that the Terror was a necessary phase and ingredient of the Revolution influential and dangerous enough to be opposed in detail. Terror, for Constant, reinstated the arbitrary (as opposed to the 'natural') political regime of the past by establishing a distance between the government and the people on the basis of fear.[35] Furthermore, by using misleading words (such as 'justice' for unjust actions), it contributed to the confusion of things, words, and ideas, thereby creating a gap between the sacred law of nature and the arbitrary imaginations of despotic rulers:

> [The Terror] has habituated the people to hearing the most sacred words being pronounced to motivate the most abhorrent actions. It has confused all notions, accustomed [the people's] minds to despotism, inspired disdain for manners (*formes*), and prepared the ground for acts of violence and crimes in all directions.[36]

The impetus for Constant's criticism was a book by Adrien Lezay-Marnésia (1769–1814) entitled *Of the causes of the Revolution and of its results* (1797), which defended the Terror as a necessary episode of the Revolution. Like Petit, Lezay considered the Revolution a 'complete change of customs, habits, circumstances, properties'.[37] He situated his analysis of the shock of the Terror within a broader interpretation of historical forces, that is, the progress of enlightenment, which he believed had led to Revolution. In his own words, 'enlightenment and corruption progress together, which is why every popular revolution brought about by the progress of enlightenment is necessarily violent'.[38] Lezay-Marnésia was convinced that in order to destroy ancient customs ('anciennes habitudes'), an excessive despotism ('despotisme outré') had been necessary to prepare the ground for a free constitution.[39] Drawing once again on the field of medicine to furnish an analogy, the Terror was for Lezay-Marnésia a kind of 'fever', whose tremors would be felt even after the actual political event had subsided.[40] The despotism of the Terror had in this way made a 'new people' who could only attain liberty through 'shocks', even if those shocks were inflicted by 'criminals'.[41]

After the *coup d'état* in 1799

Dominant figures in the burgeoning field of the human sciences after the establishment of the National Institute in 1795 presented a rather different analysis of the people in periods of violent political circumstances. The physiologist and materialist philosopher Pierre-Jean-Georges Cabanis (1757–1808), for example, believed that the practice of the human sciences could contribute to avoiding revolutionary violence and that it was only the anachronism of the political regime, as compared to the progress of enlightenment, that caused the excesses of the revolutionary struggle. Indeed, this violence could be avoided through careful attention to the people's state of mind (*état des esprits*).[42] For Cabanis, the human sciences would provide a means of governing that would allow social institutions to avoid friction between the people's state of mind and the nature of the social institutions that had produced the revolutionary violence in the first place. One way or the other, these advocates of the human sciences sought to produce situations in which the progress of the mind and the state of societal institutions did not show any difference in development. These could be called 'regimes of contemporaneity', and such regimes were regarded as the foundation of a harmonious society.

In these circumstances, a heterogeneous group of actors gathered in Paris to establish a learned society, the Society of the Observers of Man (*Société des observateurs de l'homme* (1799–1804)). Its forty-five resident and sixteen corresponding members included physicians (Félix Vicq d'Azyr and Philippe Pinel), orientalists (Antoine-Isaac Silvestre de Sacy (1758–1838)), mathematicians (Auguste-Savinien Leblond (1760–1811)), naturalists (Aubin-Louis Millin de Grandmaison (1759–1818)), and philosophers (Pierre Laromiguière (1756–1837)). The society was established just after Napoleon's *coup d'état* in 1799 and promised to generate a range of useful knowledge for safeguarding the new political regime against instability. One of its main actors, Joseph Marie de Gérando (1772–1842), believed that the general shock to 'all beliefs' that had been caused by the Revolution necessitated a profound reflection upon the rights and duties of human beings and the place of each being in French society.[43] Therefore, he argued, a new and universal science of human beings should form the basis of a harmonising knowledge system, providing insight into the workings of the human mind, and the effects of education and various external influences, such as climate.[44]

The most visible activities of the Society were concentrated at Paris's *Institution nationale des sourds-muets*, which was a central revolutionary institution because it could demonstrate the moral power of education in very tangible ways during the public sessions which were attended by many, sometimes famous, visitors (such as the Pope, who attended a public session in 1805).[45] Visitors to the school could admire its realisation of the Enlightenment's educational utopia, which promised to render every human being equally rational.[46] This programme was based on a conception of human beings as naturally good and virtuous, and it maintained that only the aberrations of history, that is, arbitrary developments, could corrupt these natural qualities. One of the more remarkable means of corrupting people was the above-mentioned misuse of words, the *abus des mots*, which is why advocates of this position were highly interested in reforming language.

The school's director, Roch Ambroise Sicard (1742–1822), claimed to have developed a 'methodical sign language' that was able to replace the sign language normally used by *sourds-muets*, by which he meant that every sign would unequivocally represent only one idea, which, in turn, was connected to only one type of thing in the world.[47] While there is not space to discuss this idea in detail here, Sicard's basic strategy was to base the signs of the methodical sign language on what he thought to be a natural analysis of the parts of speech, a natural grammar, which therefore represented the structure of things in the world perfectly in language. Hence, Sicard believed he could translate the order of things into an order of words and preserve this order in a language unobstructed by tradition, creating a new language of a new people, the methodical sign language. Contemporary critics of Sicard pointed out that he had entirely overlooked the fact that *sourds-muets* generally already had an elaborate language and that he failed to sufficiently deal with its structure – a disregard that remained a characteristic aspect of the marginalisation of the Deaf Community.[48]

For Sicard's admirers, on the other hand, his methodical sign language seemed ideally suited to eliminating the *abus des mots*, which, for Tallien as well, was crucial to explaining the power accumulated during the Terror. He enjoyed significant success with his programme. A high-ranking official of the Interior Ministry, Jean-Pierre Barbier de Neuville

(1754–1822), mentioned Sicard's public lessons and 'discovery' of the methodical sign language in a letter of recommendation to the Interior Minister, because Sicard was hoping for a pay rise: 'Mr Sicard is well known to the learned foreigners who all frequent his lessons, and who rank his discovery among the achievements upon which our nation prides itself and which elevate it above the others.'[49] One admirer of his work, the Abbé Pierre David, claimed that Sicard's methodical sign language could form the basis for a much needed clarification and purification of the political vocabulary. Terror, he argued, had managed to deceive people through the misuse and perversion of words such as 'equality' and 'democracy', which would not be possible in a 'natural' language such as Sicard's.[50] Sicard had influential supporters from the outset. Charles-Maurice Talleyrand (1754–1838) surmised in his 1791 report on public education that Sicard's methodical sign language might help create a universal language 'which will be for thinking what algebra is for calculation'.[51] An archival report of the Committee of Public Assistance in 1796 proposed that 'the analytical signs of the school of the *sourd-muets* might become 'the universal language of educated men of all nations'.[52]

Sicard was also active, under the pseudonym of 'Dracis', as a writer for the *Annales religieuses*, where, in 1797, an account was published of his experiences during the September Massacres of 1792. This piece described a riot involving the slaughter of imprisoned enemies of the Revolution, including so-called 'refractory priests' like Sicard who had refused the civil constitution of the clergy. Here as well, Sicard painted a picture of an 'irascible' people whose misguided actions stemmed solely from their dependence on the opinions of their leaders.[53] The people were susceptible to the voice of reason, but they also listened to those who wanted to inflame unjust passions – they were, ultimately, dependent on the whims of the elite.

Sicard believed that *sourds-muets* represented a perfect natural state prior to the onset of education. They were therefore ideal objects for an 'experimental metaphysics', which he believed could demonstrate how, from the raw, natural state of humanity, an enlightened educational practice would produce enlightened and peaceful citizens.[54] Sicard's project effectively responded to the Consulate's need to build up a coherent system of knowledge that allowed for the creation of a functioning society through a series of prudent educational and administrative interventions.[55] The figure of the *sourd-muet*, also referred to at this time as the 'savage' or the 'automaton'[56] because of an alleged lack of communication, was conceived as a being without history and therefore deemed suitable for the implementation of a perfect system of customs, habits, and signs. Many audience members at Sicard's regular public lessons at the *Institution nationale des sourds-muets* shared this conviction; one of them even believed he had attended the 'creation of man'.[57] Sicard's perspective also existed in governmental contexts, as demonstrated by this unpublished report of the *Director General of Public Instruction* (c. 1795–99):

> It is less by communicating words that are only ever used to signal ideas, than by helping to beget ideas themselves, that it is possible to proceed with some success in the teaching [of *sourds-muets*]. It is as if there is a sort of world map on which the philosophical genius of the teacher establishes, between the ideas that are supposed to be covering the surface, connections that tie them together.[58]

Sicard's experimental metaphysics was an answer to the challenge of regeneration, that is, of how a society with a history, with traditional customs and habits, might be regenerated without violence or shock, on the sole basis of the laws of nature, thereby avoiding the arbitrary abuse of power witnessed during the Terror. He framed this reference to nature within a sentimental narrative depicting education as an unimpeded discovery and development of immanent abilities through the enjoyment and admiration of nature. In Sicard, we therefore often find emotional descriptions of Jean Massieu (1772–1846) – one of his most famous pupils – hard at work classifying various natural phenomena, but we are very seldom privy to scenes of conflict.[59] Sicard here reflects the wide-ranging discourse about 'nature' that blossomed during the French Revolution, a discourse that highlighted its harmonious, normative, and tender aspects. Roederer, one of the architects of Napoleon's *coup d'état* and an outspoken champion of Sicard's method, shared Tallien's perspective on the Terror, regarding it as a 'disease where the moral and the physical constantly influence each other'.[60] Since that system had relied on the 'arbitrary' whim of despots, the appeal of an educational technique that promised to reinstate the 'natural' order had a special appeal. If, as Roederer believed, the 'natural' was intimately tied to the good and the beautiful, then a concrete technique for attaining the 'natural' was a way to avoid the regression to Terror and the moral and physical distress associated with it. In 1799, he was therefore already staunchly critical of any approach to interpreting the Terror as a necessary phase of the Revolution, regarding it instead as the work of 'some villains' who had merely seized the opportunity to deceive an 'impatient and blind people'.[61] Sicard's version of enlightened education thus fulfilled at least two functions: first, it served as a rhetorical device to criticise the regime of the Terror as 'unnatural'; second it created the possibility to relate to a positive concept of 'nature' serving as a tool to preserve a normative stance towards the concept of 'humanity' without giving up the securalised anthropology. While this latter provided orientational knowledge to situate the new 'citizen' within a sphere of new possibilities for action, it defined human beings as self-referential and developing systems of processing sense perceptions. In order still to be able to claim for ethical norms the actors followed different paths: one, Sicard's and Roederer's, was to add to this self-referential image a concept of 'nature' that already implied the values in question; another, Gérando's and Maine de Biran's, was to define a centre, which was at the same time empty and invisible and could be used to found and legitimate ethical and political norms. Both options were taken to deal with the challenge of a human being as part of nature without transcendence, but which should at the same time serve as a means to formulate a knowledge system for creating a new society. Winfried Wehle has put forward the thesis, that it was precisely this latter conflict (*Zerrissenheit*) to form a centre but not to fill it out that formed the basic concern of the 'modern subject.'[62]

Victor, the 'wild boy'

So far, I have shown that protagonists of the *coup d'état* of 1799 rejected the interpretation of the Terror as a necessary phase of the Revolution. However, the year 1800 saw a different version of shock within the human sciences emerge in rather local circumstances, when a so-called feral, or 'savage' ('sauvage') child was transferred to Paris's school for deaf mutes.[63] This child, approximately twelve years of age, who was later named Victor, initially served the same functional role as the figure of the *sourd-muet*. The Society of the Observers of Man had high hopes that Sicard's educational methods would succeed in integrating him into society.[64]

Sicard withdrew from the case the same year. Eventually, the task of educating Victor was taken over by Jean Marc Gaspard Itard (1774–1838), the school physician and a student of Pinel, who worked with the boy for five years, gave him his name, and wrote reports on his progress for the Interior Minister. His reports of 1801 and 1806 stand out in the history of feral children because, compared to other cases, they are quite long and very precise in their descriptions of his educational interventions.[65] Itard started out in his education of Victor from Sicard's conviction that Victor's supposedly natural condition would allow for the 'creation of man', the harmonious unfolding of his pupil's faculties through his classifications of nature. Since, for Sicard and Itard, nature was generally good and virtuous, transferring the natural order to an order of signs and ideas meant safeguarding nature for society.

It is clear from his early report that Itard, like Sicard, began his work assuming that education was the most powerful means of moulding human beings and, furthermore, that humanity owed everything it had to education.[66] It is clear from his later report of 1806, however, that Itard increasingly deviated from his initial convictions. He saw Victor more and more as a particular, unique research object, who could not serve as a model for all human beings, for he could be compared only to himself.[67] Within this new framework, the once joyful classification activities were abandoned in favour of a new ensemble of techniques designed to act on Victor's mind, including punishing and surprising Victor, as well as traditional medical treatments such as hot and cold baths. Itard's report of 1806 illustrates how a different version of the sensualist self was taking shape in educational and research practices. While he still believed that sense perception was highly important in moulding human beings, he also used techniques aimed at producing unexpected results, an approach we do not find in Sicard. The kind of self Itard tried to act on was therefore defined at least in part as an area that could only be made visible by an experimental approach in the modern sense. In some way or the other, Itard had to shock Victor's inner self; for while the self itself may be invisible, its effects could, in Itard's view, be made observable. In carefully designed experimental spaces, moral shock thus made perfect sense. Sometimes, Itard also used his personal bond with Victor to experiment with the effects of emotions:

> I approached Victor; I spoke affectionately to him, expressing myself in terms suitable for him to grasp their meaning, and adding even more intelligible signs of friendship. His tears redoubled, accompanied by sighs and sobs. Increasing the intensity of my caresses, I drove the emotion to its highest point and, if I may say so, made tremble the moral Man unto his last fibre.[68]

With interventions like these, Itard was trying to stimulate Victor into active and inventive, especially linguistic, performances. His strong focus on Victor's activity was due to his reading of Gérando's book on the generation of ideas, in which Gérando proposed a transformation of Condillac's conceptualisation of the human mind.[69] The focal point of this transformation was the mind's passivity or activity.[70] Gérando concentrated here particularly on the faculty of attention. One of the central claims of his philosophy is that the human being has an active ability to create hitherto unknown combinations of ideas. Attention and invention were means of staking out a specific terrain proper to being human, for – as Michel Foucault has shown – classical sensualist philosophy lacked an argumentational device for defining a particular being called 'man': every totality capable of processing sense perception, of generating ideas and signs was indistinguishable from 'man' (this also partially explains the excitement about 'automatons' and the question of whether they could potentially become human).[71] Gérando chose a path that enabled him to define the essence of human beings within a sensualist vocabulary while dispensing with Condillac's commitment to the absolute emptiness of the mind before education. He called this essence the *Moi*, the ego. It was consciously characterised as an active principle. In the first lines of his *Des signes* (*On signs*), Gérando thus defines the verb 'to think' as analogous to the verb 'to act'.[72] This activity of the ego begins with the faculty of attention, which is the moral counterpart of physical sensation. While sensation comes from the outside, Gérando claims, attention comes from 'us', meaning that there is a structuring principle which we cannot alter (the system of the nerves, the sense organs etc.) and an active principle dependent on the ego. On the first pages of his prize-winning essay, Gérando observes that both principles had to be treated as unknown variables. This was attractive for philosophers like Victor Cousin (1792–1867), who embraced this concept of the human being with a specifically human core, as well as for other researchers, since the existence of such a core ultimately called for the existence of a research programme.

I contend that it was precisely this human core that also underpinned Itard's subsequent research activities at the *Institution nationale des sourds-muets*. Sicard's ideal rational Enlightenment subject was replaced by a subject whose rich interiority was difficult to locate and to expound.[73] This was also the interpretative framework that Itard used in his larger work on the education of *sourds-muets*.[74] Itard thereby particularised the notion of 'civilisation', so important for revolutionary discourse, and applied it to partially discrete zones of action. The *Institution nationale des sourds-muets* was one such zone, characterised by its unique progress of reason and sensibility. As in the 1806 report on Victor, this particular civilisation of the school's pupils could only be measured against its own zone of action; there could be no comparison with the universal progress of enlightenment.[75]

This version of modern subjectivity as a local challenge of negotiation within local developments necessitated a concomitant interpretation of the place of individuals within their wider social collective. In an 1802 manuscript about insanity, Itard introduced a concept he called the 'spirit of the present time' ('esprit du temps actuel'), which, he argued, constituted the most basic measure of mental health and illness.[76] Sanity could thus only be defined as a function of the development of a more general, sometimes national, spirit. Political revolutions were comparable to the 'blind anger of a maniac during the most terrible attack', a 'universal and contagious exaltation of every human passion' to the level of 'national mania'.[77] At the same time, Itard assumed that a diagnosis of mental illness was closely linked to the ensemble of 'national customs'.[78] Cabanis and Itard shared a perspective on the historicity of nations and of individuals that diverged from the universal narratives of progressive enlightenment.[79] In their view, the prerequisite for a morally and physically sound relationship between the individual and their more or less extensive community was the synchronous development of their mental progress.[80]

Esquirol and the insane

Itard's friend Jean-Étienne Esquirol (1772–1840), who also was a student of Pinel, published his influential medical dissertation on the human passions in 1805. Esquirol was one of the first physicians in France to reflect systematically on how the passions might be used to cure the insane.[81] In addition, he introduced the concept of 'moral shock' ('sécousse morale') to this framework and added to the history of medicine several striking case studies of moral shock at work.[82] Esquirol believed that the Revolution, and especially the Terror, had produced devastating effects on the mental, emotional, and physical state of the French people:

> The political shocks, by bringing all the passions into play, by stimulating artificial passions, by overemphasising violent passions, by multiplying the needs of certain individuals, by depriving the others of the fortune which had become necessary for their habits, the political upheavals have increased the number of the insane. It is what was observed after the revolution in England, it is what has been observed in France since our revolutionary turmoil.[83]

Throughout his dissertation, Esquirol generally criticises the effects of every sort of disturbance, such as the increasing levels of noise produced within European cities; but at the same time, he believes that the calculated interventions of medical experts in the form of moral shocks may have salutary effects. In many cases, these interventions are arranged analogically to theatrical plays, in order to convey to the insane an understanding of their illness and escort them back to their rational selves. Esquirol uses every means of dissimulation and disguise to induce the necessary moral shock and to break the delusions of insanity:

> We have never pretended we could cure [the insane] by arguing with them. This pretension would be contradicted by daily experience. Do the passions give way to reasoning? […] [T]o treat them with dialectical formulas and syllogisms would be to misunderstand the course of the passions and the clinical history of insanity.

Esquirol argues that it is 'only by giving a moral shock, by placing the insane in a state opposite and contrary to that in which they were before' that they can be cured.[84]

In 1816, Esquirol drew on his intellectual and medical forebears – the physicians Cabanis, Moreau de la Sarthe, and Pinel – in order to strengthen his hypothesis that insanity was caused by an imaginary passion, which, by means of moral shock, could be substituted with a real passion.[85] To achieve this, the physician first had to master the art of reading the signs of physical and moral disorders (physiognomic signs, for example, but also specific kinds of fever etc.) in order to contrive a specific and individual form of intervention. This would result in breaking the 'veil' that separated the interior world of a 'vicious chain of ideas' from the outer world.[86] While individually tailored moral shock could be a legitimate means when carefully controlled by a medical expert, Esquirol considered abrupt changes of habits, 'dangerous innovations', and the loss of ancient forms, especially among the lower classes, to be particularly dangerous.[87] Republican and democratic regimes, in particular, encouraged insanity, according to Esquirol, who, in this particular text of 1816, criticised the whole course of the Revolution.[88]

In summary, in the texts describing the medical interventions of Itard and Esquirol, two types of shock can be distinguished: a political shock, which is harmful, and a therapeutic shock induced by a medical expert, which can be helpful. In the texts of both doctors, the invention of a certain relationship between experts of the mind (psychiatrists, physicians, educators) and objects of this expertise can be retraced. This relationship was characterised by the reification of the objects of medical intervention and the attempt to confine the use of the passions to controlled spaces, while the more general and public zones of action were to be kept free of the excessive shocks linked especially to the Terror. An article by Michel Gourevitch tells of a case that illustrates this dissipation, in the new expert regime, of the Enlightenment's conviction that every human being is a rational decision-maker with regard to her or his own mind. In 1812, Gourevitch notes, a dispute between the administrator and the physician of the asylum for the insane at Charenton was brought before the police commissioner. The two men disagreed on the question of whether only the physician or also the administrator had a right to make decisions on curing insanity. The police commissioner decided in favour of the physician and thus, as Gourevitch argues, in favour of the consequential growth of 'medical power'.[89]

Conclusion: modern subjectivity and moral shock

By using moral shocks physicians such as Itard and Esquirol adopted a perspective on the relationship between the individual and society that entailed specific assessment of the individual's capacity for freedom and the right of social and scientific elites to exert control over individuals. This type of scientific and therapeutic activity was marked by constant reflection on the regime of the Terror. In 1789, Pinel had put his trust in the justice of the heated passions of the people, which had shaken off a 'long lethargy' through an eruption of the human spirit, and 'could no longer be oppressed'.[90] But the Terror had shown human scientists that the moulding of a republican people was not as easy a task as they had hoped. The people were understood to have proven themselves deceivable and seducible, and their passions had been easily manipulated by the leaders of the Terror.

Itard and Esquirol are only two examples of an array of administrators, physicians, and educators (such as Gérando, Pinel, and Cabanis) who were active in discussions about the human and social sciences around 1800, who, especially after the downfall of the universalist hope for a unified *science de l'homme*, helped to develop new medical and scientific spaces for controlling and adjusting the passions. They mistrusted the naturalistic narrative espoused by figures such as Lezay-Marnésia and Petit, who tried to include the Terror in a civilising story of progress. Instead, they advocated an elitist regime that would harmonise the violent passions of the people. For this reason, institutions like the asylum and the school – and, as Michel Foucault has shown, the prison – became important centres comparable to laboratories, where experiments on the control and analysis of the passions could be carried out.[91] Within these spaces, a system of control was established that might be labelled an 'elitist regime', as it was based on the figure of the expert who controlled different aspects of the people's behaviour. This elitist approach held that the people may have a rational and, to some degree, free will, but in cases of deviance, an administrative or scientific expertise is needed to explain, control, and limit the discrepancies.

There are, of course, other anthropological reactions to the challenges of the restructuring of French society, such as clearly mystical or religious answers, that, like the ones presented in this chapter, took up the modern challenge to define human beings as part of nature and at the same time to formulate normative (ethical and political) claims. This chapter has pointed out that the kind of subjectivity espoused by the human sciences around 1800 explicitly reacted to the experiences of the French Revolution and the anxiety that the people might again fall prey to an instrumentalisation of their easily heated passions. The advocates of Napoleon's *coup d'état* of 1799 therefore rejected the universalist hope for a complete regeneration of 'the people' and 'the mind' and instead tried to install spaces of control within which subjects might exercise their rights freely as long as they did not conflict with basic governmental interests. These spaces made possible a transformed concept of *difference*: at a governmental level, a single, homogeneous layer of education, wealth, or power was no longer necessary; there could be differences everywhere, as long as they were kept within a certain tolerance range. Within these zones of action, attempts were undertaken to establish regimes of contemporaneity. The idea of the civilising mission, so important for the eighteenth century, was thus transformed and used to establish a general scheme of administration.

Another expert, who has been the focus of this chapter, was the medical expert. As pointed out, medical experts like Pinel, Itard, or Esquirol built on a discourse about the effects of the shock of the Revolution to formulate a new version of medical intervention. Esquirol thereby distinguished the political and harmful shock from the medically controlled and curative shock. The kind of modern subjectivity informing this stance towards shock rested upon the figure of the vulnerable and unstable subject on the one hand and the medical, administrative, and political expert systems taking care of mitigating the impact of unstable political and social constellations on the other. Thus, this version of the modern subject was basically semi-autonomous, being unobstructed as long as kept within a tolerance range, and becoming the object of expert systems of control when transgressing the boundaries of situatively defined norms of the tolerable. As Herrnstadt has shown at length, the establishment of the Napoleonic version of authoritarian administration was based on a comparable concept of semi-autonomous units, which was itself based on a transformed version of sensualism.[92] We thus find the same kind of shift – from transparency predicated upon a universal scheme towards opacity predicated upon a semi-particularised scheme – at the level of the individual, as well. On this individual level, the education of the passions within controlled spaces was supposed to form the basis for a general harmonisation and pacification. There emerged in this regard a new type of experimental object within the traditional field of the 'analysis of ideas', a specifically human being, with an opaque inner zone called the *Moi*, which enabled the renewed application, now in the context of 'moral treatment', of an old approach to curing physical diseases through shock. We can therefore distinguish two kinds of shock: a universal and revolutionary shock, which is uncontrolled and therefore extremely harmful, and a local shock used to heal the mind or to find out something about the interdependence of the physical and the moral. The kind of subject proffered by the human sciences was marked by an authoritarian relation between experts and the human beings whom they viewed as objects of research, who were at once potentially dangerous and in need of care. This combination of anxiety and care enabled the emergence of two approaches to the problem of control: welfare and the human sciences. And this modern subject, conceived on the basis of mistrust, accordingly reappears as an object of research and as an administrative unit.

Notes

1 'Les révolutions sont au corps politique qu'elles agitent, ce que sont au corps humain altéré les médicamens qui doivent y rétablir l'harmonie. Dans l'un comme dans l'autre, le premier effet est un désordre, la première sensation une douleur'. M. A. Petit, *Essai sur la médecine du cœur* (Lyon: Chez Garnier/Chez Reymann, 1806), 116. If not otherwise stated, the translations provided in the text are my own.
2 *Ibid.*, 122.
3 *Ibid.*, 123.
4 *Ibid.*, 127–8. Petit tried to show that there was a range of illnesses that had arisen from weakness. Although he did not explicitly limit these cases to women, most of the case studies he presented related to women with forms of diseases stemming from weakness that were cured by the revolutionary shock. In his speech Petit therefore gives various examples of women being cured during the Revolution, but also some of feeble men. It is not easy to say whether Petit was assuming an essential difference here. But I think he was more inclined to believe that there was a difference between men and women based on education. Thus, on p. 124, he explained that women had been brought up in softness and idleness and that the Revolution had put

these harmful habits aside. According to Petit, women had been 'transformed' into 'new beings' who faced the new demands.
5   N. Gelbart, 'The French Revolution as medical event: the journalistic gaze', *History of European Ideas*, 10:4 (1989), 417–27 (p. 417).
6   G. Rosen, 'Social stress and mental disease from the eighteenth century to the present: some origins of social psychiatry', *Millibank Memorial Fund Quarterly*, 37:1 (1959), 5–32.
7   R. Wokler, 'From the moral and political sciences to the sciences of society by way of the French Revolution', *Annual Review of Law and Ethics*, 8 (2000), 33–45 (p. 35).
8   See I. Wallerstein, 'Citizens all? Citizens some! The making of the citizen', *Comparative Studies in Society and History*, 45:4 (2003), 650–79.
9   J. Goldstein, *The Post-Revolutionary Self: Politics and Psyche in France, 1750–1850* (Cambridge, MA: Harvard University Press, 2005).
10 *Tableau des opérations de l'Assemblée nationale d'après le Journal de Paris*, 2 vols (Lausanne: Chez Hignou & Comp., 1789), vol. 2, 227.
11 For a comprehensive overview, see J. Goldstein, *Console and Classify: The French Psychiatric Profession in the Nineteenth Century* (New York: Cambridge University Press, 1987).
12 J. É. D. Esquirol, *Des passions considérées comme causes, symptômes et moyens curatifs de l'aliénation mentale* (Paris: Didot jeune, 1805), 82.
13 For Robespierre's idea of the *tabula rasa* see D. Wahrmann, *The Making of the Modern Self: Identity and Culture in Eighteenth-Century England* (New Haven, CT: Yale University Press, 2004). According to Wahrmann, 'The notions of "regeneration" and the "new man", after all, stood at the center of the French revolutionary project. No one was a better spokesman for the malleability of identity than Maximilien Robespierre, who in true Lockean fashion proclaimed children to be mere tabulae rasae that the revolution could fashion as it pleased. It was also Robespierre who remarked that the revolution had transformed the French, in comparison to other European powers, "as if they had become a different species"' (313).
14 S. Wahnich, *Les Émotions, la Révolution française et le présent. Exercices pratiques de conscience historique* (Paris: CNRS Éd., 2009).
15 As Martin Herrnstadt has shown, on a governmental level, the administration was no longer interested in generating an absolutely homogeneous framework, but tolerated zones that were partially independent. See M. Herrnstadt, 'Verwaltung des Selbst – Epistemologie des Staates. Joseph-Marie de Gérando, die Wissenschaft vom Menschen & der 18. Brumaire des Jahres VIII' (PhD dissertation, Frankfurt am Main, 2017).
16 J. Goldstein, *The Post-Revolutionary Self: Politics and Psyche in France, 1750–1850* (Cambridge, MA: Harvard University Press, 2005), 104.

17 E.-J. Sieyès, 'Qu'est-ce que le tiers-état?' (s.l., 1789), 172–3.
18 This allowed for the famous advent of the 'human', which Michel Foucault analysed in *The Order of Things: An Archaeology of the Human Sciences* (New York: Pantheon, 1970). See, in particular, Chapter 10.
19 Within Deaf History, the concept of the 'sourd-muet' – the 'deaf-mute' has been considered offensive. In this text I therefore use the original French name as a quotation.
20 As Marcel Gauchet argues, it was exactly this concept of the rational self that in this period also made it possible to believe in the curability of insanity. It was possible to establish a discourse with the insane because behind their insanity, the rational self was believed to be still intact. See M. Gauchet, 'De Pinel à Freud', in G. Swain (ed.), *Le Sujet de la folie. Naissance de la psychiatrie* (Paris: Calmann-Lévy, 1997), 7–57 (p. 23).
21 Goldstein argues that after the Revolution, the philosophy of Cousin provided the opportunity to establish a new regime of the 'self' that differed from that of Condillac and Destutt de Tracy. See Goldstein, *Post-Revolutionary Self*, 11. See also pp. 80ff. concerning the implementation of the sensualist philosophy in public education.
22 *Ibid.*, 21–60.
23 A. L. C. Destutt de Tracy, *Quels sont les moyens de fonder la morale chez un peuple* (Paris: Agasse, 1798), 19.
24 *Ibid.*, 10.
25 J. O. Schacht, *Dissertatio medica inauguralis de terrore ejusque effectis in corpus humanum* [...] (Utrecht: Alexander van Megen, 1733), 2; 35.
26 See E. Williams, *The Physical and the Moral: Anthropology, Physiology, and Philosophical Medicine in France, 1750–1850* (Cambridge: Cambridge University Press, 1994). On the history of the 'moral treatment', see A. Benzaquén, *Encounters with Wild Children: Temptation and Disappointment in the Study of Human Nature* (Montreal: McGill-Queen's University Press, 2006), 147ff.
27 Roederer therefore claimed that the positive aspects of recent history had been caused by philosophy, whereas revolution was harmful. P. L. Roederer, *De la philosophie moderne et de la part qu'elle a eue a la Révolution française* (Paris: Imprimerie de Journal de Paris, 1799), 23–4.
28 B. Baczko, *Ending the Terror: The French Revolution after Robespierre* (Cambridge: Cambridge University Press, 1994 [1989]), 41.
29 A. Jainchill, *Reimagining Politics after the Terror* (Ithaca, NY: Cornell University Press, 2008), 204. See also K. Margerison, 'P. L. Roederer: political thought and practice during the French Revolution', *Transactions of the American Philosophical Society*, 73:1 (1983), 1–166.

30 'La terreur est un tremblement habituel, général, un tremblement extérieur qui affecte les fibres les plus cachées, qui dégrade l'homme et l'assimile à la brute; c'est l'ébranlement de toutes les forces physiques, la commmotion de toutes les facultés morales, le dérangement de toutes les idées, le renversement de toutes les affections; c'est une véritable désorganisation de l'âme, qui, ne lui laissant que la faculté de souffrir, lui enlève dans ses maux et les douceurs de l'espérance et les ressources du désespoir'. J. L. Tallien, 'Speech before the *Comité de salut public*', *Moniteur* (Tridi, 13 fructidor an II = 30 August 1794, no. 343), 613.

31 See L. Formigari, 'Les Idéologues. Philosophie du langage et hégémonie bourgeoise', in W. Busse and J. Trabant (eds), *Les Idéologues. Sémiotique, théories et politiques linguistiques pendant la Révolution française* (Amsterdam: John Benjamins, 1986); S. Rosenfeld, *A Revolution in Language: The Problems of Signs in Late Eighteenth-Century France* (Stanford, CA: Stanford University Press, 2001).

32 M. Staum, 'The Class of Moral and Political Sciences, 1795–1803', *French Historical Studies*, 11:3 (1980), 371–97.

33 Destutt de Tracy, *Quels sont les moyens*, 12; 15.

34 *Ibid.*, 5.

35 B. Constant, *Des effets de la terreur* (s.l., 1797).

36 '[La terreur] a accoutumé le peuple à entendre proférer les noms les plus saints pour motiver les actes les plus exécrables. Elle a confondu toutes les notions, faconné les esprits à l'arbitraire, inspiré le mépris des formes, préparé les violences et les forfaits en tous sens'. Constant, *Des effets de la terreur*, 31–2.

37 'changement total de mœurs, d'habitudes, de conditions, d'intérêts, de propriétés', A. Lezay-Marnésia, *Des causes de la Révolution et de ses résultats* (Paris: Imprimerie du Journal d'économie publique, 1797), 5.

38 'Les lumières et la corruption font leur progrès ensemble: c'est pourquoi toute révolution populaire, amenée par le progrès des lumières, est nécessairement violente'. Lezay-Marnésia, *Des causes*, 20.

39 *Ibid.*, 43–4.

40 *Ibid.*, 31; 35.

41 *Ibid.*, 44–5; 65–6. On the widespread idea of the 'new people' see M. Ozouf, 'La Révolution rançaise et l'idée de l'homme nouveau', in C. Lucas (ed.), *The Political Culture of the French Revolution* (Oxford: Pergamon, 1988), 213–32.

42 'Les chocs révolutionnaires ne sont points, comme quelques personnes semblent le croire, occasionnés par le libre développement des idées: ils ont toujours [...] été le produit inévitable des vains obstacles qu'on lui oppose imprudemment; du défaut d'accord entre la marche des affaires et

celle de l'opinion, entre les institutions sociales et l'état des esprits'. ('Revolutionary upheavals are not, as some appear to believe, caused by the free development of ideas: they have always [...] been the inevitable product of the vain obstacles which are imprudently opposed to it; of the dissonance between the development of affairs and that of opinion, between social institutions and the collective state of mind'.) P. J. G. Cabanis, *Rapports du physique et du moral de l'homme* (Paris: J. B. Baillière, 1844 [1798]), 50.
43 J. M. Gérando, *Des signes et de l'art de penser considérés dans leur rapports mutuels*, 4 vols (Paris: Chez Goujon, 1800), vol. 3, p. 20.
44 The most comprehensive interpretation of the Society of the Observers of Man is J. L. Chappey, *La Société des observateurs de l'homme (1799–1804). Des anthropologues au temps de Bonaparte* (Paris: Société des Études Robespierristes, 2002). On Gérando see Herrnstadt, *Verwaltung des Selbst* and J. L. Chappey, C. Christen, I. Mouiller (eds), *Joseph-Marie de Gérando. Connaître et réformer la société* (Rennes: Presses Universitaires de Rennes, 2014).
45 With regard to the school's public sessions, see S. Rosenfeld, 'The political uses of sign language: the case of the French Revolution', *Sign Language Studies*, 6:1 (2005), 1–37.
46 This trust is especially visible in Claude Adrian Helvétius' (1715–71) book *De l'homme*. Helvétius wanted to reveal a 'great truth to the nations', that is, that human beings were merely the product of education. C. A. Helvétius, *De l'homme, de ses facultés intellectuelles et de son éducation* (London: Société typographique, 1773), 5–6.
47 See Rosenfeld, *A Revolution in Language*.
48 See A. Quartararo, *Deaf Identity and Social Images in Nineteenth-Century France* (Washington: Gallaudet University Press, 2008).
49 'Mr Sicard est très connu des étrangers instruits qui tous fréquentent ses leçons, et comptent sa découverte parmi les titres dont notre nation s'honore et qui l'élèvent au dessus des *autres*'. Archives nationales, Paris, F/17/1145, Dossier 7.
50 See, for example, P. David, *Epître à l'abbé Sicard, sur les mots avec lesquels on nous a gouverné pendant la Révolution* (Paris: Chez les Marchands de Nouveautés, 1801), 10.
51 'qui devint pour la pensée ce que l'algèbre est pour les calculs', C. M. Talleyrand-Périgord, *Rapport sur l'instruction publique fait au nom du Comité de constitution a l'assemblée nationale* (Paris: Baudouin/Du Pont, 1791), 99.
52 'les signes analytiques de l'école des muets à devenir la langue universelle des hommes instruits de toutes les nations'. Archives nationales, Paris, FN/15/2584.

53 R. A. Sicard, 'Relation adressée par M. Abbé Sicard, Instituteur des sourds et muets, à un de ses amis, sur les dangers qu'il a courus les 2 et 3 septembre 1792', in P. J. B. Buchez and P. C. Roux (eds), *Histoire parlamentaire de la Révolution française* (Paris: Paulin, vol. 18, 1835 [1797]), 72–103 (p. 101).
54 This expression stems from the editor of Sicard's *Cours d'instruction*; see R. A. Sicard, *Cours d'instruction d'un sourd-muet de naissance, pour servir a l'éducation des sourds-muets* (Paris: Le Cere, 1799/1800), Avertissement de l'éditeur, p. x. The word 'metaphysics' might be misleading for the modern reader. Gérando, for example, believed that metaphysics was nothing else than an 'art to produce an inventory of our knowledge', Gérando, *Le génération des connoissances humaines*, 23. For Sicard, metaphysics was most probably the art of analysing the association of ideas.
55 Which is why, as Baczko shows, the Thermidorians' reaction already assumed a technical attitude towards the use of the passions and of rumours in controlling the people. Baczko, *Ending the Terror*, 17–32.
56 'c'est un être parfaitement nul dans la société, un automate vivant, une statue, telle que la présente Charles Bonnet, et d'après lui, Condillac; une statue dont il faut ouvrir, l'un après l'autre, et diriger tous les sens, et supléer à celui dont il est malheureusement privé'. ('it is a being entirely null within society, a living automaton, a statue, as described by Charles Bonnet and, following him, Condillac; a statue whose senses must be opened up one by one and guided, and compensate for the one of which it has unfortunately been deprived'.) Sicard, *Cours d'instruction*, pp. vi–vii.
57 Cf., e.g., a report of a public lesson in the *Bulletin de l'Europe*: 'J'ai assisté aux leçons de Sicard, c'étoit assister à la création de l'homme [...]. Au milieu des discussions les plus abstraites, lorsque Sicard faisoit entrer dans la tête de ses jeunes élèves les idées les plus subtiles de la métaphysique, il les ramenoit toujours d'un monde idéal dans le monde que doivent habiter des enfans, des frères et des amis [...]', *Bulletin de l'Europe* (26 fructidor an VII = 12 September 1799).
58 'C'est moins en communiquant des mots qui ne doivent jamais arriver qu'au signal des idées, qu'en faisant naître les idées qu'on procède avec quelque succès dans cet enseignement [of the deaf mutes]. C'est là que comme sur une sorte de Mappe monde le génie philosophique de l'Instituteur établit entre les idées qui sont censées en couvrir la surface, les rapports qui les lient entr'elles'. Archives nationales, Paris, F/17/2500: École des sourds-muets.
59 'Ah! combien la nature lui [Massieu] paroissoit grande et superbe dans ses reproductions! Il classa donc les plantes des jardins, les arbres des vergers, ceux des forêts; chaque genre dans un feuillet particulier, chaque série dans sa colonne, comme les noms d'autant d'amis avec lesquels il étoit empressé

de former une liaison qui devoit durer autant que le sens qui en avoit remarqué les analogies et les différences.' ('Ah! how great and magnificent nature seemed to him [Massieu] in his reproductions! And so he classified the garden plants, the trees of the orchards and those of the forests; each genus in an individual leaflet, each series in its own column, like the names of as many friends with whom he was eager to establish a relationship which should last for as long as the very intuition which had identified the analogies and differences'.) Sicard, *Cours d'instruction*, p. 32.

60 'Maladie où le moral et le physique étaient continuellement en action l'un sur l'autre'. P. L. Roederer, *L'Esprit de la Révolution de 1789* (Paris: Chez les principaux libraires, 1831), 201.

61 Roederer, *De la Philosophie moderne*, 30, 31.

62 W. Wehle, 'Kunst und Subjektivität. Von der Geburt ästhetischer Anthropologie aus dem Leiden an Modernität – Nodier, Chateaubriand', in R. Fetz, R. Hagenbüchle, and P. Schulz (eds), *Geschichte und Vorgeschichte der modernen Subjektivität* (Berlin/New York: De Gruyter 1998), vol. 2, 901–41 (p. 931).

63 There exists an extensive literature on Victor; I want to point to two books which are based on a wealth of material: T. Gineste, *Victor de l'Aveyron. Dernier enfant sauvage, premier enfant fou* (Paris: Hachette Littératures, 2004 [1981]); A. Benzaquén, *Encounters with Wild Children: Temptation and Disappointment in the Study of Human Nature* (Montreal: Queen's University Press, 2006).

64 This section is highly indebted to the work of Jean-Luc Chappey, in particular his thesis that the perspective on human beings after 1800 is characterised by what he calls 'fixism', that is, the idea that the identity (of 'women', 'men', *sourds-muets*, 'idiots') cannot change easily or in fact at all. See J. L. Chappey, *Sauvagerie et civilisation. Une histoire politique de Victor de l'Aveyron* (Paris: Fayard, 2017).

65 Bonnaterre, who wrote the first report on Victor, supplemented the list of *homini feri* given by Carl Linné in different editions of his Natural History. None of these cases was documented extensively; sometimes there were only a few lines testifying to the existence of a supposedly 'wild' individual. See Benzaquén, *Encounters with Wild Children*, part one.

66 See Helvétius, *De l'homme*, 5–6.

67 J. M. G. Itard, 'Second rapport fait au Ministre de l'intérieur sur les nouveaux développements et l'état actuel du sauvage de l'Aveyron', in J. M. G. Itard, *Rapports et mémoires sur le sauvage de l'Aveyron, l'idiotie et la surdi-mutité* (Paris: Progrès Médical, 1894 [1806]), 60.

68 'Je me rapprochai de Victor; je lui fis entendre des paroles affectueuses, que je prononçai dans des termes propres à lui en faire saisir le sens, et

que j'accompagnai de témoignages d'amitié plus intelligibles encore. Ses pleurs redoublèrent, accompagnées de soupirs et de sanglots; tandis que redoublant moi-même de caresses, je portai l'émotion au plus haut point, et faisais, si je puis m'exprimer, frémir jusqu'à la dernière fibre sensible l'homme moral', Itard, 'Second rapport', 80–1.
69 This is at least what Gérando himself says in a letter to Roederer (22 May 1802), Archives nationales, Paris, 29AP/10.
70 Herrnstadt, *Verwaltung des Selbst*, 56–8.
71 See S. Klinge and L. Schlicht, 'Differenz Automat. Ein Ausschnitt aus der Geschichte des Menschen: Taubstummenforschung (um 1800) und Kybernetik (1946–1953)', in M. C. Gruber, J. Bung, and S. Ziemann (eds), *Autonome Automaten. Künstliche Körper und artifizielle Agenten in der technisierten Gesellschaft* (Berlin: trafo, 2014), 103–34.
72 Gérando, *Des signes*, vol. 1, p. 2.
73 'One trajectory of the argument of Isolate Cases follows the self-sufficient inward subject who is the protagonist of Locke's Essay from an enlightenment origin as a figure of normativity, a theoretical model for all minds, to its nineteenth-century manifestations as tragic anomaly – as a monster who has the upbringing of a philosopher as a philosopher made monstrous by preternatural cultivation of the mind alone.' N. Yousef, *Isolated Cases: The Anxieties of Autonomy in Enlightenment Philosophy and Romantic Literature* (Ithaca, NY: Cornell University Press, 2004), 8.
74 J. Itard, *Traité des maladies de l'oreille et de l'audition* (Paris: Chez Méquignon-Marvis, 1821).
75 Ibid., 427–9.
76 J. Itard, 'Vésanies', in Gineste, *Victor de l'Aveyron*, 431.
77 Ibid., 431.
78 Ibid., 433.
79 One of the most explicit versions of this unidirectional narrative can be found in M. J. Condorcet, *Esquisse d'un tableau historique des progrès de l'esprit humain. Ouvrage posthume de Condorcet* (Paris: Agasse, 1795).
80 At the same time, as Fritzsche argues, the category of 'contemporaneity' gained prominence: P. Fritzsche, *Stranded in the Present: Modern Time and the Melancholy of History* (Cambridge MA: Harvard University Press, 2004).
81 There are in fact some earlier texts, e.g. F. C. G. Scheidemantel, *Die Leidenschaften als Heilmittel betrachtet* (Hildburghausen: Johann Gottfried Hanisch, 1787).
82 Esquirol, *Des passions*, 82; see also Scheidemantel, *Die Leidenschaften*. Scheidemantel states that in earlier times the 'passions' were regarded as a cause rather than as a means of treating illness (p. ii).

83 'Les sécousses politiques en mettant en jeu toutes les passions, en donnant plus d'essor aux passions factices, en exagérant les passions haineuses, en multipliant les besoins de certains individus, en privant les autres d'une fortune devenue nécessaire à leurs habitudes, les commotions politiques augmentent le nombre des aliénés; c'est ce qu'on a observé après la révolution d'Angleterre; c'est ce qu'on observe en France depuis notre tourmente révolutionnaire'. Esquirol, *Des passions*, 15.
84 'on n'a jamais prétendu les guérir en argumentant avec eux, cette prétention serait démentie par l'expérience journalière: les passions cèdent-elles aux raisonnemens? [...] les traiter avec des formules dialectiques et des syllogismes, ce serait mal connaître la marche des passions et l'histoire clinique de l'aliénation mentale. [...] [C]e n'est qu'en donnant une secousse morale, en plaçant l'aliéné dans un état opposé et contraire à celui dans lequel il était avant de recourir à ce moyen'. Esquirol, *Des passions*, 82.
85 J. É. D. Esquirol, 'De la folie', in J. É. D. Esquirol, *Des maladies mentales considérées sous les rapports médical, hygiénique et médico-légal* (Paris: Baillière 1838 [1816]), 133.
86 *Ibid.*, 133.
87 *Ibid.*, 49–50.
88 *Ibid.*, 54.
89 M. Gourevitch, 'La Psychiatrie sous l'empire', *Histoire des sciences medicales*, 23:1 (1989), 27–32 (p. 31).
90 *Tableau des opérations de l'Assemblée nationale d'après le Journal de Paris*, 228.
91 For prison see M. Foucault, *Surveiller et punir. Naissance de la prison* (Paris: Gallimard, 1975).
92 Herrnstadt, *Verwaltung des Selbst*, 272–3.

2

Medical negligence in nineteenth-century Germany

Torsten Riotte

In 1933, the German lawyer Friedrich Franz König published an essay on medical negligence.[1] He pointed out that the number of negligence cases in Germany had risen to unprecedented heights in recent times. The years 1927–29 had seen an increase of close to 50% of negligence cases, as the insurance statistics demonstrated. König suggested that such a rise was due to the global economic crisis that had hit Germany hard.[2] As a second argument for this growth, König referred to the doctor–patient relationship. He saw patients as increasingly estranged from their doctors and lacking confidence in the representatives of the medical profession.[3] Finally, König claimed that the popularisation of medical sciences had made patients less reluctant to sue doctors. He wrote: 'The traditional belief in the authority of doctors has vanished.'[4] Although such arguments seem plausible, it remains to be discussed whether (and to what extent) broader social trends had an impact on the figures of negligence cases.[5] The democratisation of scientific knowledge, and the availability of data and information, as well as the rise in popularity of so-called alternative medicines and hence the contestation of general medical practice, all seem to have encouraged patients to sue doctors more readily for negligence.[6]

This chapter discusses medical jurisdiction in Germany as a case study to explain how professional accountability changed during the nineteenth century. It examines the transformation that occurred in medical jurisdiction, in order to discuss how doctors were held responsible for professional malpractice and how legal procedures changed. The transformation of medical jurisdiction is understood as the result of changing patterns of accountability in more general terms. The French sociologist François Ewald sees a shift in accountability in the workplace, from the idea of individual liability to the collectivisation of personal risk, as an indicator of modern European society. While an individual would traditionally be accountable for his or her performance at work and possible injury or damage in the workplace, the complexity of labour in an industrialised society created a new idea of accountability that Ewald links to the emergence of the term 'accident'.[7] In the course of the nineteenth century, most employers learnt to accept that work, particularly in the new industrial workplaces, had become too complex generally for workers to avoid making mistakes.[8] By the end of this development, the strict liability of the employer became a common feature for occupations in European nation states – hence Ewald's argument that such a transition from individual accountability to social insurance should be understood as the beginning or the origin of modernity.[9]

In practical terms, the emergence of the concept of the 'accident' meant that employers and employees no longer faced legal persecution in cases of professional misconduct. This is why Ewald's interpretation is closely linked to the emergence of the welfare state in Europe. From the late nineteenth century, most accidents in the workplace were covered by insurance policies, with a rising number of states introducing compulsory insurance systems for employees.[10] To explain such a transition, historiography has emphasised the evolving relationship between risk, responsibility, and statehood. Julia Moses writes in her comparative study of social states in Europe: 'to contemporaries in the late nineteenth century, accidents had seemed a shadowside of industrial modernity that would require a thoroughly modern solution: national social policy managed by a modern bureaucracy.'[11]

Although the state as the manager of 'risks'[12] became a key player in modern industries, such interpretation appears to be more difficult to translate into the medical profession. The introduction of the term 'medical negligence' around 1800 can be seen as indicative of a renegotiation of doctors' accountability. Due to the increasing complexity and sophistication of medical therapies, it became increasingly unlikely that a single medical authority could provide reliable, consistent, and long-lasting guidelines for medical jurisdiction. Negotiating the legal frameworks included arbitrating professional, scientific, and legal politics. The question arose as to whether the state would need to act as legislator or institutional innovator to master the challenges of medicine and modernity. A substantial number of doctors in Germany argued in favour of medical disciplinary courts, but it took until the last third of the century before so-called courts of honour were introduced. Until this period, doctors, politicians, and the public discussed whether medical negligence should be treated as a civil or criminal offence.

The chapter also addresses institutional responses to the challenges of modernity. The late Napoleonic and Restoration periods saw the birth of medical commissions in most German states. Such medical advisory boards were intended to ensure the quality of medical training. They also advised the ministries in the German states in cases of medical negligence.[13] Exploring the archival material produced by the medical commission in Hanover, the chapter explores different cases of negligence. While the need for expertise in cases of medical negligence had been identified by the authorities at the beginning of the nineteenth century, legal reform was delayed until the last third of it.

Finally, the chapter points to an additional element that constituted the transformation of liability in the workplace. In accordance with the so-called risk historiography, it is argued that collectivising professional accountability not only meant the rise of the state as the manager of 'risks' but also, and arguably more importantly, the commodification of the latter.[14] The invention of liability insurance for doctors in the 1880s will be used as a point in case. While the traditional idea of individual accountability prevailed in modern medicine, the opportunities to tackle the economic consequences of professional liability changed fundamentally.

The first popular court case and the discourse on medical negligence from 1800

Until around 1800, the German term used for medical misconduct was *Unkunst*, a word that went back to the criminal code established by the German emperor Charles V in 1532, known under its Latin name of *Constitutio Criminalis Carolina*.[15] The *Carolina* sanctioned the suing of a doctor for compensation in cases of serious professional misconduct.

It distinguished between cases where doctors were accused of failing to meet professional medical standards (*Unkunst*) and those where patients suffered due to carelessness or neglect (*Unfleiss*).[16] The *Carolina* listed a number of prerequisites necessary to sue a doctor. It laid down that medical experts should advise the judge in his decision, and also regulated the amounts of compensation for different forms of misconduct.[17]

With regard to German medicine, a new word entered the medical, legal, and political discourse around 1800. At the turn of the nineteenth century, medical professional misconduct began to be referred to as *Kunstfehler*, which translates as 'medical negligence'. The first mention in a German encyclopedia dates to 1797, but it was the first prominent court case a few years later that sparked wider public discussion.[18] In December 1811, Ernst Horn, a Professor at the Berlin Charité hospital was sued over the death of one of his patients. The twenty-one-year-old Louise Thiele had been hospitalised in August 1811 and diagnosed with hysteria. The doctor recommended the full variety of applications commonly prescribed at the time. Cold water baths were applied with doses of a hundred buckets of cold water. The patient was put in a rotating bed, an apparatus inspired by the English swing machine, restrained and rotated with a cadence of 120 times per minute.[19] After an additional number of other treatments that all failed to calm her, Thiele was finally put in a restraining jacket, covered in two woollen sacks and left to herself. Unattended for a couple of hours, she died of a heart attack on 1 September 1811.[20]

Heinrich Kohlrausch, one of Horn's colleagues at the hospital, filed a complaint against the doctor to the Prussian Ministry of Justice, blaming him for professional misconduct and cruelty.[21] Kohlrausch and Horn had been at odds over several other professional and also personal issues beforehand. It was well known that the two did not show any sympathy towards each other.[22] The Prussian Ministry of Justice considered whether Kohlrausch's complaint should be moved to a criminal court. Johann Christian Reil, one of the experts who acted as medical consultant to the ministry, argued against a prosecution. In a private letter to a colleague, Reil criticised Kohlrausch as stupid, mean, and devious.[23] By some mysterious route, Reil's private correspondence found its way into the hands of Kohlrausch who forwarded it to the ministry.[24] The Prussian Ministry of Justice finally decided that the case should be moved to court. Further evidence was collected, experts consulted, and witnesses heard. In November 1812, Horn was acquitted and found not guilty. Kohlrausch left the Charité the following year.[25]

The conflict between Horn and Kohlrausch counts as the first modern court case of medical negligence, not least due to the prominence it gathered in the public reaction. To a certain extent, it appears to be a personal feud between colleagues. The medical historian Moritz Kalisch, who published a number of documents on the case in 1860, argued in favour of a conspiracy against Horn.[26] However, this was only part of the story. The political authorities had felt the necessity to respond to Kohlrausch's accusations because they had caused public interest.[27] In this context, it is important to consider that an earlier complaint by a relative of Louise Thiele had been turned down by the ministry.[28] As the trial gained more prominence, the Prussian authorities acted out of necessity.[29] Independent of Kohlrausch's motivation and the outcome of the trial, the Thiele case also caused a public debate about medical negligence.[30] The following decades saw a substantial number of publications on the topic. While there were more theoretical tracts about doctors' accountability until approximately the 1850s, case studies in medical negligence increasingly appeared during the second half of the century.[31]

The expanding nature of medical knowledge and its impact on medical therapy was perceived as a fundamental problem in defining doctors' accountability in fixed legal terms. As the German pathologist Rudolph Virchow argued, what was regarded as established medical therapy at one time could become serious professional misconduct at another.[32] How should the law respond? Contemporary medical authors did not grow tired of pointing out that the rising body of medical research showed many examples of groundbreaking innovations that challenged traditional assumptions about medical care.[33] Virchow wrote that there was no authority in science that could lay down once and for all what should be allowed in medical care and what should be banned.[34] With regard to medical jurisdiction, he argued against medical negligence as a criminal offence and in favour of civil legislation that would refer to the leading medical authorities for advice in such cases.[35]

The core of Virchow's argument advances a generally optimistic outlook on the benefits of medical research and the expansion of scientific knowledge.[36] He argued that 'there are certain types of surgery that nowadays save the lives of thousands of people that used to be seen as daring and foolhardy in the past'.[37] In the context of the more general question of state interference in cases of professional accountability, two aspects seem worth elaborating upon. Firstly, a codification of good medical practice seemed restrictive with regard to innovation in medical sciences. As a general principle, scientific research needed to transgress boundaries in order to innovate. Hence, doctors depended on the liberty to experiment beyond established practices.[38] In its most extreme form, such an understanding of medical science as innovation included human experimentation.[39] One of the most notorious cases of medical jurisdiction in Germany involved the German doctor Albert Neisser, who injected nine female patients with blood serum from syphilis patients in 1892. Four patients developed syphilis. After a delay of several years, the Neisser case sparked a debate about the legality of human experimentation. As a result, the Prussian Ministry for Religious, Educational, and Medical Affairs passed instructions to the heads of clinics and hospitals laying down a list of regulations for such experiments.[40] Although historiography has justly claimed that the doctor–patient relationship during this period was characterised by the disregard of medical researchers for the safety and consent of their patients,[41] the publicity of the Neisser case demonstrates that negligence cases could provide a patient (or more generally, the public) with the means to challenge doctors' authority.

Secondly, and despite such notorious cases as the syphilis experiment, doctors claimed enormous successes in treating patients, particularly during the last decades of the nineteenth century. While, in the example of the German federal state Baden, only three out of ten babies survived a birth by Caesarean section in the period from 1865 to 1874, these figures rose to almost nine out of ten in the 1890s (with the total number of Caesareans increasing substantially).[42] To be hospitalised would have posed a serious risk to health in the 1850s and 1860s, but this was clearly not the case by the 1890s.[43] This breakthrough in hospital surgery can be dated to the last third of the nineteenth century, when asepsis and antisepsis helped to fight gangrene, which had been a contributing factor to high mortality rates after operations. Claudia Huerkamp argues that due to more reliable practices in several fields of medicine, doctors were no longer challenged as the most reliable experts in treating illnesses from the 1850s onwards. Medical pluralism progressively disappeared and the expert status of doctors became increasingly uncontested.[44]

In the light of such successes, the inability to cure a patient began to appear as a failure of the individual doctor, rather than being attributed to the incapability of wider medical practice. This meant that increasing success in medical and surgical procedures at large correlated with a rise in the number of negligence cases brought against individual doctors.[45] Doctors, and the medical associations of which they were members, had to defend their professional status and they worried that individual failure would damage the reputation of the wider medical profession.[46] Patients increasingly expected to be fully and swiftly cured by a doctor, and, as patient or client, demanded successful and reliable treatment. In Germany, patients showed more readiness to sue if doctors failed to help.[47] Finally, an increase in competition within the health sector (particularly since the 1880s) made it necessary for doctors to appear superior to lay healers and other medical personnel.[48] As medical historiography has emphasised, growing success made the profession not less but more controversial – at least on the level of individual accountability.[49] In this sense, the doctor–state relationship proved ambivalent. While the medical profession relied on state protection to establish university-trained doctors as the dominant and indisputable authority in the health sector, its growing self-confidence based on more successful treatment led to a cry for institutional reform and professional autonomy.

Responsibility in transition: an institutional perspective

During the second half of the nineteenth century, state-of-the-art laboratory sciences and the latest medical innovations were only reluctantly introduced into medical practice on a broader scale. Although the leading authorities could point to great successes within the profession, doctors with limited financial resources or without access to modern medical training centres had difficulties in keeping up with the latest research or in applying such breakthrough innovations to medical practice.[50] Therefore, the image of the doctor during the second half of the nineteenth century was characterised by a certain ambiguity. What qualification, training, and performance could be expected from the 'average' doctor? German medical discourse referred to the idea of a generally accepted and commonly agreed upon medical expertise as a standard for doctors and as a benchmark for cases of medical negligence.[51] But who was to judge?

Since the sixteenth century, early modern German legislation offered the means to sue doctors in civil and criminal court cases. German doctors could be liable for criminal offences if a patient under their care died. They could also be sued for compensation in civil court cases for injuries or neglect. However, no specific law on medical liability existed. Instead, doctors were charged with manslaughter or bodily harm with some qualifying remarks on professions with close contact to clients or patients.[52] For a substantial time during the nineteenth century, German doctors argued against the practice of treating negligence as a 'common' crime, and hoped to establish professional courts that would treat negligence as a disciplinary offence.[53]

German doctors had been state-controlled and legislated since the early modern period (and with increasing intensity since the second half of the eighteenth century). Whether or not doctors were allowed to settle and practice at a specific place depended on an official licence issued by the so-called medical police.[54] In addition, until the trade ordinances of 1869, doctors were legally bound to provide professional help to patients within their assigned district and could be forced to take on public functions.[55] As the historian Andreas Holger Maehle writes: 'Since the early nineteenth century German doctors had virtually been treated as civil servants. Governments could discipline them with reprimands and fines, or even withdraw their license if they showed a lack of professional competence and reliability'.[56] The medical police were part of the ministry of the interior, which generally acted on a regional level; its members are best understood as representatives of the local or regional bureaucracy. They dealt with complaints about individual doctors, but only occasionally compiled statistical data. In essence, they represented a tool of state bureaucracy and administration – though with an exclusively regional outlook.

Due to an increasing demand for professional medical expertise, the majority of German federal states set up advisory boards, or commissions, to the (often reorganised) ministries of the interior in the first two decades of the nineteenth century.[57] In the case of the Kingdom of Hanover (which will be used as a case study in this chapter), the commission consisted of two directors, three permanent members, and three extraordinary members, as well as two members of the pharmaceutical profession.[58] These were all university-trained doctors (sometimes pharmacists), whose expertise was more medical than legal. The commission supervised medical training standards (including medical exams), and its members acted as consultants to the government (including the medical police) for complaints against doctors. It was the introduction of the medical commissions that coincided with the 'invention' of the term 'negligence' in the first third of the nineteenth century. Their introduction points to a new awareness on the part of German governments of the increasing complexity of modern medicine, but also to an increasing self-confidence in the medical profession: doctors could not be judged by a legal expert alone.[59] In more general terms, the medical commissions appear as an institutional equivalent to the invention of the term 'negligence' and coincided with the renegotiation of the state–doctor relationship.

Although the available data overwhelmingly concerns local or regional incidents and lacks the quantity of twentieth-century statistical data, a survey of the cases dealt with by the commission in Hanover gives an indication of how medical jurisdiction and doctors' accountability were debated in the period before 1900.[60] A large number of files deal with disciplinary aspects that had little to do with medical expertise. Doctors were reprimanded for drunkenness or other forms of misbehaviour in public.[61] In the period between 1848 and 1850, an additional motive for disciplinary action can be identified. The 1848 European revolutions are generally understood as a turning point in doctors' political engagement. The historian Tobias Weidner argues that medicine became an 'un-political' profession in the aftermath of the revolutions.[62] In accordance with such an interpretation, several incidents can be identified where doctors were disciplined due to political engagement. In the closing decades of the nineteenth century, political offences referred more often to socialist doctors than to their liberal colleagues. Medical jurisdiction looked beyond professional practice and towards the doctor as a public person.[63]

Conflicts between individual doctors can equally be found in the files of the medical commission. Senior doctors regularly complained about the government's licensing of their younger colleagues.[64] The medical profession as a whole experienced increasing competition in the course of the century.[65] When applying for a licence from the medical police,

Medical negligence

doctors would refer to their qualification, but also to their knowledge of the region to which they applied. Often, doctors who had just qualified would apply for a licence in their home town or somewhere close by.[66] Such arguments of familiarity became increasingly obsolete after the medical commissions started advising on the granting of licences. However, personal networks still mattered enormously for a doctor's career.

Early modern medicine had encompassed different types of medical practitioners with distinct forms of training and social function.[67] Physicians with university training competed with surgeons who conducted a smaller range of medical practices. Such distinctions continued into the nineteenth century and did not disappear until the early twentieth century. In a number of complaints to the medical commission of Hanover, university-trained doctors accused surgeons of carrying out practices for which they were not qualified.[68]

Although a substantial number of cases point towards the interpretation of medical courts as watchdogs for professional honour and habitus, about half of the cases in Hanover refer to medical negligence. A husband sued a doctor over the death of his wife after she died giving birth.[69] An employer sued another doctor for an incorrect certificate for one of his employees.[70] Although the figures are in no way representative, the Hanoverian cases allow for the conclusion that there was indeed some interest in the performance of doctors, which could lead to accusations by private persons. In some instances, however, it was the government that interfered. This could be the case when a law had been broken. In 1850, for example, a surgeon was accused of performing an abortion, which was illegal (and continued to be so throughout the century).[71] The medical commission gathered six volumes of files for its statement on the case to the ministry.[72]

Despite such activity, the medical authority was lacking the legal means to discipline doctors in the majority of cases. This is best illustrated by a case study.[73] In the Prussian town of Pollitz, a thirty-four-year-old pregnant woman had gone into labour in May 1854. It turned out to be a breech birth and she was unable to deliver the baby's head. A surgeon was called and after some unsuccessful efforts to assist in delivering the baby, he pulled at the baby's legs so hard that he tore the baby's head from its body. The head was retained within the woman's body. Instead of completing the surgery, the surgeon gave the mother a laxative and left her with the assurance that the continuing contractions would expel the head. It was only due to a physician being called that the life of the mother was saved. Shortly after this incident, the surgeon moved from Prussia to Hanover, which explains why the case received special attention. In response to a Prussian enquiry, the local authorities in Hanover consulted the federal state's general medical commission. In its report, the commission suggested that the surgeon should receive a formal warning for failing to use the forceps correctly. No other disciplinary measures were advised.[74] The Prussian authorities thought such a decision too lax, and applied for a second opinion, inviting their own (regional) medical commission to supply a statement.[75] In accordance with their ministry, the Prussian medical commission argued that the surgeon's licence should be withdrawn. As their report stated, the surgeon had not only shown insufficient skill, but far more importantly, his behaviour showed disregard for the scientific standards of gynaecological care.

The commission particularly criticised the fact that the surgeon had shifted some of the blame on to the attending midwife. In his defending statement, the surgeon argued that the latter had already damaged the spine of the unborn baby before he arrived. However, the Prussian commission wrote that there existed no possibility for any doctor (surgeon or physician) to delegate responsibility (and hence accountability) to some other (subordinate) person.[76] The surgeon was responsible for the accident. If the midwife had caused damage to the spine, the doctor should have shown even greater attention in treating baby and mother. The surgeon was also criticised for leaving his patient unattended for more than eighteen hours. The surgeon's fatigue and exhaustion (a point he had referred to in his defence) would not suffice as an excuse for the failure in treatment. Instead, the commission argued that the surgeon's behaviour should be regarded as serious professional misconduct and be punished accordingly.

In response to the second statement, the Prussian ministry banned the surgeon from practising in Prussia.[77] Despite Prussian protest, he was allowed to continue working as a surgeon in Hanover. With regard to medical jurisdiction, a closer look thus seems necessary. The Prussian ministry disallowed the licensing of the surgeon in Prussia. Should he ever want to return to his former workplace, no Prussian ministry would grant a licence. The Hanoverian commission discussed the jurisdictional options open to its own authorities.[78] Although the baby had died, the mother survived. As a request by the ministry to a Hanoverian court confirmed, such a case would not count as a criminal offence. There was no reason for a police investigation, either. Hence, according to the existing legislation, a withdrawal of the granted licence was not justified. The surgeon was not under the government's direct disciplinary jurisdiction. Only surgeons (or physicians) in public offices would fall under government disciplinary control.[79] The medical commission, on the other hand, did not possess the authority to punish the surgeon. Instead, a formal warning was the maximum penalty it could issue.[80]

As to medical negligence, the case demonstrates the intensity with which the state – in collaboration with the medical experts of the medical commissions – discussed medical legislation and the limits of possible disciplinary action. In another case, in which a doctor refused to look after a patient, the commission stated that the licence could not be withdrawn. Again, no criminal offence existed that would legitimate the withdrawal of the licence. Instead, the medical commission suggested that the government should issue additional licences to doctors within the district: an increase in competition as a form of punishment.[81] In a further case, a doctor had lost his licence because he had spent time in a penitentiary. The medical commission raised some doubts as to whether the medical police's withdrawal of the licence on such grounds (which had nothing to do with medical practice) was lawful.[82] The medical commission's reports confirm that the Hanoverian government debated the shortcomings of existing medical jurisdiction.

To clarify: it is not sufficient to describe the process of medico-legal reform as the rise of state control. Instead, a more complex transition occurred in which the state and medical profession collaborated and negotiated optional changes. It was the lack of coercive means that caused disciplinary professional courts to be introduced in the German states from 1864 onwards. In order to fully understand the difficulties in establishing these courts, we must consider Germany's federal tradition. German doctors became part of a national organisation (*Deutscher Ärztevereinsbund*) in the early 1870s.[83] Legislation concerning doctors, however, was not negotiated on a national level. Neither the German Confederation (post-1815) nor the German Empire (post-1871) passed national laws on medical jurisdiction.[84] Instead, the (at times more than thirty) federal states oversaw medical societies, medical boards, and professional courts individually.[85] The early medical societies founded in the German federal states of Baden, Brunswick, and Saxony in the 1860s, for example, included disciplinary bodies with the right to issue fines.[86] In Prussia, negligence was treated as a civil or criminal offence until the end of the nineteenth century. It was not until 1899 that the Prussian government introduced medical courts of honour.[87] In Bavaria, medical chambers with some disciplinary control were established in 1871, but professional courts were not introduced until 1927.[88] In institutional terms, German medical jurisdiction remained diverse and heterogeneous.

The introduction of medical courts of honour led to a more systematic approach to medical negligence. From 1903, the Prussian medical authorities compiled statistical data on court cases. The historian Andreas-Holger Maehle has examined the files for the period between 1903 and 1921.[89] His results for doctors in Prussia are revealing with regard to the specific character of the medical courts of honour. In the majority of cases, and this represents a central argument in Maehle's analysis, it was not the patient who sued the doctor. Instead, the largest number of trials involved conflicts within the profession itself, brought against individuals by their colleagues and peers.[90] With regard to the registered offences, medical negligence proved the exception. Most complaints (in Maehle's case study of the medical court of honour for Brandenburg and Berlin between 1903 and 1920) concerned issues like advertising, financial misconduct, slander or libel, and sexual offences.[91] Unfair competition or lack of collegiality could also be found amongst the reasons for disciplinary punishment.[92] A much smaller number of accusations referred to issues that would nowadays be considered medical negligence. False certifying, negligent certifying, and maltreatment do not rank high in the court's statistics.[93] Hence, the main argument in Maehle's publication is that medical courts of honour were introduced to discipline doctors and to ensure the coherence of the medical profession, rather than to improve patient safety.[94]

By 1900, the overwhelming majority of cases of medical misconduct would be treated by a professional disciplinary court. Criminal court cases proved the exception. Instead, national organisation and professional institutionalisation of doctors had increased throughout the century. Medical courts of honour existed exclusively on the level of federal jurisdiction with differences between the federal German states. Honour and habitus appear as the key to understanding medical courts in Germany. With regard to the time-gap that existed between the early court cases of medical negligence and the introduction of the professional courts, it appears noteworthy that medical commissions had already provided scientific medical advice since the beginning of the nineteenth century. However, they did so without any disciplinary authority. Questions of medical misconduct were more prominent in the commissions' cases than in Maehle's case study. More importantly, the period from 1810 to 1900 showed representatives of the state (in our case study from Hanover) pointing towards the limits of medical jurisdiction. The intensifying debate about the shortcomings of the existing legislation and the introduction of disciplinary courts are an indicator of such change. However, the result of such involvement led to professional courts with a high degree of autonomy. The overwhelming majority of cases of medical negligence would not be considered by a legally trained judge but by representatives of the profession itself. Professional autonomy went so far that the legal historian Peter Collin has described medical courts of honour as resulting in multinormativity in a mononormative legal order.[95] With regard to the question of professional accountability and modernity, medical experts did not argue in favour of a no-fault compensation scheme. Instead, they insisted on sole responsibility based on expertise. They themselves were to judge their colleagues in the profession. But who was to pay for fines and penalties?

Commodifying risk: a German case study in international perspective

As the example of medical negligence in nineteenth-century Germany has amply demonstrated, the social and legal status of the expert is best understood as the result of a process of negotiation – a process that can hardly be regarded as uniform, and knows several stages and multiple agents. Negotiating accountability could be an international enterprise. German efforts to establish disciplinary courts were inspired by similar institutions in Britain. The foundation of the General Medical Council in 1858 introduced mechanisms for disciplining practitioners for misconduct and negligence.[96] With regard to the difficulties in translating leading scientific research into medical practice, German authors also referred to their British colleagues. The British medical directory of 1881 had laid down that in considering medical conduct a doctor was not expected 'to use the highest possible degree of skill' when treating a patient.[97] Instead, he was expected 'to bring a fair, reasonable, and competent degree of skill'.[98] The majority of medical authors in Germany agreed with the British approach and stipulated in accordance that each case of medical negligence required due consideration of individual circumstances such as the availability of equipment.[99]

There were also substantial differences in medical legislation between European nation states. German doctors longed for state recognition to a much larger degree than their British colleagues, emphasising doctors' special status in comparison to other professions.[100] The most peculiar differences can be noted between German and Austrian legislation. The Austrian criminal code of 1852 stated that doctors who had caused 'severe bodily harm' to a patient under their care were banned from practising only until passing an additional exam to justify the renewal of their medical licence. As very few doctors failed such a test, legal historiography treats this section of the criminal code under the heading of 'doctors' privilege' (*Ärzteprivileg*).[101] Unlike their German colleagues, Austrian doctors did not face legal prosecution in cases of negligence.

This difference in legislation reminds us that questions of accountability were a matter of negotiation between state authorities and professional representatives. From the perspective of medical jurisdiction in Germany, the individual accountability of doctors remained of great importance. The court cases explicitly stress doctors' responsibility for the content and performance of medical therapy. The concept of the employer's (or in the case of German doctors, the state's) strict liability (*Gefährdungshaftung*) was never introduced into the medical profession.[102] The idea of reduced accountability due to a special privilege, as in the Austrian case, did not come up. The prominence of personal honour in medical jurisdiction reinforced the idea of individual accountability with all its consequences. Few doubts appear to have existed in the public mind that German doctors remained legally accountable for the results of their treatment.[103] Instead, such responsibility, the sophistication of medical knowledge (i.e. expertise) and the complexity of medical therapy were used to legitimise status and privilege.

There exists, however, an important reservation to the idea of full individual accountability. As a closer look at the private insurance

Medical negligence

sector demonstrates, professionals, including doctors, could rely on private liability insurances minimalising the practical consequences of individual accountability from around 1880 onwards. The German government passed a law on liability (*Reichshaftpflichtgesetz*) in 1871 that laid down under what conditions compensation had to be paid in railway industries. Questions of accountability were further defined with the introduction of employers' strict liability as part of the German law on social insurance of 1884. Only three years later, in 1887, the first private liability insurance for doctors was advertised, covering costs for fines issued for medical negligence. Although liability insurance for doctors was criticised in public discourse, 6,500 doctors had signed up for this kind of insurance with the largest German insurance house (the *Stuttgarter Versicherungsverein*) by 1901.[104] A glance at the numbers of liability policies for all professions in the *Stuttgarter* insurance company overall supports such an interpretation. It rose from 41,000 in 1892 to almost 270,000 in 1900. The price for individual policies had to be renegotiated several times, sometimes doubling in consecutive years. This was due to the doubling of liability cases from 1889 to 1898.[105] The majority of workplaces saw an increase in reported accidents. In this sense, the emergence of private liability insurance for doctors can be seen as a complementary development to the emergence of the welfare state. Accidents in the workplace were increasingly covered by insurance for wage labour (by the state) and the professions (privately) alike.

Although this chapter has been concerned with demonstrating the importance of doctors' legal accountability in negligence cases (and hence contests Ewald's claim of collective accountability in modernity), with some caveats Ewald's interpretation can help us to understand the transformation of medical jurisdiction. While doctors remained accountable in legal terms, they benefitted from the commodification of risk.[106] The German phrase *Verantwortung* embraces two very distinct meanings. On the one hand, it can describe the 'authority', 'command', or 'entitlement' of a person, in German legal terms 'ex ante responsibility'. On the other hand, the German phrase can equally be translated as 'accountability' or 'liability', the German legal expression of 'ex post responsibility'. Although German doctors were legally accountable for negligence and malpractice, the private insurance business collectivised the potential danger of being economically liable.[107] With reference to the discussion of risk it is stipulated that it was less the rise of the state as manager of risks that constituted modernity than the disentanglement of professional accountability and private/personal risk. In opposition to Ewald, this chapter has demonstrated that the latter did not replace the former. Instead, the two interacted within different spheres – such as the legal, the professional, and the economical.

Notes

1. F. F. König, 'Geschichte und Begriff des Kunstfehlers', *Zeitschrift für die gesamte gerichtliche Medizin*, 20 (1933), 161–72.
2. *Ibid.*, 161–2.
3. *Ibid.*
4. *Ibid.*
5. O. Jürgens, *Die Beschränkung der strafrechtlichen Haftung für ärztliche Behandlungsfehler* (Frankfurt am Main: Lang, 2005), 23–5.
6. Variations in the number of cases are generally far more consistent than König's examples imply. Next to the figures in A.-H. Maehle, *Doctors, Honour, and the Law: Medical Ethics in Imperial Germany* (Basingstoke: Palgrave Macmillan, 2009), 32; see also Jürgens, *Beschränkung der strafrechtlichen Haftung*, 28–9.
7. F. Ewald, *Der Vorsorgestaat* (Frankfurt am Main: Suhrkamp, 1993).
8. R. Ogorek, *Untersuchungen zur Entwicklung der Gefährdungshaftung im 19. Jahrhundert* (Köln and Wien: Böhlau, 1975), 48–68; D. Murswiek, *Die staatliche Verantwortung für die Risiken der Technik. Verfassungsrechtliche Grundlagen und immissionsschutzrechtliche Ausformung* (Berlin: Duncker & Humblot, 1985).
9. Ewald, *Der Vorsorgestaat*, 21–6.
10. W. U. Eckart and R. Jütte (eds), *Das europäische Gesundheitssystem. Gemeinsamkeiten und Unterschiede in historischer Perspektive* (Stuttgart: Franz Steiner Verlag, 1994).
11. Julia Moses, *The First Modern Risk: Workplace Accidents and the Origins of European Social States* (Cambridge: Cambridge University Press, 2018), 3–4.
12. *Ibid.*
13. H. Deichert, *Geschichte des Medizinalwesens im Gebiet des ehemaligen Königreichs Hannover* (Hanover and Leipzig: Hahn, 1908), 41.
14. A. Mohun, *Risk: Negotiating Safety in American Society* (Baltimore, MD: Johns Hopkins University Press, 2013), 7–8.

15 Krähe, *Ärztlicher Kunstfehler*, 25–30; F. F. König, 'Geschichte und Begriff des Kunstfehlers', *Zeitschrift für die gesamte gerichtliche Medizin*, 20 (1933), 161–72 (pp. 162–3).
16 *Ibid.*
17 Krähe, *Ärztlicher Kunstfehler*, 25–30; König, 'Geschichte und Begriff des Kunstfehlers', 162–3.
18 Krähe, *Ärztlicher Kunstfehler*, 109.
19 Kohlrausch to Langermann, 2 September 1811, in M. Kalisch, *Die Kunstfehler der Ärzte* (Leipzig: Veit und Comp., 1860), 6.
20 Kalisch, *Kunstfehler der Ärzte*, 4.
21 Kohlrausch to Langermann, 2 September 1811, in Kalisch, *Kunstfehler der Ärzte*, 6.
22 Krähe, *Ärztlicher Kunstfehler*, 37.
23 Reil to Schmalz, n.d., quoted in Kalisch, *Kunstfehler der Ärzte*, 12.
24 Kohlrausch to the Prussian police department, 16 February 1812, quoted in Kalisch, *Kunstfehler der Ärzte*, 12–13
25 Krähe, *Ärztlicher Kunstfehler*, 37.
26 Krähe, *Ärztlicher Kunstfehler*, 37 with reference to Kalisch, *Kunstfehler der Ärzte*, *passim*.
27 Kalisch, *Kunstfehler der Ärzte*, 13–14.
28 *Ibid.*, 35–6.
29 *Ibid.*, 38–9.
30 *Ibid.*, 40.
31 See the bibliography in O. A. Oesterlen, 'Kunstfehler der Ärzte und Wundärzte', in J. Maschka (ed.), *Handbuch der gerichtlichen Medizin*, vol. 3 (Tübingen: Verlag der H. Laupp'schen Buchhandlung, 1882), 589–647 (p. 592).
32 Kühner, *Kunstfehler der Ärzte vor dem Forum der Juristen* (Frankfurt am Main: Knauer, 1886), 4.
33 Kalisch, *Kunstfehler der Ärzte*; Kühner, *Kunstfehler der Ärzte*.
34 Kühner, *Kunstfehler der Ärzte*, 4.
35 R. Virchow, 'Kunstfehler der Aerzte', in R. Virchow, *Gesammelte Abhandlunge aus dem Gebiet der Öffentlichen Medizin*, vol. 2 (Berlin, 1879), 514–22.
36 On Virchow, see C. Goschler, *Rudolf Virchow. Mediziner – Anthropologe – Politiker*, 2nd edn (Köln/Weimar/Wien: Böhlau, 2009); on the postmodern turn in medical discourse, R. Cooter, 'Medicine and Modernity', in M. Jackson (ed.), *The Oxford Handbook of the History of Medicine* (Oxford: Oxford University Press, 2011), 100–16 (pp. 109–13).
37 Kühner, *Kunstfehler der Ärzte*, 4.
38 This is the central argument in Virchow, 'Kunstfehler der Aerzte', 514–22.

39 B. Elkeles, *Der moralische Diskurs über das medizinische Menschenexperiment im 19. Jahrhundert* (Stuttgart: Fischer, 1996).
40 Ibid., 180–217; Maehle, *Doctors, Honour, and the Law*, 82–3.
41 Maehle, *Doctors, Honour, and the Law*, 67–94.
42 C. Huerkamp, *Aufstieg der Ärzte im 19. Jahrhundert. Vom gelehrten Stand zum professionellen Experten. Das Beispiel Preußens* (Göttingen: Vandenhoeck und Ruprecht, 1985), 132–7.
43 C. Hudemann-Simon, *Die Eroberung der Gesundheit 1750–1900* (Frankfurt am Main: Fischer-Taschenbuch-Verlag, 2000), 115–69.
44 Huerkamp, *Aufstieg der Ärzte*, 132–7.
45 Jürgens, *Die Beschränkung der strafrechtlichen Haftung*, 23–5.
46 Maehle, *Doctors, Honour, and the Law*, passim.
47 Krähe, *Ärztlicher Kunstfehler*, 107; König, 'Geschichte und Begriff des Kunstfehlers', 4.
48 Huerkamp, *Aufstieg der Ärzte*, 110–18; a contemporary voice: A. Kühner, *Der ärztliche Stand und dessen besondere Gefahren. Supplement zu der Abhandlung über 'Die Kunstfehler der Aerzte' nebst einer Casuistik* (Frankfurt am Main: Knauer, 1889), 3–4.
49 Krähe, *Ärztlicher Kunstfehler*, 107.
50 Hudemann-Simon, *Eroberung der Gesundheit*, 68–73; Huerkamp, *Aufstieg der Ärzte*, 185–9.
51 Krähe, *Ärztlicher Kunstfehler*, 106–7, for German jurisprudence on this idea, E. Barnert, *Der eingebildete Dritte. Eine Argumentationsfigur im Zivilrecht* (Tübingen: Mohr Siebeck, 2008).
52 D. Püster, *Entwicklungen der Arzthaftpflichtversicherung* (Berlin: Springer, 2013), 5–8; J. Möhle, *Die Haftpflichtversicherung im Heilwesen. Eine Studie über die versicherungsrechtliche Deckung medizinischer Haftpflichtschäden* (Frankfurt am Main: Lang, 1992), 5–11; C. Katzenmeier, *Arzthaftung* (Tübingen: Mohr-Siebeck, 2002), 151–6; for the contemporary discourse, see Krähe, *Ärztlicher Kunstfehler*, 91.
53 Maehle, *Doctors, Honour, and the Law*, 6–46.
54 U. Frevert, *Krankheit als politisches Problem 1770–1880. Soziale Unterschichten in Preußen zwischen medizinischer Polizei und staatlicher Sozialversicherung* (Göttingen: Vandenhoeck und Ruprecht, 1984), 23–44, G. Göckenjan, *Kurieren und Staat machen. Gesundheit und Medizin in der bürgerlichen Welt* (Frankfurt am Main: Suhrkamp, 1985), 94–109.
55 Huerkamp, *Aufstieg der Ärzte*, 254–61; Maehle, *Doctors, Honour, and the Law*, 8.
56 A.-H. Maehle, 'Professional ethics and discipline: the Prussian medical courts of honour, 1899–1920', *Medizinhistorisches Journal*, 34 (1999), 309–38 (p. 313).

Medical negligence 75

57 Ibid.
58 Ibid.
59 Gedrucktes Zirkularschreiben der Provinzial-Regierung (gez. Nieper), Hanover, 15 April 1817, NLA Hanover, Hann. 74 Calenberg Nr. 550.
60 The reports can be found in NLA Hanover, Hann. 134, Nr. 2113–2130.
61 Anonyme Anklage gegen den Dr. Stiepel zu Lindau, 1847, NLA Hanover, Hann. 134, Nr. 2114. Die Entziehung der Concession des Dr. med Gravel zu Aschendorf in Folge der wider denselben anhängig gewesenen Criminal-Untersuchung, 1848, NLA Hanover, Hann. 134, Nr. 2115.
62 T. Weidner, *Die unpolitische Profession. Deutsche Mediziner im langen 19. Jahrhundert* (Frankfurt am Main: Campus, 2012); for doctors in 1848, see also Göckenjan, *Kurieren und Staat machen*, 267–86.
63 Disziplinaruntersuchungssache der Landrostei Osnabrück gegen den Bürgermeister und Arzt Miquel zu Emlichheim, 1849, NLA Hanover, Hann. 134, Nr. 2119; for political biases see B. Rabi, *Ärztliche Ethik – eine Frage der Ehre? Die Prozesse und Urteile der ärztlichen Ehrengerichtshöfe in Preußen und Sachsen 1918–1933* (Frankfurt am Main: Lang, 2002), 182–4.
64 Beschwerdeschrift des Dr. Frerich zu Lengerich und Dr. Vaal zu Schapen über die Anstellung des Dr. Niemann zu Nordhorn, 1848, NLA Hanover, Hann. 134, Nr. 2116; Eingabe des Landphysikus Dr. von Hahn und des Landchirurgus Dr. van Nes, beide zu Lingen, in Beziehung auf deren unangemessenen Inhalt, 1849, NLA Hanover, Hann. 134, Nr. 2117.
65 Huerkamp, *Aufstieg der Ärzte*, 110–18.
66 For the difference between the arguments of the medical police and the medical commissions see Anweisungen und Verordnungen über die Medizinalpolizeit im Amt Münden, NLA HA Hann. 74 Münden, Nr. 7538.
67 Huerkamp, *Aufstieg der Ärzte*, 22–40; T. Rütten, 'Early Modern Medicine', in M. Jackson (ed.), *The Oxford Handbook of the History of Medicine* (Oxford: Oxford University Press, 2011), 60–81.
68 Die von dem Magistrat zu Celle wider den Landchirurgen Brandmüller zur Sprache gebrachte Überschreitung seiner Befugnisse, NLA Hanover, Hann.134, Nr. 2121; Gutachten über eine wider den Wundarzt Koch zu Wallensen erhobenen Beschuldigung wegen Überschreitung seiner Befugnis, 1850, NLA Hanover, Hann. 134, Nr. 2122.
69 Die von dem Medizinalrat Tiedemann beantragte zurechtweisende Erinnerung und Ermahnung des Dr. Dankwerts wegen des üblen Ausganges eines Geburtsfalles, 1850, NLA Hanover, Hann. 134, Nr. 2123.
70 Unterstellung des Dr. Fontheim zu Hannover unter die Beaufsichtigung und Beachtung der hiesigen Physici wegen eines mit großer

Gewissenlosigkeit ausgestellten Gesundheitszeugnisses, 1850–51, NLA Hanover, Hann. 134, Nr. 2120.
71 S. Putzke, *Die Strafbarkeit der Abtreibung in der Kaiserzeit und in der Weimarer Zeit. Eine Analyse der Reformdiskussion und der Straftatbestände in den Reformentwürfen (1908–1931)* (Berlin: Berliner Wissenschafts-Verlag, 2003).
72 Gutachten über eine wider den Wundarzt Koch zu Wallensen erhobenen Beschuldigung wegen Überschreitung seiner Befugnis, 1850, NLA Hanover, Hann. 134, Nr. 2122.
73 Landdrostei in Lüneburg to the Königliche Obermedizinalkollegium in Hanover, Lüneburg, 20 March 1855, NLA Hanover, Hann. 134, Nr. 2128.
74 Statement of the Obermedizinalkollegium (draft), Hanover, 19 April 1855, NLA Hanover, Hann. 134, Nr. 2128.
75 Königlich Preußische Regierung (Fleischmann) to the Königlich Hannöversche Landdrostei Lüneburg, Magdeburg, 14 August 1855 (copy), NLA Hanover, Hann. 134, Nr. 2128.
76 Königliches Medicinal-Collegium der Provinz Sachsen (v. Weitzleben, Andreae, Niemann, Schulze] to the Prussian Innenministerium (copy), Magdeburg, 28 June 1855, NLA Hanover, Hann. 134, Nr. 2128.
77 Königlich Preußische Regierung (Fleischmann) to the Königlich Hannöversche Landdrostei Lüneburg, Magdeburg, 14 August 1855 (copy), NLA Hanover, Hann. 134, Nr. 2128.
78 Landdrostei in Lüneburg to the Königliche Obermedizinalkollegium in Hanover, Lüneburg, 20 March 1855, NLA Hanover, Hann. 134, Nr. 2128.
79 In one case, a doctor was fined and lost his licence because he occupied the position of the mayor of a Prussian village and hence of a public servant: Disziplinaruntersuchungssache der Landrostei Osnabrück gegen den Bürgermeister und Arzt Miquel zu Emlichheim, 1849, NLA Hanover, Hann. 134, Nr. 2119.
80 Deichert, *Geschichte des Medizinalwesens*, 41.
81 Landdrostei Lüneburg an das Ober-Medicinalcollegium zu Hanover, 30.6.1847, NLA Hanover, Hann. 134, Nr. 2113.
82 Zurücknahme der Konzession des Dr. Heye Albertus Molter zu Norden wegen seiner Verurteilung zu einer Arbeitshausstrafe, 1849, NLA Hanover, Hann. 134, Nr. 2118.
83 Göckenjan, *Kurieren und Staat machen*, 315–27; Huerkamp, *Aufstieg der Ärzte*, 241–55.
84 Maehle, *Doctors, Honour, and the Law*, 6–46; Rabi, *Ärztliche Ethik*, 37–57.
85 A. Gabriel, *Die staatliche Organisation des Deutschen Ärztestandes* (Berlin, 1920).
86 Ibid., 21–7; for Saxony also Rabi, *Ärztliche Ethik*, 44–7.

87 Ibid., 146–62; Maehle, *Doctors, Honour, and the Law*, 6–46.
88 Maehle, *Doctors, Honour, and the Law*, 21–30; for the earlier legislation in Bavaria Gabriel, *Die staatliche Organisation*, 167–97.
89 Maehle, *Doctors, Honour, and the Law*, 32.
90 Ibid.
91 Ibid., 37.
92 Ibid.
93 Ibid.
94 For both the Prussian and British medical associations this has already been stated in Maehle, 'Professional ethics and discipline', 330–2.
95 Peter Collin, 'Ehrengerichtliche Rechtssprechung im Kaiserreich und der Weimarer Republik. Mulitnormativität in einer mononormativen Rechtsordnung?' *Rechtsgeschichte/Legal History*, 25 (2017), 138–50.
96 Maehle, *Doctors, Honour, and the Law*, 16; Maehle, 'Professional ethics and discipline', 330–2.
97 Kühner, *Kunstfehler der Ärzte*.
98 Ibid.
99 Ibid. For the GMB: R. Smith, *Medical Discipline: The Professional Conduct Jurisdiction of the General Medical Council, 1858–1990* (Oxford: Clarendon Press, 1994).
100 Maehle, *Doctors, Honour, and the Law*, 6–46; Huerkamp, *Aufstieg der Ärzte*, 265–72.
101 Jürgens, *Beschränkung der strafrechtlichen Haftung*.
102 Ibid.; S. Yoon, *Die Gefährdungshaftung für moderne Techniken. Zugleich eine Stellungnahme zum neuen Schadensersatzrecht* (Frankfurt am Main: Lang, 2002).
103 Hudemann-Simon, *Eroberung der Gesundheit*, 225–31.
104 Möhle, *Haftpflichtversicherung im Heilwesen*, 8–9.
105 Ludwig Arps, *Auf sicheren Pfeilern: Deutsche Versicherungswirtschaft vor 1914* (Göttingen: Vandenhoeck & Ruprecht, 1965), 267–85 (p. 275).
106 Inspiring, though addressing the American rather than the German situation: Mohun, *Risk: Negotiating Safety in American Society*.
107 Jan Henrick Klement, *Verantwortung. Funktion und Legitimation eines Begriffs im Öffentlichen Recht* (Tübingen: Mohr Siebeck, 2006); Kurt Bayertz (ed.), *Verantwortung. Prinzip oder Problem?* (Darmstadt: Wissenschaftliche Buchgesellschaft, 1995).

3

Imperfect bodies: the 'pathology' of childhood in late nineteenth-century London[1]

Steven Taylor

[S]ocial institutions are those that best know how to denature a man, to take his absolute existence from him in order to give him a relative one and transport the I into the common unity.[2]

This quote, taken from Jean-Jacques Rousseau's influential text *Émile* (1762), serves to outline the overarching objective of this chapter: to assess whether charitable interventions directed at children living with impairment in the late nineteenth century, over a hundred years after the publication of *Émile*, were designed to 'denature' their subjects for the benefit of society or instead served as an attempt at improving and integrating youngsters, so as to develop them into independent and productive adults. A raft of work has focused on the nature of social institutions. The most enduring and compelling arguments have been espoused by Michel Foucault who presented them as vehicles for supervising, controlling, and disciplining individual bodies.[3] With regard to 'child rescue', the moniker given to evangelical attempts at 'improving' the lives of children living in poverty in the late nineteenth century, the scholarship is less complete, especially when it comes to the sick and disabled.[4] By considering the treatment and experience of the impaired/disabled child in a voluntary organisation, the Church of England-sponsored Waifs and Strays Society, this chapter embarks on a significant departure from the current literature, navigating through the successes and failures of reform and the subsequent categorisation of the non-normal child.

The late nineteenth century was a significant time in the formulation of ideas about welfare and childhood. The socio-economic landscapes of urban environments were shaped by industrial depression and severe cholera outbreaks during the late 1860s. These factors fed into an evangelical movement that became prominent in the same period. It was primarily led by influential middle-class women, eager to expand beyond the well-defined gender roles of the period, and whose moralising gaze focused on the amelioration of children who were perceived to be helpless and deserving.[5] The Goschen Minute of 1869, issued by the President of the Poor Law Board, George Goschen, signalled a renewed focus on reducing poor law expenditure and stricter adherence to the principals of the Poor Law Amendment Act (1834). His core demand was for a closer relationship between welfare and philanthropy, with the workhouse dealing with the truly destitute, and charities supporting the needs of families that were just about managing. This shift legitimised and energised the efforts of evangelical reformers who were increasingly worried by the perceived ubiquity of 'ragged' children on the streets of British cities. With the average population being much younger than it is today, these children, often orientalised as 'arabs' or 'urchins', came to symbolise a fear of national decline and social degeneration.[6] This fed into a proto-eugenic discourse, adopted by evangelical reformers, aimed at breaking the ties between urban families accustomed to immorality (such as intemperance, promiscuity, and criminality) and their children.[7] Evidently, the last three decades of the century are of crucial significance to historians, as philanthropic practice changed from intervention aimed at improving the living conditions of the urban poor child (and family), to intrusive attempts at rescuing and removing them.[8]

As the core themes of this volume highlight, self-conscious reflections on 'modern life' in Britain and its social, cultural, and political consequences, increased concerns about urban environments and the place of individuals within them, as well as raising broader questions about the nature of identity, nation, and social development. Subsequently, within this climate the elevation of children's health to a national concern should be unsurprising as they represented the future of state and empire.[9] Legislation in the form of the Factory Acts (1833–1901), Education Acts (1870–1902), Prevention of Cruelty to Children Act (1889), and later free school meals (1906) and medical inspection (1907) reinforced this position. Increased state investment in the education and improvement of children worked in tandem with reduced welfare options offered by the Poor Law Crusade[10] to create a vacuum in which the child rescue movement flourished. Yet despite the perception of children being vulnerable and in need of amelioration in this nascent 'modern' ideal, Harry Hendrick notes that the child victim was 'nearly always seen as harbouring the possibility of another condition, one that was sensed to be threatening: to moral fibre, sexual propriety, the sanctity of the family, the preservation of the race, law and order, and the wider reaches of citizenship'.[11] In essence childhood was a battleground where the future success of the 'modern' state would be decided.

This chapter focuses on the 'unacceptable', 'unideal' children, who lived with physical impairments and were understood to be incapable of 'improving' without charitable intervention. Later they were considered to be beyond help or, as Hendrick outlines, 'threats' to society. The failure of reformers to meet the needs of these youngsters meant they were subsequently constructed as 'pathologically' different from the norm.

Two core issues sit at the heart of this chapter: firstly the nature of childhood in late nineteenth-century England, and, secondly, definitions and concepts of impairment. At a rudimentary level, Rousseau provided a framework in which to consider ideas of childhood. On the one hand there is the 'sheltered' or 'innocent' childhood that features in *Émile* that still has resonance today as an idealised, and quintessentially 'modern', notion of the 'perfect' child. Yet this paradigm was challenged by another category of youngster, one that has been labelled here the 'pathologically' different child. Of course, this is an imperfect and polarised model and the majority of children, according to medical, social, cultural, and familial viewpoints, would fit somewhere between these binaries. This chapter concentrates on those that congregated around notions and conceptions of 'imperfection'. It is therefore important to delve a little deeper into what is meant by the idea of 'pathology' in this context.

In its strictest definition the term refers to the scientific process of exploring the causes of disease through the inspection of bodily materials. However, the phrase has evolved into common usage and developed a pseudo-scientific social meaning. Those whom we consider to be pathological behave in a habitual way that does not comply to an accepted social norm. Yet, pathology in this instance is not synonymous with impairment. Therefore, children who were not physically impaired could be pathologised by philanthropic reformers and vice versa. Louise Jackson has argued that the 'ugly twin' of the modern, romantic, child was the juvenile delinquent.[12] Similarly, Pam Cox has demonstrated that two distinct discourses functioned within the criminal justice system of the early twentieth century: the first concerned with care and protection, and the second control and punishment.[13] Whilst these assessments have furthered our understanding of transgressive childhoods, the concept needs to be refined and expanded to include children of the poor more generally. For children whose childhoods were 'pathologised', and not necessarily criminalised, they were constructed as distinct and separate from the norm and in need of specialised help and intervention; this may have been through physical or mental impairment, knowledge of sexual activity, questionable morality, or criminality. Pathology refers to ideas about improvability in a non-medical charitable institution, the Waifs and Strays Society. Yet, the spectre of the pathologically different youngster haunts the academic literature dealing with childhood in the past.

It has been argued that social groups became of interest to authorities when they posed particular problems or threats.[14] Such a chronology fits with increased state and philanthropic focus on children from the 1870s.[15] Consequently a discourse was constructed by philanthropists and reformers at a time when the welfare, physical condition, and health of youngsters appeared to reflect the moral and physical fibre of the empire.[16] Ideas about normalcy and abnormality took on a scientific form by the turn of the twentieth century. 'Technologies' such as height and weight charts in the first instance and then more specific tools, such as intelligence tests, made it possible to count, measure, and evaluate children, with the result of both reinforcing and visualising concepts of normality/abnormality.[17] Early physical checks conducted on newborn babies from the mid-twentieth century, Cathy Urwin has suggested, were efforts designed to identify potential deviance.[18] In the years following the First World War, child mental well-being was a particular concern and John Stewart has explored the child guidance movement that grew in the British welfare system. Its underlying principle – that any child might experience emotional or psychological disturbance, regardless of how 'normal' they might be considered, and demonstrating that the idea of a pathologically different child, or indeed of childhood itself as a pathology – perpetuated into the twentieth century.[19] The sample of impaired/disabled children used in this chapter adds to this scholarship and provides a particularly useful vehicle for this analysis, primarily because it has been convenient to blame a lack of 'progress' on physical (and visible) defects rather than carefully analysing the experiences of these individuals. This chapter outlines the conception, growth, and coming to maturity of childhood as pathology in and of itself. By the late nineteenth century children were thought capable of causing familial, social, and moral instability. Hence the pathological childhood needs to be considered within broader histories of childhood.

The Waifs and Strays Society

The historical records of the Church of England Waifs and Strays Society provide rich source material to better understand how pathologised children were cared for by philanthropic institutions in the late nineteenth century. The Society was founded by Edward Rudolf in 1881 and offered residential childcare to families facing poverty-induced crises. Alongside Dr Stephenson's Homes (founded in 1868) and Dr Barnardo's Homes (founded in 1870), it was one of the major voluntary organisations of the period that made up a mosaic of welfare options which were developing for children in the late nineteenth century.[20] When a child was admitted, they were accompanied by an application form that explained their personal, family, and health circumstances. These documents have been used initially to identify those admitted with physical 'impairments' and thus more likely to be pathologised. As a cohort, they reveal much about Victorian attitudes towards childhood and disability. When entering the Waifs and Strays Society, children were usually seen by two doctors for diagnostic purposes before being moved to a residential home run by the society. Two of these homes, St Agnes and St Nicholas, functioned solely as homes for 'crippled' children. The application, along with both medical forms, was then placed in a casefile where the experience, movements, and interactions of that child with the charity were kept.[21] These records, now held by the Children's Society, contain a wealth of information and, much like the children whose stories they reveal, are diverse in both content and detail.

Between the years 1882 and 1899, there were 7,400 successful applications made to the Waifs and Strays Society. Of these, there were roughly 300 children, aged between one and seventeen years old, who were living with some form of physical impairment or deformity.[22] The age classification deployed here is that defined by the Waifs and Strays Society as an institution exclusively for children.[23] The recorded impairments were varied, and included mental disabilities, epilepsy, amputations of digits, arms, and legs, those suffering from burns, paralysis, and sensory impairments of sight and hearing. Most common were those described as 'crippled' who had experienced some kind of physical deformity usually caused by rickets, scoliosis, tuberculosis of the bones, or acquired through an injury. This is in line with the broader population and supports Ashley Mathisen's research into the London Foundling Hospital during the eighteenth century, where physical deformity and the loss of a limb were the most recorded disabilities amongst children there.[24]

The cohort of impaired children at the Waifs and Strays Society included both sexes but girls were in the overwhelming majority, accounting for 78% of those admitted with impairments. This is at variance with other studies of the period where impaired boys were more commonly institutionalised,[25] a state of affairs explained by the usefulness of young girls in the domestic environments of poor families where they were capable of completing simple household chores or caring for younger siblings while their parents were at work.[26] In the case of this particular charitable home it might be assumed that the number of girls was a reflection of a middle-class desire to improve the respectability of the working poor and 'improve' the life chances of these individuals. Comments such as those that accompanied Annie C. who was impaired 'owing to the careless habits of the mother – who drinks',[27] or the statement that Catherine W.'s 'home is quite unfit for an invalid' and she only ever was seen 'wearing one dirty garment' were not uncommon.[28] The institutional concerns about these girls were directly related to broader ideas about what it meant to be 'modern': in the near future there was a strong possibility that they would be responsible for their own households and their progeny would be the men and women that the British Empire relied on as industrial workers and members of the armed forces.

Childhood and the welfare experience

Able-bodied children of the working poor were regularly found in the workplace throughout the eighteenth and nineteenth centuries.[29] In line with increasingly Rousseauesque views of childhood, however, their economic role was gradually questioned by authorities, and the first effective government inspectorates into child workers were introduced in the 1830s.[30] From the mid-nineteenth century, it can be observed that the legislative agenda towards children reinforced the dichotomy between the innocent and the pathologically different child. Workplace and education reforms, such as the numerous Factory and Elementary Education Acts, were all geared towards the protection of the innocent, and by the turn of the century education was being provided up to the age of twelve, even if it was on a half-time basis in some circumstances. The criminal justice system, however, lagged behind. The age of criminal responsibility was set at seven in the seventeenth century and it remained so until it was raised to eight with the Children and Young Person's Act of 1933, and was finally increased to ten by an Act of the same name in 1963. In comparison, during the medieval period, often considered a time when children were treated as protoadults, the criminal trial of children under the age of twelve was banned because they could not be held responsible for their actions. We might consider such a young age in the nineteenth and twentieth centuries as a legal mechanism to manage those who did not conform to accepted social norms.[31]

The children who came into contact with the Waifs and Strays Society were most commonly orphans or those who had been deserted, and thus they were often filtered towards philanthropy via the institutions of the poor law system. From its inception in the Tudor period, the poor law sought to distinguish between the deserving and undeserving poor. It was implemented at a local level so that officials could use knowledge of their catchment area to identify those truly in need of assistance, usually defined in relation to 'usefulness' in the workplace.[32] In 1697, John Locke stated that the poor law should consider using the malleability of children to mould them into well rounded adults and he, in particular, highlighted the benefits of education for them.[33] Doing so, he argued, would break the cycle of dependence, an obsession that extends into modern times. This was a somewhat different view from that of Rousseau, who later argued that children should be at liberty to enjoy childhood before entering the adult world. Despite their differing philosophies regarding the nature of childhood, their influence reshaped understandings of what it meant to be a child in the modern world.

The belief that children deserved support in varying degrees was a political and cultural subtext throughout the eighteenth and nineteenth centuries.[34] The majority of children under public care in the nineteenth century were there because of their parental situations. However, Frank Crompton has also stated that Poor Law Guardians were eager to remove the influence of parents who had proved themselves unsuitable.[35] Thus, there was a particular awareness, both in the poor law and charitable spheres, that children were not responsible for their poverty; rather families, the nature of parenting, and the environments in which they lived, were the fundamental elements in constructing the need for intervention. These are themes that have persisted through to the present day.[36] Similar attitudes are evident in the sample of children admitted to the Waifs and Strays Society, demonstrating the fluidity of ideas between the state and voluntary sectors. James T., for example, was three years old when he was admitted to the care of the Waifs and Strays Society from his home in east London where he was said to 'live in an unhealthy neighbourhood'.[37] In this situation we can observe the environment in which the child was living as the key negative factor, and it was a widely held view that parents, at the very minimum, were supposed to provide for their children. Those parents unable to do so upset the social order.

In a different case, Lucy F. was taken into the Society's St Chads home in 1889 at the age of fourteen. The catalyst for her admission was the death of her mother and 'her father [wa]s a good for nothing, ignorant man, with no idea of looking after his children, though he would not wilfully injure them'.[38] We are thus provided with a picture of working-class parenting that did not comply with middle-class expectations. Interestingly, this case makes no reference to drunkenness, idleness, or criminality, which so often occurred in the records for other children. In contrast to the father's ignorance of child-rearing, Lucy F. was described as 'a bright, happy-tempered child by nature, responding readily to kindness – very quick and intelligent – and has made great efforts to keep her father's house tidy'.[39] Two important threads emerge here. First, there was a parent in danger of tainting a child who had the potential to fit with the ideal of a respectable childhood, that being one who would grow into an independent and productive adult. She was eager to learn and evidently a hard worker. Secondly, there was the underlying tension created by an adolescent girl living with a working man who, because of his status, could be a physical or sexual threat to her. This fear was elucidated later in the application where it was stated that, 'so far we have every reason to believe that the child has escaped moral injury, but that she is in grave danger there can be no doubt'.[40] Despite no actual harm coming to the child, this danger was perceived to be ever present in homes of the poor, especially when there was no mother figure available to prevent potentially abusive behaviour.

The perceived unsuitability of working-class homes for young children is further evident in the case of Minnie K. who was aged just two, and diagnosed with a curvature of the spine, when she came under the care of the Waifs and Strays Society in 1890.[41] Twelve years later, in 1902, her mother wrote to Edward Rudolf asking for Minnie to be returned to her care. This letter to the society is important as it makes a wider point about the nature of disability during the period. It has often been assumed that those with impairments were cast aside or ignored by their families, but here we witness a parent requesting that their child is returned to them after an extensive period of separation. While Rudolf initially agreed to the mother's demands, Katherine Warton in the St Agnes Home, Croydon, put up more resistance and wrote the following statement back to Rudolf at Society Headquarters:

> We shall be very sorry to lose Minnie K., as she is a nice child, Miss Carling quite hoped she was going to be of great use in the Home, as she grew older. She is very delicate, and very backward at school, and Mrs Pereira wondered if it could not be arranged for her to stay with us up to Christmas, for the childs [sic] own sake. If Mrs K. has the means would she not be willing to pay something, as it would be so much to the childs [sic] advantage to stay on with us, as I understand the mother is out at work all day so suppose Minnie is going to keep house for her. Minnie is attending the Church day school, and having been so long we should be very sorry for her to leave at such short notice. Should I write to Mrs K. about it?[42]

Numerous strategies are deployed by Warton in this letter to emphasise the benefits to the child of remaining in the care of the society, rather than being returned to the family home. There was a clear expectation that she would be a productive and useful worker in the charity home, despite her slow progress at a church school. The irony of the letter is that Warton expected Minnie to do nothing more than 'keep house' for her mother once back home, a role considered negatively in comparison to the similar work she was most probably carrying out in the St Agnes Home. Furthermore, Katherine Warton felt so strongly about the benefits of the charitable institution for the child that she was willing to ask her mother for a contribution to her maintenance, despite the mother clearly stating that she wanted her returned to the family home. Rudolf encouraged Warton to write but later conceded that the mother 'appears to be very respectable, and although I did what I could to persuade her to leave the daughter under the society's care, she still reiterated her desire to have her under her control'.[43] Here we witness two significant elements in the care of children during the late nineteenth century. The first is the agency that poor parents could exert when faced with philanthropic interference in their lives; the second is an unwavering belief on the part of middle-class philanthropists that intervention into the lives of the poor had moral and economic value, both for the individual and wider society. From the three cases presented thus far it can be seen that middle-class expectations regarding child-rearing, environment, and acceptable behaviour were integral to the construction of pathologically different children.

Children who were cared for within the state welfare system of the poor law were expensive and were often dependent on tax-payer support for a good number of years. Therefore, keeping families together was often a pragmatic decision made by overseers and guardians.[44] This philosophy, however, was often complicated by issues such as parental disability, ill-health, or premature death. Moreover, there was a prevailing belief that children under the age of seven were entitled to parental care. Children occupied a unique place in the poor law system and were not always subject to harsh conditions, especially after the Poor Law Amendment Act of 1834. The New Poor Law introduced a welfare system whereby the position of those receiving state help had to be in situations that were deemed 'less eligible' than the lowest labourers.[45] Such punitive measures were not usually applied to children who were directed to 'improvement' through schooling, apprenticeship, and eventually employment, contradicting and inverting the eligibility test.

Childhood disability and pathological difference

Scholars of disability have painted a bleak picture of the exclusion, separation, and incarceration of individuals living with impairment in the past. Those working in the field have argued that disability was a social construction imposed on the biologically impaired through architecture, stigma, and socio-economic structures, all of which were shaped by an able-bodied society.[46] Much literature in this field has concentrated on the twentieth century, with the experience of earlier periods being relatively neglected. When a child, with what today would be called a disability, was admitted to the Waifs and Strays Society, their application forms usually described them as being impaired, crippled, or lame. The term disability did not feature, and therefore this chapter uses the linguistic register of the time.

Recently, there has been a growing historiographical interest in children living with impairment in the past. David Turner has observed an increased concern with 'problem' children in the eighteenth century, who were growing up with impairments existing from birth or acquired through mismanagement and were inevitably a burden, either on their families or the state.[47] Ashley Mathisen has also demonstrated a more nuanced understanding of the 'disabled' child body deployed at the London Foundling Hospital in this period.[48] She outlines how individual development through work (and work-associated activities such as apprenticeship), within the hospital itself and beyond, instilled ideas about adult independence. A picture of equal complexity is presented by Steve King in the context of nineteenth-century England. He contends that the experience of impairment for the young was often negotiated, between families, employers, and relieving officers, and the nature of relief depended on the able-bodiedness of the individual. It might thus be suggested that an imperfect body was not necessarily socially or economically liminal.[49] Furthermore, Dale and Borsay's collection of essays exploring experiential and definitional concepts of childhood disability have raised the profile of this subject further.[50] Their volume begins by linking general concerns about childhood health with an emerging professional interest in the disabled child in the mid-nineteenth century.

The impaired child was thus, by the 1870s, a subject of attention for a range of observers and commentators that led to numerous judgements about their abilities and potential future lives.

Rescuing children of the poor – The Waifs and Strays Society

By the late nineteenth century, children had acquired a wider social significance and were seen by authorities and those in philanthropic circles as the future of the nation and imperial project.[51] The terminology used to describe those who sought to protect and improve children in the late nineteenth century is particularly telling. They were 'child rescuers' or 'child savers' and thus were guardians of the discourse. They alone were supposedly responsible for bringing children back into the folds of acceptability and respectability. What is particularly interesting is the class gulf between those intervening and the children themselves. The philanthropists making judgements on the habits and cultures of the working poor had limited understanding and no lived experience of the circumstances of their subjects. The likes of Barnardo, Stephenson, Rudolf, and Rye were, without exception, raised and educated in very different conditions.[52]

To emphasise the key arguments of this chapter, examples have been chosen to reflect the complexities of how pathological difference was constructed. These are distinct cases, but all evidence the intricate nature of this process. In 1889, Albert C., a six-year-old boy whose mother had died and whose father had deserted him, entered the care of the Waifs and Strays Society. Not only was he an orphan but he had been 'crippled' after having his right leg amputated due to 'a palsy disease of the knee joint'.[53] Albert was thus representative of deservingness in Victorian society through two avenues, first through his youthfulness and secondly through his physical impairment. It might have been expected that he would have lived his life dependent on state welfare and charitable assistance but, despite his condition, he was apprenticed eight years after entering the charity to a tailor in Frome, Norfolk, and a note was placed in his file that stated 'he will not be able to maintain himself until the end of his apprenticeship'.[54] While this reveals the poor wages he received as an impaired apprentice, it also makes clear that following the completion of his term he was expected to be independent. A similar case was that of Edward M. who was taken into the care of the Waifs and Strays Society in 1883 at the age of five from the home of his mother and stepfather.[55] His impairment was from ankylosis (stiffening of the joints due to fusion of the bone) and a deformity of the vertebrae: he had not attended school because it was three-quarters of a mile away and he could not walk there. Yet on his arrival it was stated that he 'is a bright intelligent child and provided his health keeps well will be capable of earning his living in some way with either his hands or his head'. Edward did not go into an apprenticeship like Albert, but from his file it is clear that the organisation had an expectation of him developing into an independent and productive adult, a core facet of the modern idea of childhood where individuals were expected to support themselves into adulthood. While these children may have lost the sheltered innocence that was only available in a family home, philanthropy was enthusiastic about moulding them into responsible and respectable future citizens.

The situation was different, however, for children viewed through a lens of pathological difference. Annie B. was taken into the care of the Waifs and Strays Society on 9 October 1888. She was aged thirteen and had been an orphan for almost three months.[56] The aunt with whom she had been staying following the death of her mother had agreed to bring up her two younger siblings, but could not afford to keep the older girl and provide for her own family. Annie was noted to be in good health and had attended the Harrow Board School for five years, reaching the Standard of Level IV which was in line with academic expectations of the time. At admission, she was described as 'a rough uncouth girl but there is every reason to believe that under the good training she would get in the Home she would turn out well'.[57] At this point the girl fulfils the established modern model of a child of the working poor ripe for improvement. The notes from the case file continue: 'whereas were she sent to the workhouse (which is the only alternative) she would probably become quite unfit for respectable service'.[58] Here we can see recognition of the two models of childhood in operation. There was deservingness, respectability, and potential for improvement in the philanthropic home of the Waifs and Strays Society on the one hand and the undeserving dependence found in the publicly funded workhouse, a place to be avoided at all costs, on the other. Upon her admission Annie was initially sent to the Society's Arnold Grove Home but while there it soon became apparent that 'she is a very dull girl, and will not be fit for domestic service.'⁵⁹ Following this judgement she was then passed through numerous homes for industrial training before eventually being taken into St Chads where she was to learn machine knitting. However, by 1894, Annie had grown into an adult and her lack of development and progress led officials to decide that nothing more could be done with her. In a letter to Rudolf, Mr Stansfield at the St Chads Home lamented that 'this girl will be on the society's hands all her life unless she is sent to the workhouse.'⁶⁰ He continued that she is 'not quite all there' implying that she had some form of mental or learning disability and he complained that 'she is simply taking the place of a girl who might be learning a trade', before signing off by observing that she was 'particularly dull and stupid'. To Stansfield, the girl was clearly different from the norm and she was destined to not fulfil the expectations of a deserving childhood or adulthood. The only option, in his opinion, was to send the girl back to the workhouse, so that somebody more deserving might take her place in the home.

Sending Annie B. to the workhouse though was not as simple a task as it might appear. In order to receive relief an individual had to have earned a settlement. This could be achieved through birth, apprenticeship, marriage, or continuous employment for twelve months. Annie, however, had been touring the institutional provision of the Waifs and Strays Society and not been in one place long enough to earn a settlement. Stansfield had assessed that she was most likely to live out an existence dependent on ratepayer assistance. She was thus expensive and a burden to whichever workhouse in which she was placed. The Leeds Poor Law Guardians refused to take her and, following discussions of her settlement, Annie was eventually placed in the Edgware Workhouse, where we lose track of her narrative. This case demonstrates that both models of childhood could operate in tandem. First, there was the ideal of improvability that was applied until it became clear that a productive and independent future was unlikely. Then the child was pathologised because she was considered to be mentally incapable, even though before becoming orphaned she had reached Standard IV in the education system. Nevertheless, she had not met the requirements for trainable childhood and she was cast aside into the workhouse.

Mary B.'s experience further underscores how compounding conditions shaped reform attempts. She was admitted to the Society aged ten in 1889 having suffered severe burns to her hands. Her home was a poor one, with her father earning just eighteen shillings a week and the mother unable to work due to blindness.[61] In this situation the child was unable to help around the home due to her injuries; she was unproductive and constituted a drain on the limited household economy. The Waifs and Strays Society took the girl in with the objective of teaching her a trade. However, she soon was 'returned to her mother ... being crippled in her hands consequently not able to learn the knitting machine'. Again we see evidence of a child not being able to progress vocationally and being sent back to conditions that were considered unfavourable and dangerous prior to their interaction with philanthropy. This was a similar fate to that experienced by Jane M., aged fifteen, who was admitted to the St Chads Home to learn industrial knitting. It was said though that she was 'simply filling a bed that might be occupied by a capable girl'.[62]

The experience of Annie B., Mary B., and Jane M. were evidently not isolated examples. Now we turn to the case of Annie M., which provides a slightly different situation. Annie M. was admitted to the Waifs and Strays Society aged fourteen with both of her parents still alive.[63] She had been suffering from spinal disease and had received medical attention and care intermittently in a hospital for seven years. By way of treatment she wore a plaster jacket that was designed to aid the straightening of her spine. It might be assumed that physical deformity in itself was enough to establish difference but the situation was far more complex. Regardless of impairment, the Waifs and Strays Society sought and found occupations for children suffering from a range of conditions; it was not simply that disability equalled difference.

The construction of Annie M.'s pathological difference was multifactorial. Her father had been certified a lunatic and confined in the Cane Hill Pauper Lunatic Asylum for twelve months. He was seen to demonstrate family weakness and proto-eugenic bad heredity, while her mother worked at bookbinding earning a meagre two shillings per week, which was subsidised with three shillings on a temporary, yet ongoing, basis by the Poor Law Guardians, and consequently incurring the stigma attached to it. Furthermore, the girl displayed a lack of potential for improvement and was sent back to her mother on 7 October 1888, less than a month after being admitted, even though the

Guardians had committed to paying £13 a year for her care. The pathologically different were evidently constructed according to their ability to fit the established expectations of the 'modern' model. When this was not possible, evidence from family, occupation, and domestic spheres was used to demonstrate undeservingness and difference.

Further complexity in the construction of pathologically different childhoods is observed with the case of Frederick F.[64] He was taken into the care of the Waifs and Strays Society aged just eighteen months old. At this young stage of development it was more difficult to construct the child as falling outside of the parameters of a 'normal' childhood, so instead there was an increased emphasis on his background. Such actions highlight the expectation that individuals in some circumstances would always be marginal to acceptable society. In this case, the boy had been conceived as a result of a sexual assault committed against his mother by his uncle. The mother admitted herself to the poor law union workhouse to escape the familial and social repercussions associated with bearing an illegitimate child and sought a space in the Waifs and Strays Society for her 'innocent' infant. In these circumstances, the pathological difference was directly related to the criminal tendencies and bad heredity of the father. The initial response of the Waifs and Strays Society was to attempt emigrating the child to Canada but this was not an option because of his age. Here, we see another example of how childhood difference was created and the various methods of dealing with it. Frederick was never sent to Canada, but he eventually moved away from London to Warwickshire where he was apprenticed and then later employed as a tailor.

Conclusion

The formative years in establishing pathologically different childhood as a distinct conceptual entity were the thirty years after 1870, what one might label the high watermark of child rescue efforts. The archive of the Waifs and Strays Society provides a valuable window into the lives of children living with disability and in poverty at this time. From their records we can glean insights into the everyday lives of working families and the relationships that were developed between them and those doing charitable work. Furthermore, the records reveal important discourses about attempts to mould children's lives based around ideals of dependence and 'modern' citizenship. Moving into the twentieth century, many of the historical sentiments still persist but interventions into the lives of children have shifted from lay do-gooders to scientifically informed professionals. This has been achieved particularly through the medicalisation of children, primarily via the education system, that sees early intervention into diet, sensory impairment, and mental/behavioural disorders.

A continuity that is fairly well hidden is the widespread practice of child removal, albeit by the state rather than a voluntary sector today. Little has changed over the past hundred or so years. A child in an economically deprived area is more likely to be taken into care than a child living in an affluent one. This practice is surprisingly common. In the UK, youngsters are more likely to be removed from their families than anywhere else in Europe; there were nearly 28,000 children removed from their families in the UK in 2015 compared to 200 in Germany and twenty-eight in the Netherlands, a process supported by government policy and that can be completed within twenty-six weeks.[65] Furthermore, a child from a poor background is more likely to receive a diagnosis of behavioural or learning disorder such as attention deficit hyperactivity disorder (ADHD), oppositional defiant disorder (ODD), or autism spectrum disorder (ASD). Add into this the complex issue of race and ethnicity and it becomes apparent that the pathologically different child remains in the twenty-first century, even if the nomenclature and categories have altered somewhat.

Notes

1 The research for this chapter would not have been possible without the help of Ian Wakeling and the archives team at the Children's Society and the financial support of the Wellcome Trust, WT108624MA. I would also like to thank the editors of this volume for their thought-provoking and insightful comments, and Dr Annmarie Valdes for reading early versions of the chapter.
2 J.-J. Rousseau, *Émile, or on Education*, trans. Allan Bloom (New York: Basic Books, 1979), 49.
3 M. Foucault, *Discipline and Punish: The Birth of the Prison* (New York: Random House, 1975); M. Foucault, *Madness and Civilization* (London:

Routledge, 2009 [1961]); M. Foucault, *Power/Knowledge: Selected Interviews and Other Writings, 1972–1977* (New York: Random House, 1980).
4 P. Bean and J. Melville, *Lost Children of the Empire* (London: Unwin Hyman, 1989); E. Boucher, *Empire's Children: Child Emigration, Welfare, and the Decline of the British World, 1869–1967* (Cambridge: Cambridge University Press, 2014); R. Parker, *Away from Home: A History of Childcare* (Ilford: Barnardo's, 1990); S. Swain and M. Hillel, *Child, Nation, Race and Empire: Child Rescue Discourse, England, Canada and Australia, 1850–1915* (Manchester: Manchester University Press, 2010); C. Soares, 'Neither Waif nor Stray: Home, Family and Belonging in the Victorian Children's Institution, 1881–1914' (PhD dissertation, University of Manchester, 2014); S. J. Taylor, 'Insanity, philanthropy and emigration: dealing with insane children in late-nineteenth-century north-West England', *History of Psychiatry*, 25:2 (2014), 224–36; S. J. Taylor, 'Poverty, emigration and family: experiencing childhood poverty in late-nineteenth-century Manchester', *Family and Community History*, 18:2 (2015), 89–103.
5 M. Diamond, *Emigration and Empire: The Life of Maria S. Rye* (New York: Routledge, 2016).
6 A. Davin, 'Imperialism and motherhood', *History Workshop Journal*, 5 (1978), 9–65. A. Davin, *Growing up Poor: Home, School and Street in London, 1870–1914* (London: Rivers Oram, 1995), 15.
7 L. Murdoch, *Imagined Orphans: Poor Families, Child Welfare, and Contested Citizenship in London* (New Brunswick: Rutgers University Press, 2006).
8 H. Cunningham, *Children of the Poor: Representations of Childhood since the Seventeenth Century* (London: Blackwell, 1991), 134–5.
9 H. Hendrick, *Child Welfare in England, 1872–1989* (London: Routledge, 1994), 7.
10 The Poor Law Crusade was the name given to the campaign to reduce welfare spending according to the vision of Goschen. See E. Hurren, *Protesting about Pauperism* (Woodbridge: Boydell and Brewer, 2007).
11 *Ibid.*
12 L. Jackson, *Child Sexual Abuse in Victorian England* (London: Routledge, 2000), 6.
13 P. Cox, *Bad Girls in Britain: Gender, Justice and Welfare, 1900–1950* (Basingstoke: Palgrave Macmillan, 2013), 6.
14 J. Zinneker, 'What Does the Future Hold? Youth and Sociocultural Change in the FRG', in L. Chisholm, P. Büchner, H. H. Krüger, and P. Brown (eds), *Childhood, Youth and Social Change: A Comparative Perspective* (Basingstoke: Falmer Press, 1990), 17–32.
15 Hendrick, *Child Welfare*, 1–42.
16 *Ibid.*, ch. 2.

17 A. Turmel, *A Historical Sociology of Childhood* (Cambridge: Cambridge University Press 2008), ch. 3; E. Burman, *Deconstructing Developmental Psychology* (London: Routledge, 1994), 11.
18 C. Urwin, 'Constructing Motherhood: The Persuasion of Normal Development', in C. Steedman, C. Urwin, and V. Walkerdine (eds), *Language, Gender and Childhood* (London: Routledge, 1985), 164–202 (p. 166).
19 J. Stewart, '"The dangerous age of childhood": child guidance and the "normal" child in Great Britain, 1920–1950', *Paedagogica Historica*, 47:6 (2011), 785–803.
20 For a detailed discussion of the various welfare avenues available for children living with mental impairment, see S. J. Taylor, *Child Insanity in England, 1845–1907* (Basingstoke: Palgrave Macmillan, 2016), ch. 5.
21 J. Stroud, *Thirteen Penny Stamps: The Story of the Church of England Children's Society (Waifs and Strays) from 1881 to the 1970s* (London: Hodder and Stoughton, 1971) is a useful insight into the management and operation of the society.
22 A. Skinner, 'Overview of applications for care to the Waifs and Strays Society from 1882–1899' (unpublished paper 2016), 1; A. Skinner and N. Thomas, '"A pest to society": the Charity Organisation Society's domiciliary assessments into the circumstances of poor families and children', *Children & Society*, doi 10.111/chso.12237.
23 For a more detailed discussion of age classification and childhood, see: Taylor, *Child Insanity*, ch. 1.
24 A. Mathisen, '"So that they may be useful to themselves and the community": charting childhood disability in an eighteenth-century institution', *The Journal of the History of Childhood and Youth*, 8:2 (2015), 191–210 (p. 197).
25 Taylor, *Child Insanity*, 29; A. Borsay, *Disability and Social Policy in Britain since 1750* (Basingstoke: Palgrave Macmillan, 2005), 39; D. Wright, *Mental Disability in Victorian England: The Earlswood Asylum, 1847–1901* (Oxford: Clarendon 2001); Wright, 'Familial Care of "Idiot" Children in Victorian England', in P. Horden and R. Smith (eds), *The Locus of Care: Families, Communities, Institutions and the Provision of Welfare since Antiquity* (London: Routledge, 1997), 176–97 (p. 183).
26 J. Parr, *Labouring Children: British Immigrant Apprentices to Canada, 1869–1924* (London: Croom Helm, 1980), 16–19.
27 Children's Society (hereafter CS), Casefiles, CF/01565, Annie C.
28 CS, Casefiles, CF/06259, Catherine W.
29 J. Humphries, *Childhood and Child Labour in the British Industrial Revolution* (Cambridge: Cambridge University Press, 2010).
30 P. Kirby, *Child Workers and Industrial Health in Britain 1780–1850* (Woodbridge: The Boydell Press, 2013), 3.

31 H. Cunningham, *The Invention of Childhood* (London: BBC Books, 2006), 242.
32 Mathisen, 'Charting childhood disability', 192.
33 J. Locke, *Memorandum on Poor Relief for Board of Education*, quoted in F. Crompton, *Workhouse Children* (Stroud: Sutton, 1997), 8–9.
34 *Ibid.*
35 *Ibid.*, 7.
36 For a twentieth-century perspective, see J. Crane, '"The bones tell a story the child is too young or too frightened to tell": the battered child syndrome in Post-War Britain and America', *Social History of Medicine*, 28:4 (2015), 767–88.
37 CS, Casefiles, CF/01976, James T.
38 CS, Casefiles, CF/02173, Lucy F.
39 *Ibid.*
40 *Ibid.*
41 CS, Casefiles, CF/02271, Minnie K.
42 Minnie K., CF/02271/9.
43 Minnie K., CF/02271/13.
44 A. Levene, *The Childhood of the Poor: Welfare in Eighteenth-Century London* (Basingstoke: Palgrave Macmillan e-book, 2012), Location 208.
45 Historians have debated the impact and implementation of the Poor Law Amendment act; see S. King, *Poverty and Welfare in England 1700–1850: A Regional Perspective* (Manchester: Manchester University Press, 2000); D. Englander, *Poverty and Poor Law Reform in Nineteenth-Century Britain, 1834–1914, from Chadwick to Booth* (Florence: Taylor and Francis, 2013).
46 B. Linker, 'On the borderland of medical and disability history', *Bulletin of the History of Medicine*, 87:4 (2013), 540–59 (p. 54); T. Shakespeare, *Disability Rights and Wrongs* (London: Routledge, 2006).
47 D. M. Turner, 'Impaired children in eighteenth-century England', *Social History of Medicine* 30:4 (2017), 788–806.
48 Mathisen, 'Charting childhood disability'.
49 S. King, 'Constructing the disabled child in England, 1800–1860', *Family and Community History*, 18:2 (2015), 104–21.
50 A. Borsay and P. Dale, *Disabled Children: Contested Caring, 1850–1979* (London: Pickering and Chatto, 2012).
51 Davin, 'Imperialism and motherhood'.
52 This has a remarkable resemblance with the modern day. In Britain the coalition government of 2010 introduced a 'fast track' programme into social work. This scheme sought to attract the 'brightest' graduates from Britain's best universities to be accelerated into working with the country's most vulnerable children often in deprived areas. Again, these were rarely those with experience of living in urban poverty and so the

class gulf between perceived helpers on one hand and constructions of those in need on the other remains; www.gov.uk/government/news/talented-graduates-wanted-for-career-in-social-work.
53 Waifs and Strays Society (WSS), Albert C., CF/001647/3.
54 CS, Casefiles, CF/01647/16, Albert C.
55 CS, Casefiles, CF/01771/1, Edward M.
56 CS, Casefiles, CF/01646, Annie B.
57 *Ibid.*
58 *Ibid.*
59 *Ibid.*
60 *Ibid.*
61 CS, Casefiles, CF/02194, Mary B.
62 CS, Casefiles, CF/01786, Jane M.
63 CS, Casefiles, CF001581/1–6, Annie M.
64 CS, Casefiles, CF004828/1–3, Frederick F.
65 UK Government Statistics, *Children Looked After in England*, SFR41/2016, available at www.gov.uk/government/statistics/children-looked-after-in-england-including-adoption-2015-to-2016.

4

Phrenology as neurodiversity: the Fowlers and modern brain disorder

Kristine Swenson

In *Self-Culture and the Perfection of Character* (1847), the American phrenologist, Orson Fowler, offered phrenology as a remedy for those who 'are daily and earnestly inquiring –"How can I REMEDY my defects? By what MEANS can I increase my deficient organs, and diminish or regulate those that are too large? … How can I make my children better?"'[1] Orson and his brother, Lorenzo, founded a phrenological and publishing empire in mid-nineteenth-century America that revitalised and popularised this heterodox medical practice. Phrenology had enjoyed widespread, if controversial, application within Western medicine in the century's first decades, but by the 1840s, it had been marginalised and largely branded as quackery, as laboratory-based biomedicine increasingly monopolised the medical marketplace.

Phrenology began in the late eighteenth century under the Viennese physician Franz Joseph Gall, who argued that the brain is an aggregate of mental 'organs', each with localised and specific functions such as fidelity, ambition, or poetic talent. The larger the organ, the greater the corresponding faculty, which could be measured by the size and shape of the skull. Thus, phrenology could explain the relative strengths and weaknesses of a person's mind and character. Although phrenology's claims were not substantiated by experimental scientific method, historians of science have traced the real and lasting impact of Gall's thinking, from the diffusion of scientific naturalism that prepared the public for Darwinian evolution, to its influence upon fields as diverse as psychology, physical anthropology, and neuroanatomy.[2] However, the cultural impact of phrenology is more complicated. Roger Cooter argues that phrenology first gained traction among physicians in the 1820s and 1830s not because of its scientific validity but as a way to gain social power and assert meritocratic values over traditional forms of authority.[3] Once bourgeois-liberal thought became dominant, it lost this particular power of social aggrandisement, but took on other roles.[4] Alternative medical practices such as phrenology gained popularity after 1840 in part because they were more responsive than laboratory-based medicine to nineteenth-century culture and politics. If, as Stanley Finger asserts, phrenology as a science was finished by 1840,[5] it nevertheless left its mark on 'virtually every cultural province of Victorian life'.[6] Phrenology was integral to the fabric of mid-century Anglo-American culture, from major literary works such as Charlotte Brontë's *Jane Eyre* (1847) and Walt Whitman's *Leaves of Grass* (1855), to the educational reforms of Horace Mann, and the workings of the criminal justice systems of both countries. If the scientific and intellectual elite were sceptical of phrenology by the mid-century, the 'doctrine served as a cohesive cultural factor',[7] and in the second half of the nineteenth century, it 'became in many ways more deeply entrenched than ever in everyday thought and expression'.[8]

This chapter will examine how the Fowlers, as entrepreneurial popularisers, revitalised phrenology in the US and, to a lesser degree in Britain, in the mid-nineteenth century, by the masterful dissemination of their ideas and products and their direct appeal to consumer-patients who sought alternatives to mainstream medicine through self-help and self-culture. 'Practical' phrenologists such as the Fowlers responded to the supposed ills of modern, industrialised capitalism by touting progressive self-improvement through phrenological self-knowledge. The Fowlers' 'nonintellectualist' and 'healthean'[9] brand of phrenology enabled a populist response to perceptions of 'epidemic' health issues and, in particular, to what mainstream medicine considered largely innate and untreatable conditions. It was working-class Victorians who bore the brunt of widespread cultural fears of degeneration and race suicide, while the middle classes were increasingly diagnosed with the 'modern' illnesses of neurasthenia and dyspepsia. The Lamarckism of nineteenth-century practical phrenology, which promised personal improvement through proper living habits and exercising the faculties, served as a response to the harsh consequences of modernity, Darwinian evolution, and hereditary conditions. The Fowlers' phrenology also prospered from a popular distrust of the newly orthodox laboratory-based medicine. Though dismissed by nineteenth-century intellectuals as pseudoscience or as a 'vulgarisation' of earlier European and British phrenology, its appeal is perhaps less surprising given that working-class patients were disproportionately subject to the experimentation of laboratory-based medicine that often caused more immediate harm than good to their families.[10] The Fowlers' phrenology ultimately sustained the essentialist taxonomies from which it promised to liberate its adherents. Their programme of individualistic self-culture was also a means of self-regulation within a normative social code.

Phrenology has remained an undercurrent in Western medicine and culture, resurfacing recently in relation to diagnosing neurological conditions.[11] In the twenty-first-century press, duelling headlines proclaim that the 'Brains of Those with Autism are Not Shaped Differently'[12] and that 'Kids with ADHD Have Some Brain Regions that are Smaller than Normal'.[13] In response to such studies and the sharp rise in children diagnosed with neurological disorders, the cerebral self-help industry is alive and well with works such as *The Whole-Brain Child* and *Brain Rules for Baby*.[14] After analysing the Fowlers' phrenological practice, this chapter will draw parallels between the Fowlers' phrenology of the nineteenth century, and the twenty-first-century neuro-information campaign which, like practical phrenology, resists orthodox medicine's theories about the mind and brain. Both movements demonstrate the broad public appeal of alternative medical theories and treatments in the face of modernity's 'mass medicine',[15] with its drive toward a normativised body and brain. And both demonstrate the pitfalls as well as the advantages of populist medical movements that respond to cultural exigencies.

Early phrenology

Phrenology in both theory and practice evolved significantly between Gall's initial formulation and the Fowlers' publications in the 1840s. Young calls Gall the 'first modern empirical psychologist of character and personality' because he rejected the idea of normative mental faculties, an assertion that has been vital to thinking about cognitive difference to the present day.[16] However, Gall was a pre-evolutionary thinker who assumed that organisms, placed within the Great Chain of Being, were static.[17] In contrast, Gall's dissectionist, Johann Gaspar Spurzheim, introduced 'practical phrenology' to Britain in the 1810s, with a new emphasis on training and education as a way to develop positive faculties and support social reform.[18] In an argument that prefigures the later eugenics movement, Spurzheim regrets that 'the laws of hereditary descent are so much neglected, whilst ... whole nations, might be improved beyond imagination, in figure, stature, complexion, health, talents and moral feelings.'[19] It was Spurzheim's follower, George Combe, a Scottish lawyer and philosopher, who was most responsible for the transformation of phrenology from an 'arcane theory' to a 'socially respectable scientific vehicle of "progressive" ideas'.[20] Combe was a 'moralizing popularizer', who combined Spurzheim's phrenology with the social reform of Jeremy Bentham and James Mill.[21] At mid-century, Combe's *Constitution of Man* was the third most likely text to appear on shelves in English-speaking homes after the *Bible* and *Pilgrim's Progress*.[22] Because, like Spurzheim, Combe believed the size and shape of the phrenological organs were inherited, he perpetuated race and class prejudices in pseudo-scientific language, for instance asserting that working-class and racially 'primitive' women feel less pain in childbirth than middle- and upper-class white women.[23] A 'practical' benefit of phrenological knowledge was the ability to choose appropriate servants.[24] At the same time, Combe advocated a phrenological Larmarckism that encouraged self-improvement and protected against transmitting negative traits to offspring through the proper application of the 'Natural Laws' as established by the Creator and revealed through phrenology.[25] Under the guidance of the phrenologically knowledgeable, inherited faculties would be directed to 'proper objects' and their 'action [would] become good'.[26] Cooter reads *Constitution of Man* as a 'secular revival' of Scottish Calvinism, 'sacralizing the social norms and values most appropriate to the industrially modified and modifying economic order'.[27] Spurzheim and Combe brought practical phrenology, with its promise of personal and social betterment, to the United States in the 1820s, where it soon became even more popular under the Fowlers.

The Fowlers' practical phrenology

The Fowler family – led by the brothers Orson and Lorenzo, their sister Charlotte, and her husband, Samuel Wells – were among the first fully to exploit the potential of phrenology as practical self-help (or 'self-culture'). Their motto was 'self-made or never made'.[28] Heeding their own advice, they built an empire of phrenological lecture tours, publishing, and therapeutics that kept phrenology, broadly defined, profitable and in the public eye into the twentieth century. Orson and Lorenzo Fowler, like George Combe, were not medical men by training but they saw in phrenology a way to combine their oratorical skills with their commitment to progressive reform. The brothers began as itinerant phrenologists in the 1830s, lecturing and giving demonstrations on the heads of audience members and taking plaster casts of the prominent or interesting. Sometimes performing blindfolded or giving 'double-test' examinations, the theatrical brothers thrived in front of local audiences, pronouncing noted painters as possessing 'small Color' or well-loved clergymen as having 'an utter absence of Conscientiousness'.[29] The brothers defended 'the science' and their readings, even when local audiences disagreed with them, revelling especially when some secret life or bad behaviour was revealed to confirm an earlier diagnosis. By the late 1830s, Orson had established an office and examination room in Philadelphia, which housed many of the busts and their *Phrenological Journal*, which ran from 1838 to 1911.[30] Meanwhile, Lorenzo opened offices in New York, where Orson and the bust collection joined him in 1842. This Phrenological Depot became the centre of the Fowler empire. There they offered private examinations and clinical instruction, sold books, charts, porcelain busts, and other phrenological paraphernalia, and ran a large publishing house that printed not only the Fowlers' own tracts but works by many ancillary progressive health and social reformers. These publications were widely disseminated in Britain as well through the Fowlers' agent in London.[31] In the 1860s, Samuel Wells, Lorenzo Fowler, and Fowler's wife, Lydia Folger Fowler, exported their American style of practical phrenology directly to Britain with highly successful lecture tours; in London, they opened the Fowler Phrenological Institute, published *The Phrenologist*, and founded the British Phrenological Society which remained active until 1967.[32]

At least some of the Fowlers' great success must be attributed to how much their programme of self-study and exertion was in keeping with the mind-set of the mid-nineteenth century. The idea of self-improvement was foundational to the American republic, with Benjamin Franklin – Lydia's cousin through the Folger line[33] – a much cited exemplar.[34] However, the phrase 'self-made man', which the Fowlers appropriated for their motto, is generally attributed to US senator, Henry Clay, who, in 1832, used it explicitly in the context of entrepreneurial capitalism.[35] By the 1830s, the pressures of new urban populations, market capitalism, and abolitionist rhetoric saw the liberalism of the Enlightenment give way to an emphasis on differences and hierarchies within the social body. '[N]ew statistical practices' in science and social science 'divided society into masses of standardized or deviant individual bodies', with the aim of creating a 'fit' citizenry; the rhetoric of natural rights was replaced by an emphasis on natural laws that must be understood and followed for the good of the self and the nation.[36] In the United States, antebellum reform movements promised the 'moral transformation' of the individual and thus the nation.[37] Cynthia Eagle Russett cites phrenology as an example of a new scientific practice that nevertheless served social reform, at least for a time.[38] She singles out the Fowlers' phrenology, in particular, as the 'crescendo' of American optimism in scientific reform before the rise of physical anthropology with its explicit emphases on biological differences and human limitations rather than aptitudes and possibilities.[39] Within the Fowlers' programme, the entrepreneurial capitalism of being 'self-made' was in tension with the religious idea of 'self-culture', introduced to the American public by the Unitarian theologian William Ellery Channing and then spread through the writings of nineteenth-century transcendentalists and progressives, such as Ralph Waldo Emerson and James Russell Lowell. Channing defined self-culture as the 'care which every man owes to himself, to the unfolding and perfecting of his nature', and noted that Americans held the 'means of improvement, of self-culture, possessed no where else'.[40] Nevertheless, the Fowlers managed to persuade many in Britain that they, too, had the means and the duty of phrenological self-culture. In 'A Farewell Entertainment to Mr and Mrs Fowler' during their Scottish lecture tour in 1863, a working man from Glasgow explained that in contrast to earlier, British phrenologists, Lorenzo Fowler 'gives us higher and more ennobling views of the mission and destiny of the human race … .[N]ot only are we privileged, but it is our duty, so to use them [mental faculties] for the purpose of raising ourselves mentally and morally.'[41]

In contrast to their European and British counterparts, and very much in keeping with mid-nineteenth-century American thought, the Fowlers' phrenological programme was self-directed and, with notable exceptions, largely egalitarian. Whereas Combe denied that 'original propensities can be *eradicated* by education and other means' and trusted only the most morally and intellectually virtuous to guide their own phrenological improvement,[42] the Fowlers promised 'self-improvement' to 'every individual' with publications such as *The Illustrated Self-Instructor in Phrenology and Physiology* (1857) and *Education and Self-Improvement, Founded on Physiology and Phrenology* (1843).[43] The Fowlers were not unique among phrenologists in advocating a self-help doctrine, but they were certainly the most successful. Historian Mary Miles credits this achievement to the Fowlers' drive to commodify phrenology via public lectures and their publishing house.[44] For the Fowlers, 'self-made' meant body and mind, but it also meant an unapologetic entrepreneurialism. Orson Fowler's preface to the first edition of *Education and Self-Improvement* champions the Fowler programme over that of earlier phrenologists: 'Too long ... have Phrenologists been content with *knowing* themselves by this science. It is now high time for them to *apply* it to their own mental cultivation, and to the intellectual and moral improvement of mankind.'[45] To that end, the Fowlers' self-help texts often include tables listing the phrenological organs keyed to their full descriptions in the text and with space for charting family members. The Fowlers translated complex scientific language and a physical examination into simple images on the page (see figures 4.1 and 4.2)[46] and adopted the language of an accessible photorealism to win their audience: phrenology was 'the camera through which we may look at ourselves', wrote Samuel Wells.[47] Ironically, this accessibility, which purported to bring the mental and moral self to the easily readable surface, made categorising and discriminating against groups and individuals a simpler process. Allan Sekula has argued that the conjunction of photography and phrenology in the nineteenth century 'contributed to the ideological hegemony of capitalism' by their 'taxonomic ordering'.[48]

Combe and phrenologists who aspired to scientific acceptance were cautious about making claims for phrenology's ability to alter the brain physically. Orson Fowler, however, asserts unequivocally that one may

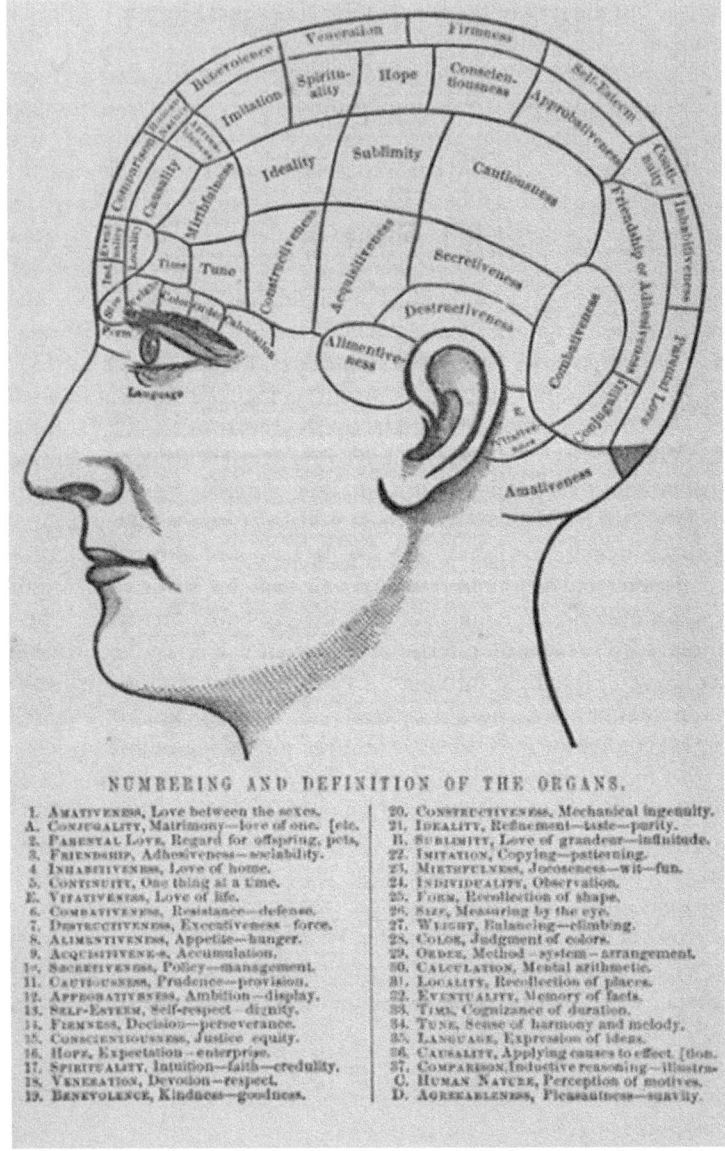

Figure 4.1 'Numbering and Definition of the Organs', O. S. Fowler and L. N. Fowler, *The Illustrated Self-Instructor in Phrenology and Physiology with over One Hundred Engravings*.

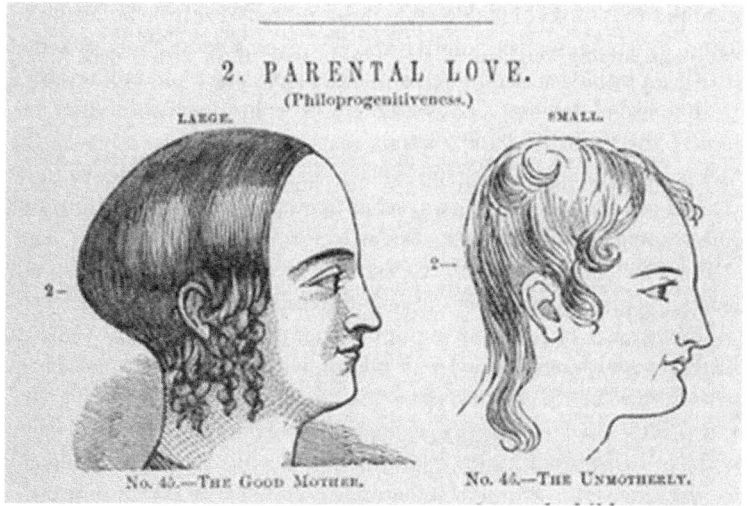

Figure 4.2 'Parental Love', O. S. Fowler and L. N. Fowler, *The Illustrated Self-Instructor in Phrenology and Physiology with over One Hundred Engravings.*

change not just the character of the faculties but their literal, physical size through their exercise or disuse.[49] As proof, Orson cites the 'decided increase of the whole intellectual lobe' of the plaster casts of the Reverend John Pierpont taken in 1835 and then in 1841, an increase attributed to Pierpont's 'almost continual *exercise* of his intellectual faculties' in the composition of poetry, temperance lectures, and debate with 'rum-sellers of his congregation'.[50] This example demonstrates the connection that the firm made between phrenological health and other progressive reform movements. At times, the Fowlers' politics clearly ran ahead of their science, for instance, when enumerating the cranial distinctions among members of various Christian denominations: strict Calvinists have heads that are 'tolerably wide' and rise 'rapidly from the intellectual organs' in contrast to the more balanced heads of Episcopalians, Unitarians, and Congregationalists.[51] Not surprisingly, the Fowlers were Congregationalists. These sorts of claims not only alienated scientists, but led to followers of Spurzheim and Combe criticising the Fowlers for their 'many inaccuracies' and 'Yankee go-a-head principle' that took coincidences for 'causations'.[52] Far from being intimidated by charges of popularisation, however, Orson shot back that British phrenology was 'rather too anxious to place phrenology on a *scientific* and *philosophical* basis, to the neglect of the *practical* examinations. Mere theorizing and abstract reasoning will never advance the interest of phrenology'.[53] Orson Fowler's easy dismissal of the scientific basis of phrenology suggests to what degree its scientific pretensions were waning even as its cultural relevance continued.

The Fowlers laid claim to the scientific when it suited them, but distancing phrenology from the scientific was, in fact, a shrewd rhetorical strategy, not uncommon in populist political and social movements that eschew expertise in favour of 'common sense' or the 'natural'. From the mid-nineteenth century, medicine became increasingly regularised as a profession and practice; using modern industrial and business models, it promised a new uniformity and efficiency in providing a healthy citizenry.[54] Biomedicine modernised itself by way of new technologies and laboratory-based experimentation, and sought to monopolise the market in response to a host of heterodox medicines that threatened its new power as a profession.[55] But as orthodox practitioners claimed greater authority to read and control the bodies of the public, the public themselves were drawn to heterodox practices, such as practical phrenology and homeopathy, which promised more patient control. The public resistance engendered by nineteenth-century health campaigns such as the Contagious Diseases Acts and compulsory vaccination suggest the degree to which the new biomedicine was distrusted.[56] Roberta Bivins argues that heterodox medical practices were and continue to be attractive alternatives to orthodox biomedicine insofar as they place patients' somatic experience 'at the centre of the therapeutic encounter', individualise that experience, and assume a 'dynamic relationship between bodies and their social and physical environments',[57] all characteristics of the Fowlers' practical phrenology. Moreover, 'scientificity', asserts Bivins, 'was no more the sole criterion of nineteenth-century consumers than it is today'.[58] Cooter remarks that the 'standard historical emphasis' on orthodox medicine's abandonment of phrenology is 'misplaced'.[59] Phrenology and other heterodox and self-help medical practices were, 'curatively speaking', as likely to 'deliver the goods' as orthodox medicine, given the limitations of orthodox medicine at the time.[60]

Dr Lydia Fowler and health reform

It is misguided, then, to characterise the Fowlers as charlatans. Following Combe, who was 'driven by a genuine religious commitment to improve the physiological condition of humankind',[61] the Fowlers turned phrenology into a popular and self-guided practice allied to hydropathy, dietetics, vegetarianism, dress reform, and temperance – all movements that contributed to a more health-conscious population. Practical phrenologists often achieved positive ends despite unscientific and occasionally laughable claims, and the Fowlers' facility with marketing and publishing made them particularly influential. They helped reform the treatment of criminals and the insane, were pioneers of American sex education and marriage counselling, and promoted educational ideas that were 'startling in their modernity' including promoting educational rights for children with physical and cognitive disabilities.[62] Moreover, though the brothers were not medically trained, the extended Fowler family contained several medical doctors, albeit with heterodox leanings, who practised in both phrenological and mainstream medical contexts. The Fowlers' younger half-sister, Almira Fowler Ormsbee Breakspear, received her MD in 1853 from the Female Medical College in Philadelphia, and then served on its faculty as a demonstrator of anatomy and chemistry.[63] And their younger half-brother, Edward Payson Fowler, received an MD from New York Medical College in 1855; deeply interested in spiritualism, mesmerism, and the 'phenomena of the mind', Edward set up a successful practice in New York with two homeopathic physicians.[64]

Most importantly, Lorenzo's wife, Lydia Folger Fowler, became in 1850 the second woman in the United States after Elizabeth Blackwell to receive an accredited medical degree, and the first woman professor of medicine in the country.[65] Madeleine Stern comments that 'by the mid-1850s', Lydia had 'not only exerted an influence upon the interests and publications of her husband's firm but made a niche for herself in the history of American medicine'.[66] Lydia practiced 'eclectic' medicine, 'accepting the best of the homeopathic and even a modicum of the drug-ridden allopathic system'.[67] Although allopathy became orthodox medicine in the twentieth century, eclectic practice was entirely respectable and probably the least harmful medical approach in the 1850s; it embraced all manner of health reforms from the truly efficacious to the merely faddish. Thus, the Fowlers' marriage of phrenology and medicine was mutually supportive and beneficial. Lydia accompanied her husband on his popular lecture tours across the United States, Canada, and Britain, where she preached the physiological benefits of temperance, hydropathy, and hygiene to great success. Lydia earned 'handsome sum[s] of money' and received accolades from lecture attendees as a 'true benefactress' who relieved the 'woes of the suffering' by 'her knowledge and skill in the medical profession'.[68] When at home in New York, Lydia kept daily appointments at her own office and at the Fowler Phrenological Depot, and taught medical courses at the Metropolitan Medical College and the New York Hydropathic and Physiological School.[69] After she and Lorenzo moved to London in the 1860s, Lydia continued her work as a health lecturer and district visitor; she furthered her medical studies in Paris and served three months in charge of the obstetrical department at the London Marylebone Road Hospital.[70] The early feminist periodical, *The Englishwoman's Review*, noted that the 'largest halls in England have not infrequently been filled' to hear Lydia's lectures, which encouraged women to 'study for themselves' the laws of life and health.[71] Lydia herself estimated that some '200,000 women in English-speaking countries had attended her lectures'.[72]

Lydia Folger Fowler's accomplishments place her at the forefront of early women doctors in Britain and America, alongside Elizabeth Blackwell, Elizabeth Garrett Anderson, Sophia Jex-Blake, and Mary Putnam Jacobi. Compared to these women, however, Lydia has received very little scholarly attention.[73] In part, this neglect stems from the energy with which physicians, including Blackwell and Jacobi, worked to discredit graduates of 'irregular' medical schools and practitioners such as eclectics and homeopaths.[74] This is true even when their practices were quite similar; for example, Lovejoy notes that in the 1870s, Elizabeth Blackwell and Lydia Fowler were both living and working in England as 'writers and lecturers on medicosocial subjects, and both were calling attention to the influence of the mind upon bodily ailments'.[75] That Blackwell was allowed on the Medical Register in England and Lydia was not was due to a loophole in the Medical Act of 1858 rather than because her credentials or her practice were superior. Eve Fine and others have shown that eclectic credentials did not necessarily disqualify physicians, and especially women, from professional consideration.[76]

Lovejoy suggests that Lydia's association with phrenology was as important – I would argue more important – as her eclecticism to her 'disadvantage' in the 'general eulogy of pioneer medical women'.[77] Most pointedly, when Lydia is mentioned in histories of women and medicine, her marriage to the 'phrenologist publisher' Lorenzo often precedes mention of her medical degree.[78]

That Lydia's historical neglect stems from her association with phrenology is ironic since phrenology prompted her medical studies and allowed her to develop a successful career and inspire other women to study medicine. Moreover, the Fowlers championed medical women enthusiastically and extended their reform activities to the woman's movement generally. 'The bridge was short', writes Stern, 'between the rights of women to water cure, dress reform, and health, and the rights of women to extended employment, equal pay for equal work, and full suffrage.'[79] In both the United States and Britain, Lydia was a leader in women's organisations, including her role as secretary at the Seneca Falls convention, where she won the admiration of Elizabeth Cady Stanton, and as honorary secretary of the Woman's British Temperance Society.[80] Lydia's combination of feminist politics and medicine was not unique – Elizabeth Garrett Anderson and Sophia Jex-Blake were both active suffragists, for instance. But as part of the Fowler enterprise, her feminist views received widespread publicity and were allied to more general and very popular reform movements. Of all the Fowlers, Lydia forces us to acknowledge that phrenology, however misguided as science, was integral to legitimate health and social reform of the nineteenth century. Her work also offers an example of how difficult it could be to distinguish between what we now consider heterodox and orthodox medicine. As Bivins and others have argued, the ascendancy of biomedicine was neither smooth nor inevitable. The Fowlers' phrenological theory partook of and contributed to the discourses surrounding modern disorders such as neurasthenia and dyspepsia and to the fears of racial degeneration. But their holistic practice, with its emphasis on education, self-help, and especially brain plasticity also offered the public ways to transcend the determinism of those discourses.

As did most other early women physicians, Lydia Fowler treated women and children; therefore, her publications, which included a temperance novel and volume of poetry as well as self-help medical tracts, brought phrenology and eclectic medical ideas to that audience. Her writings demonstrate the degree to which she both participated in and resisted the new medical orthodoxy that sought to organise bodies for modern society. Lydia's most widely read publication, the two-volume *Familiar Lessons on Physiology and Phrenology*, was specifically 'designed for the use of children and youth in schools and families'.[81] In her preface to this popular volume, Lydia writes to parents and teachers that physiology and phrenology should be studied together because they are 'absolutely necessary to a full understanding of the mind'.[82] She 'cheerfully' recommends that parents and teachers place her *Familiar Lessons* 'into the hands of their children as a guide to self-knowledge'.[83] From the 1830s, American physiology textbooks promoted the better health of the individual and the nation,[84] and the 1840s 'saw an extraordinary flowering of the literature of child development'.[85] The Fowlers come out of this tradition of self-help medicine and hygiene; their addition of phrenology to 'right living' brought currency to the tradition. And *Familiar Lessons* contains the sort of pious advice that one would expect from a mid-nineteenth-century text for children: 'Children, if we cultivate [the social and domestic organs] properly, life will be a source of joy and happiness' for 'we can all … enjoy the sweets of a quiet home.'[86] Characteristic of heterodox medicine, it insists that mind and body work together: 'The body must be in a healthy condition for the mind to act freely and vigorously.'[87]

However, despite its generic familiarity, *Familiar Lessons on Physiology and Phrenology* is surprising. First, in keeping with the Fowler belief in self-culture, it directs advanced medical information toward its audience of children – for instance, a detailed discussion of the nerves of the brain illustrated in cross-section.[88] Though some physiology textbooks in this period targeted students,[89] the degree of specialised information directed at young children is unusual and striking. Interestingly, the familiar phrenological skull appears only on the title-page, whereas the brains within the text appear as standard anatomical illustrations, emphasising the scientificity of Lydia's phrenological theory. Secondly, Lydia asserts the social and evolutionary advantages even of negative traits, and that phrenological organs can be resized to better advantage. Combativeness and Destructiveness, for instance, 'if rightly exercised, produce spirit, force, and energy of character'.[90] Third, *Familiar Lessons* shows awareness of how children's strengths and weaknesses exist on a spectrum. Lydia recounts how, in developing phrenology as a young man, Gall had noticed that some of his schoolmates 'were very generous and amiable, some selfish, some obstinate and cruel … He found that one liked the study of arithmetic, another could commit to memory, and so on … He became convinced that there must be a cause why he could not recite his lessons as rapidly and as freely as some of the other boys'.[91] In other words, the text eschews a normative model of child development in favour of one that allows for neurological diversity.

Phrenology and neurodiversity

Although *Familiar Lessons on Physiology and Phrenology* resists normativising children and their development, and though Lydia is writing here about all children, both what we would call neurotypical and atypical, her phrenological descriptions bear a striking resemblance to how doctors and scientists have worked to define children with neurological disorders since the nineteenth century. For instance, the passage that Lydia recounts above from Gall resembles Hans Asperger's descriptions of the autistic children he studied in the 1930s at the Children's Clinic in Vienna. Asperger has been applauded for his treatment of autistic children as 'unique personalit[ies]', whose conditions are a matter of 'degree', often with remarkable intelligence.[92] Asperger resisted normative neurological descriptions much as Lydia had in *Familiar Lessons*. As did phrenologists and other physiognomists, Asperger assumed correlation between mental make-up and appearance, generalising that 'Autistic children lose their baby features very quickly … Their early thoughtfulness has formed their faces'.[93] In his thesis on '"Autistic Psychopathy" in Childhood' (1944), Asperger praises psychotherapist Ernst Kretschmer for developing an accurate typology that matched 'in feine Einzelheiten' ('in fine detail') the physical to the psychological constitution – an idea embraced by 'der alten Physiognomik und der Phrenologie'.[94] Also like phrenologists, Asperger accepted as functionally useful a range of abilities, personalities, and behaviours. As opposed to most autism researchers of the mid-twentieth century, who thought institutionalisation was the best option for autistic children – and in contradiction to the Nazi regime under which he worked – Asperger asserted that 'autistic people have their place in the organism of the social community', particularly in fields that require single-minded focus and originality.[95] Still, Asperger and his colleagues were working to identify 'typical characteristics' of this 'highly distinctive' personality. Phrenologists claimed to read character quickly from facial features and the shape of the skull; Asperger claimed that 'Once one has properly recognised an autistic individual one can spot such children instantly'.[96]

As Edith Sheffer has shown in persuasive detail, Asperger's example demonstrates how categorising children – even with the most humane intentions – creates opportunities for systematic pathologising and discrimination of the kind discussed by Steven Taylor in the previous chapter.[97] Asperger's clinic grew out of the progressive and interventionist medical policies of socialist Vienna in the 1920s. But in the 1930s, Austrofascism and then the Nazi Anschluss saw Asperger's clinic move to the far right and participate in Nazi directives to sterilise, forcibly institutionalise, and murder children deemed socially unfit. Asperger himself, who had previously resisted pathologising children in his clinic, introduced the idea of autism as a 'psychopathy'.[98] Though not as extreme as the 'diagnosis regime' of the Third Reich, Anglo-American culture since the Victorian period offers plenty of examples of such phenomena, from Francis Galton's anthropometric laboratories, which collected anatomical data from thousands of students in public schools[99] to the ways in which intelligence testing in US schools confirmed 'nativist, racist, and antisocialist political programs'.[100]

It is important to acknowledge, then, that the relative social and neurological progressivism of the Fowlers' phrenology, like these later examples of measuring and categorising minds, is haunted by those who were excluded or diminished by its theory. With its evolutionary underpinnings and influence on physical anthropology, phrenology has been tied to the racial science that inspired the eugenics movement, even as it fostered certain forms of progressivism. Carla Bittel, for instance, has noted that although phrenology could be adapted to 'women's rights causes', it also helped white, middle-class women to distinguish themselves from 'others' and to 'naturalize their own positive qualities' and 'further engrained scientific racism in American culture'.[101] Phrenology remained implicated in and hampered by the taxonomic hierarchies of its times. Yet the Fowlers' adherence to nonnormative theories of the brain and human behaviour, belief in the efficacy of education and the possibility of full social integration, and the commitment to broad access of their ideas also contributed to their appeal and legacy.

The Fowlers' ambiguous legacy finds a parallel in the contradictions of the neuro-information campaigns of the twenty-first century and the populist political movements that resist mainstream medicine's treatment of those diagnosed with neurological conditions. These campaigns, which are driven largely by new media and in response to rising rates of diagnoses of neurological conditions, include positions that are both deeply sceptical of science and that demand cures from researchers, that are both liberationist and reactionary. What they share is a dissatisfaction with mainstream medicine's inability to adequately treat – sometimes even clearly diagnose – certain chronic or innate neurological conditions whose rates of diagnosis are perceived as 'epidemic'. The case of autism is particularly instructive in this regard. Like neurasthenia in the Victorian period, autism is a sort of cultural signpost of the present moment whose prevalence has been blamed variously upon genetics; twenty-first-century mating practices, and especially those tied to women's greater education and career advancement; environmental toxins; poor parenting; or dangerous vaccinations.[102] Regardless of cause, autism, like Victorian disorders of modernity, involves the family and extended social structures such as schools, social services, and healthcare. Similarly, the inability of modern medicine to provide a cure or even definitive therapy regimen for autism has opened the door for heterodox medical solutions and autism's commodification in the medical marketplace.

Just as Lydia Fowler's *Familiar Lessons on Phrenology* found an audience among mothers anxious for their children's brains and futures, the most driven twenty-first-century autism activists have been parents seeking alternatives to the bleak predictions of an autism diagnosis. The success of autism awareness campaigns has been driven by publicity and the broad dissemination of information beyond 'experts' to families and to autistic people themselves. The explosion of books, websites, and blogs published by and for the neurodiverse parallels the explosion of public health information in the nineteenth century, exemplified by the Fowlers' public relations machine, and with similar spectacular results. The Fowlers influenced everything from criminal reforms to sexual education to hygienic house design in the US.[103] The neurological information campaign has shaped special education services and products, paediatric practice, and even home design.

On one hand, this explosion of information has exposed families and the neurodiverse to commercial exploitation. In response to medical pronouncements that autism is 'hardwired' and incurable, families pursue expensive and sometimes dangerous alternative therapies of dubious medical value. The lobbies of many autism conferences are filled with vendors selling expensive technology or promoting risky biomedical treatments. Persuaded by faulty research such as Andrew Wakefield's 1998 study that MMR vaccines cause autism, some families have refused to vaccinate their children, despite surges in measles and pertussis. The impact on public health of the anti-vaccination movement of the twenty-first century rivals that of the nineteenth, when anti-vaccination activists argued that state-sanctioned medicine undermined individual civil liberties.[104]

An alternative wing of the neuro-information campaign, the emergent neurodiversity movement, offers a more positive and less dangerous response to mainstream medicine's stance on autism as largely untreatable. Though not a 'new phrenology', the neurodiversity movement shares certain features with the Fowlers' practical phrenology, both in theory and methods. Neurodiversity activists pursue alternatives to the 'pathology paradigm' surrounding the rise in neurological disorder diagnoses, and argue that neurodiversity is both a 'natural and a valuable form of human diversity'.[105] Neurodiversity activists argue for greater acceptance of neurological difference, that human brains exist along 'continuums of competence', and for an anthropological view of neurological 'competence' as culturally determined, all notions that were present in practical phrenology.[106] Significantly, as did the Fowlers' phrenology, the neurodiversity paradigm assumes a degree of neuroplasticity by which individuals might develop their brains through therapies, learned strategies, or assistive technologies. This is particularly the case when therapies are begun at an early age, and so children are central to the politics and therapeutics of both. And like the Fowlers, the neurodiversity movement both resists and employs science, in particular, by integrating the difficult issue of heredity/genetics into its paradigm while retaining space for individual development. Practical phrenologists such as the Fowlers found cultural and evolutionary value in certain innate but maligned traits, and neurodiversity activists use evolutionary arguments in support of their cause. For instance, Ari Ne'eman cites the warning of autism researcher, Simon Baron-Cohen, that testing for autism could 'repeat the history of eugenics' and 'inadvertently "cure" not just autism but the associated talents that are not in need of treatment'.[107]

Just as the Fowlers linked health to politics and social reform, the neurodiversity movement is closely allied with disability rights and other civil rights movements that see self-advocacy and representation as key to social justice. Their motto 'nothing about us, without us!' is not far from 'self-made or never made'.[108] However, unlike phrenologists, whose theories leant validity to racist and sexist taxonomies, neurodiversity activists have largely avoided the danger inherent in self-help strategies that ultimately place responsibility upon individuals to fit into a normative system. Cooter contends that Victorian phrenology 'mostly encouraged changing oneself to fit the system' rather than fuelling the social reform that Combes and the Fowlers sought.[109] And Julie Prebel observes that the 'digital body slices' produced by neural imaging technologies are analogous to the invasive taxonomic ordering of nineteenth-century phrenological sketches and photographs; both create 'epistemic changes in the scientific surveillance of the human body'.[110] In fact, most autism research and most parent-led autism awareness campaigns continue to emphasise cures and strategies whereby autistic people can adapt themselves to a neurotypical world. In contrast, the more radical and autistic-led neurodiversity movement asserts that our neurotypical-based culture itself needs to change. Neurodiversity activists, disseminating information on the internet, and working through parents and schools are becoming increasingly successful in their efforts to create accommodation for the neurodiverse and to make our culture more 'neurocosmopolitan'.[111]

Both the Fowlers' phrenology and the neuro-information campaigns demonstrate that pressure from the popular front – from parents, schools, and physicians – can push orthodox medical researchers to re-evaluate their assumptions and shift their paradigms. What seems possible to both scientists and the public is socially constructed in many respects. Just as phrenology opened the door for advances in brain science, neurodivergents are increasingly shaping scientific research both as activists and scientists around the lived experience of the patient.[112] Similarly, the predictive nature of diagnoses in phrenology

– 'you are X' and so will make an excellent 'Y' – often resulted in a fulfilled prophecy. Stern argues that Lorenzo Fowler's analysis of the young Walt Whitman's head in 1849 exerted 'a deep influence not only upon his character … but upon his work': 'Leading traits of character appear to be Friendship, Sympathy, Sublimity and Self-Esteem … and a certain reckless swing of animal will' wrote Fowler.[113] The American Civil War nurse, Clara Barton, recounted in her memoirs Lorenzo Fowler's predictive reading of her head when she was fifteen: 'She will never assert herself for herself –she will suffer wrong first – but for others she will be fearless.'[114] The extraordinary popularity of the Fowlers was surely enhanced by the self-fulfilling power of such optimistic readings, just as promises of neuroplasticity or an increasingly neurocosmopolitan society are reassuring to autistic people and their families in the present. In many cases, these promises will prove illusory or incomplete, but without medical cures or demonstrably effective medical therapies, they are preferable to extreme and dangerous therapies.

The Fowlers' negotiation of medicine and modernity was decidedly uneven. While not denying the diseases of modern life or the evolutionary correlation between progress and pathology, the Fowlers offered a medical paradigm and system of treatments that lessened the weight of modernity upon the individual. They triumphed in the modern arenas of market capitalism and information dissemination, advocating a radical individualism that promised greater agency in modern society through self-determination. At the same time, however, their phrenological theory reinforced neurological taxonomies of class, race, and gender that undergirded a white middle-class society. The Fowlers' medical eclecticism offers a path for postmodern consumers who can and do choose among a variety of orthodox and heterodox medical therapies – from acupuncture to chiropractic, herbalism to energy medicine – to pursue their 'healthean' goals. Their example also offers a warning not to ignore the socio-political implications of those choices and goals.

Notes

1 O. S. Fowler, *Self-Culture and the Perfection of Character* (New York: Fowler and Wells, 1853 [1847]), pp. iv–v.
2 R. M. Young, *Mind, Brain, and Adaptation in the Nineteenth Century* (London: Oxford University Press, 1970); J. D. Davies, *Phrenology Fad*

and *Science: A 19th-Century American Crusade* (New Haven, CT: Yale University Press, 1955); J. van Wyhe, *Phrenology and the Origins of Victorian Scientific Naturalism* (Aldershot: Ashgate, 2004).
3. R. Cooter, *The Cultural Meaning of Popular Science: Phrenology and the Organization of Consent in Nineteenth-Century Britain* (Cambridge: Cambridge University Press, 1984), 47.
4. *Ibid.*, 87.
5. S. Finger, *Minds Behind the Brain: A History of the Pioneers and their Discoveries* (New York: Oxford University Press, 2000), 132.
6. van Wyhe, *Phrenology*, 20.
7. C. Colbert, *A Measure of Perfection: Phrenology and the Fine Arts in America* (Chapel Hill: University of North Carolina Press, 1998), p. xiv.
8. Cooter, *Cultural Meaning*, 258.
9. *Ibid.*, 156.
10. *Ibid.*, 3.
11. S. K. Whitbourne, 'MRI's: the new phrenology?' *Psychology Today* (21 February 2011), https://psychologytoday.com/blog/fulfillment-any-age/201102/mris-the-new-phrenology?#. Accessed 30 January 2017.
12. A. Tobin, 'Brains of Those with Autism are Not Shaped Differently, Study Shows', *Times of Israel* (5 November 2014) www.timesofisrael.com/brains-of-those-with-autism-are-not-shaped-differently-study-shows/. Accessed 30 January 2017.
13. M. Cheng, 'Kids with ADHD have some brain regions that are smaller than normal, new study finds', *TIME Health* (15 February 2017) http://time.com/4670266/adhd-children-brains-study-normal/. Accessed 16 February 2017.
14. D. J. Siegel and T. Payne Bryson, *The Whole-Brain Child: Twelve Revolutionary Strategies to Nurture Your Child's Developing Mind* (New York: Bantam Books, 2011); J. Medina, *Brain Rules for Baby: How to Raise a Smart and Happy Child from Zero to Five* (Seattle, WA: Pear Press, 2014).
15. R. Cooter, 'Medicine and Modernity', *The Oxford Handbook of the History of Medicine*, ed. Mark Jackson (Oxford: Oxford University Press, 2013), 102–16.
16. Young, *Mind, Brain, and Adaptation*, 18.
17. *Ibid.*, 17.
18. Finger, *Minds Behind the Brain*, 130.
19. J. G. Spurzheim, *View of the Elementary Principles of Education* (1821), quoted in B. Jenkins, 'Phrenology, heredity and progress in George Combe's *Constitution of Man*', *British Journal for the History of Science*, 48:3 (September 2015), 460.
20. Cooter, *Cultural Meaning*, 101.
21. *Ibid.*, 102.

22 Finger, *Minds Behind the Brain*, 132.
23 G. Combe, *The Constitution of Man Considered in Relation to External Objects*, 6th edition (Edinburgh: Maclachlan and Stewart, 1851), 104.
24 Combe, *A System of Phrenology* (Boston: B. B. Mussey & Co., 1851), 555.
25 Combe, *The Constitution of Man*, 27; Jenkins, 'Phrenology', 461.
26 Combe, *A System of Phrenology*, 555.
27 Cooter, *Cultural Meaning*, 131.
28 Fowler, *Self-Culture*, title-page.
29 O. S. Fowler, 'The phrenological facts', *American Phrenological Journal* 5:1 (January 1843), 29–30.
30 M. Stern, *Heads and Headlines: The Phrenological Fowlers* (Norman: University of Oklahoma Press, 1971), 26.
31 Stern, *Heads and Headlines*, 112.
32 'Phrenology in England', Center for the History of Medicine (Harvard University, 2015). https://collections.countway.harvard.edu/onview/exhibits/show/talking-heads/phrenology-in-england. Accessed 13 July 2017.
33 Stern, *Heads and Headlines*, 55.
34 C. C. B. Seymour, *Self-Made Men* (New York: Harper and Brothers, 1858); I. G. Wyllie, *The Self-Made Man in America* (New York: Free Press, 1966); J. G. Cawelti, *Apostles of the Self-Made Man* (Chicago: University of Chicago Press, 1989).
35 J. Cullen, *The American Dream: A Short History of an Idea that Shaped a Nation* (Oxford: Oxford University Press, 2003), 73.
36 P. Gilbert, *The Citizen's Body: Desire, Health, and the Social in Victorian England* (Columbus: Ohio State University Press, 2007), 6.
37 J. Lears, *Rebirth of a Nation: The Making of Modern America, 1877–1920* (New York: Harper Collins, 2009), 6.
38 C. Russett, *Sexual Science: The Victorian Construction of Womanhood* (Cambridge, MA: Harvard University Press, 1989), 6.
39 *Ibid.*, 20.
40 W. Channing, *Self-Culture: An Address Introductory to the Franklin Lectures* (Boston: Dutton and Wentworth, 1838), 11.
41 'Farewell Entertainment to Mr and Mrs Fowler, and Presentation to Mrs Fowler', *Dundee Advertiser* (4 April 1863), quoted in Cooter, *Cultural Meaning*, 261.
42 Combe, *A System of Phrenology*, 555.
43 Fowler, *Education and Self-Improvement, Founded on Physiology and Phrenology*, 2nd edn (New York: O. S. & L. N. Fowler, 1844), 4.
44 M. Miles, 'Proselytizing for profit and consuming self-help: Fowlers and Wells phrenological and water-cure publications', *New York History*

Review (2016) http://nyhrarticles.blogspot.com/2016/08/proselytizing-for-profit-and-consuming.html. Accessed 2 November 2017.
45 Fowler, *Education and Self-Improvement*, 4. Emphasis in original.
46 Miles, 'Proselytizing for profit'.
47 S. Wells, *Phrenological Journal*, 49:1 (January 1869), 30, quoted in S. Ewen and E. Ewen, *Typecasting: On the Arts & Sciences of Human Inequality* (New York: Seven Stories Press, 2006), 33.
48 A. Sekula, 'The body and the archive', *October* 39 (Winter 1986), 3–64.
49 Fowler, *Education and Self-Improvement*, 126.
50 Ibid., 127. Emphasis in original.
51 Ibid., 116.
52 *Phrenological Almanac* (Glasgow), 2 (1843), 31–2, quoted in Davies, *Phrenology*, 63.
53 Fowler, *American Phrenological Journal*, 4 (1842), 270.
54 Cooter, 'Medicine and Modernity', 102–16.
55 R. Bivins, *Alternative Medicine? A History* (Oxford; New York: Oxford University Press, 2007), 35.
56 Durbach connects the nineteenth-century anti-vaccination movement to the protests surrounding the Contagious Diseases Acts in *Bodily Matters: The Anti-Vaccination Movement in England, 1853–1907* (Durham, NC/London: Duke University Press, 2007); see also Anne Summers, '"The constitution violated": the female body and the female subject in the campaigns of Josephine Butler', *History Workshop Journal*, 48 (1999), 1–15.
57 Bivins, *Alternative Medicine?*, 146.
58 Ibid., 179.
59 Ibid., 266.
60 Ibid.
61 S. Tomlinson, *Head Masters: Phrenology, Secular Education, and Nineteenth-Century Social Thought* (Tuscaloosa: University of Alabama Press, 2005), 99.
62 Stern, *Heads and Headlines*, 36, 37, 41–3.
63 Ibid., 125.
64 Ibid., 151.
65 F. Waite, 'Lydia Folger Fowler', *Annals of Medical History*, n.s. 4 (1932), 293.
66 Stern, *Heads and Headlines*, 156.
67 Ibid., 159.
68 Ibid., 159, 160.
69 Ibid., 160, 161.
70 Waite, 'Lydia Folger Fowler', 96; Stern, *Heads and Headlines*, 181.

71 'Lydia Folger Fowler' (obituary), *Englishwoman's Review of Social and Industrial Questions* (15 February 1879), 82–3.
72 E. Pohl Lovejoy's *Women Doctors of the World* (New York: Macmillan Company, 1957), 20.
73 Two exceptions to this claim are Waite, 'Lydia Folger Fowler', and Lovejoy, *Women Doctors*.
74 E. Fine, 'Women Physicians and Medical Sects in Nineteenth-Century Chicago', in E. S. More, E. Fee, and M. Parry (eds), *Women Physicians and the Cultures of Medicine* (Baltimore, MD: Johns Hopkins University Press, 2009), 266.
75 Lovejoy, *Women Doctors*, 20.
76 Fine, 'Women Physicians', 266.
77 Lovejoy, *Women Doctors*, 18.
78 R. Morantz-Sanchez, *Sympathy and Science: Women Physicians in American Medicine* (Oxford: Oxford University Press, 1985), 33; E. S. More, *Restoring the Balance: Women Physicians and the Profession of Medicine, 1850–1995* (Cambridge, MA: Harvard University Press, 1999), 19; C. Skinner, *Women Physicians and Professional Ethos in Nineteenth-Century America* (Carbondale, IL: Southern Illinois University Press, 2014), 80.
79 Stern, *Heads and Headlines*, 165.
80 'Wheaton Graduate Becomes Doctor', http://wheatoncollege.edu/college-history/1850s/wheaton-graduate-doctor/. Accessed 25 March 2017; Waite, 'Lydia Folger Fowler', 296.
81 L. Folger Fowler, *Familiar Lessons on Physiology and Phrenology: Designed for the Use of Children and Youth in Schools and Families* (New York: Fowler and Wells, 1847).
82 *Ibid.*, p. xiii.
83 *Ibid.*, p. xv.
84 Charles E. Rosenberg, 'Catechisms of health: the body in the prebellum classroom', *Bulletin of the History of Medicine*, 69 (Summer 1995), 175–97 (p. 181).
85 S. Shuttleworth, *The Mind of the Child: Child Development in Literature, Science, and Medicine, 1840–1900* (Oxford: Oxford University Press, 2010), 4.
86 Fowler, *Familiar Lessons*, 45.
87 *Ibid.*, 26.
88 *Ibid.*, 21.
89 Rosenberg, 'Catechisms', 181.
90 Fowler, *Familiar Lessons*, 53.
91 *Ibid.*, 23.

92 H. Asperger, '"Autistic Psychopathy" in Childhood', [1944] in Uta Frith (ed.), *Autism and Asperger Syndrome* (Cambridge: Cambridge University Press, 1991), 67.
93 *Ibid.*, 68.
94 H. Asperger, 'Die "Autischen Psychopathen" im Kindesalter', [1944], *Archiv für Psychiatrie und Nervenkrankheiten*, 117 (1994), 76–136. Asperger's reference to phrenology occurs in his preface which, as Edith Sheffer notes, was left out of Uta Frith's 1991 translation, and is therefore 'not known to an English-speaking audience' (E. Sheffer, *Asperger's Children: The Origins of Autism in Nazi Vienna* (New York/London: W. W. Norton & Company, 2018), 215). Sheffer argues that the omission of the preface 'softened the historical framework' of Asperger's work because it was there that he engaged explicitly with Nazi ideas and psychiatrists (242); the phrenological and physiognomical assumption he also references there, that one's character may be diagnosed by one's appearance, was, of course, also part of eugenic thinking in the Third Reich as well as in the nineteenth century.
95 Asperger, '"Autistic Psychopathy"', 89.
96 *Ibid.*, 68.
97 Sheffer, *Asperger's Children*.
98 *Ibid.*, 244.
99 Shuttleworth, *Mind of the Child*, 237.
100 L. Zenderland, *Measuring Minds: Henry Herbert Goddard and the Origins of American Intelligence Testing* (Cambridge: Cambridge University Press, 2001), 349.
101 C. Bittel, 'Woman, know thyself: producing and using phrenological knowledge in 19th-century America', *Centaurus*, 55 (2013), 104–30 (p. 106).
102 S. Baron-Cohen, 'Two new theories of autism: hyper-systemising and assortative mating', *Archives of Disease in Childhood*, 91 (2006), 2–5; B. Bettleheim, *The Empty Fortress: Infantile Autism and the Birth of the Self* (New York/London: Free Press, 1967); A. Wakefield, S. Murch, A. Anthony, et al., 'Ileal-lymphoid-nodular hyperplasia, non-specific colitis, and pervasive developmental disorder in children', *The Lancet*, 351 (1998), 637–41; P. Karimi, E. Kamali, et al., 'Environmental factors influencing the risk of autism', *Journal of Research in the Medical Sciences* 22:27 (February 16, 2017), doi 10.4103/1735-1995.200272.
103 O.S. Fowler, *The Octagon House: A Home for All* (New York: Dover Publications, 1973 [1848]).
104 Durbach, *Bodily Matters*, 204.

105 N. Walker, 'Throw Away the Master's Tools: Liberating Ourselves from the Pathology Paradigm', in J. Bascom (ed.), *Loud Hands: Autistic People, Speaking* (Washington: The Autistic Press, 2012), 231.
106 T. Armstrong, *The Power of Neurodiversity: Unleashing the Advantages of Your Differently Wired Brain* (Cambridge, MA: DeCapo Books, 2010), 11–12.
107 S. Baron-Cohen, 'Autism Test "Could Hit Maths Skills"', BBC News (7 January 2009), quoted in A. Ne'eman, 'The Future (and the Past) of Autism Advocacy, or why the ASA's Magazine, *The Advocate*, Wouldn't Publish This Piece', [2010] in Bascom (ed.), *Loud Hands*, 92.
108 Ne'eman, 'The Future', 88.
109 Cooter, *Cultural Meaning*, 268.
110 J. Prebel, 'Head bumps to brain scans: a visual rhetorical history of scientific surveillant looking', *Enculturation* (21 August 2015), http://enculturation.net/head-bumps-to-brain-scans. Accessed 30 January 2017.
111 R. Savarese, 'From neurodiversity to neurocosmopolitanism: beyond mere acceptance and inclusion', in A. Perry and C. Herrera (eds), *Ethics and Neurodiversity* (Newcastle upon Tyne: Cambridge Scholars Publishing, 2013), 191–205.
112 S. Silberman, *Neurotribes: The Legacy of Autism and the Future of Neurodiversity* (New York: Avery, 2015), 473.
113 Stern, *Heads and Headlines*, 102, 105.
114 M. S. Morse, 'Facing a bumpy history: the much-maligned theory of phrenology gets a tip of the hat from modern neuroscience', *The Smithsonian Magazine* (October 1997), www.smithsonianmag.com/history/facing-a-bumpy-history-144497373/. Accessed 28 March 2017.

II
Paradoxes of modern living

5

A disease-free world: the hygienic utopia in Jules Verne, Camille Flammarion, and William Morris

Manon Mathias

Modern Western societies have a complex relationship with hygiene. Since the publication of David Strachan's 1989 article, the 'hygiene hypothesis' has been taken up by both scientists and society at large as the basis for the idea that Western households are too clean.[1] Strachan's research has been further developed by immunologists such as Graham Rook, whose 'old friends' theory suggests that beneficial microbes have been eliminated through time, contributing towards today's inflammatory disorders.[2] Warnings of increasing antimicrobial resistance also seem to justify the belief that dirt is good for us.[3] But definitive answers to these questions are yet to be found, and the idea that 'somehow people should be less clean' is unhelpful, as shown by the high numbers of gastric ailments still caused every year by lack of handwashing.[4] The debate surrounding links between cleanliness, dirt, and health continues. This chapter intervenes in the debate by focusing on literary engagements with the topic and thereby challenges the narrative of a straightforward move from dirt to cleanliness by demonstrating a much more complex relationship between filth, hygiene, and modern selfhood.

Strachan's hygiene hypothesis seemed to undermine, indeed reverse, accepted wisdom regarding dirt and its nefarious qualities, which had been the broad consensus since germ theory was widely accepted. A connection between disease and filth, especially human waste, had, of course, been drawn by humans for centuries: Egyptian physicians, for instance, believed that disease was caused by the absorption of putrefying faeces,[5] and as asserted by Micaela Sullivan-Fowler, 'perhaps no other part of the body has played a longer or larger part in disease origin than the intestines and its most visible, odorous by-product, feces'.[6] Although human excrement had been valued for its positive qualities in certain periods, Western culture broadly witnessed a shift away from the valorisation of faecal matter from the 1500s.[7] Indeed, studies explicitly focused on excrement have mostly concentrated on early modern periods of English literature, when attitudes towards filth were strongly mediated by religious concerns and moral distinctions.[8] It was in the nineteenth century, however, that the fixation with dirt and its links with ill health came into prominence, as the growth of cities led to unprecedented levels of overcrowding and subsequent sanitary problems, particularly in relation to human waste.

Many explanations have been proposed for the increasing human revulsion towards excrement in modern Western society. Sociologist Paul Rozin has suggested that disgust is based on links with digestion, drawing on Darwin's position on disgust as a form of food rejection.[9] Others have posited a combination of biological and sociological factors. According to David Inglis, for instance, our attitudes towards excrement are based on both medico-scientific knowledge and moral factors.[10] Anthropologist Mary Douglas's classic study of dirt and hygiene also focuses on the social dimension, arguing that the phenomena considered as dirty are those which disrupt the moral or social order of society: 'dirt is essentially disorder'.[11] Such a line of thought plays an important role in the formulation of modern selfhood in the nineteenth century, and since the turn of the millennium, a wealth of reflection has emerged, particularly within Victorian studies, on the interconnected topics of dirt, filth, waste, and human response to these phenomena, disgust.[12]

Early nineteenth-century hygienist debates on the spread of disease targeted excrement particularly within working-class quarters, as has been noted by historians such as Christopher Hamlin and William Cohen.[13] The centrality of excrement within the broader development of modern societies, especially through attempts to control and excise the substance, is also outlined by Dominique Laporte and Alain Corbin, as well as by David Barnes in his study of the century's Great Stinks.[14] Studies highlight the last quarter of the nineteenth century, in particular, as a key moment for discussions of excrement and its links with disease,[15] as the realisation that disease spread through microbial transmission, especially human contact, intensified the fear of dirt and led to an increased obsession with cleanliness.[16]

The topic is all but absent within French studies, however, as far as the study of literature is concerned. Laporte's *Histoire de la merde* (1978), and to a lesser extent Corbin's *Le Miasme et la jonquille* (1986), are historical studies which do not focus on literary texts.[17] Scholarship on the complex nexus between dirt and hygiene and on their role in shaping modern selfhood is so far overwhelmingly historical in focus, and much of this scholarship traces a broad move from dirt to cleanliness, linked with the shift from primitivism to civilisation. This chapter, however, takes issue with the 'narrative of progress and deodorization' away from the dirty, malodorous body, and the unqualified benefits of such a development, through an investigation of specifically literary reflections on the consequences of dirt removal for human identity.[18]

This chapter analyses attitudes towards dirt and bodily waste in nineteenth-century British and French science fiction novels as a means of understanding perceptions of disease and hygiene in the early period of bacteriology. One of its aims is to consider what this tells us about the modern individual's relationship with the body, especially the ways in which the ambivalence of this relationship is distinctively explored through literary texts. To do this, I examine three utopian novels from the last decades of the century, when the emphasis on extreme cleanliness was at its height:[19] Jules Verne's *Cinq cents millions de la Bégum* (1880), Camille Flammarion's *Uranie* (1889), and William Morris's *News from Nowhere* (1890). Morris's novel is now widely recognised as an important contribution to English social and political thought, but has rarely been studied in relation to health and disease. The two French novels have also received little critical attention in relation to this topic, particularly Flammarion's *Uranie*, which has not been the focus of any sustained analysis. Through their visions of alternative societies, however, these three texts provide valuable insights into views on disease and hygiene in the 1880s and 1890s, the legacies of which continue to this day.

The decision to focus on French and British novels from this period is driven by the fact that the two largest cities in Europe, and its 'foremost urban and cultural centres' in the nineteenth century, were

London and Paris.[20] These two cities were regarded as the epicentres of modernity in the sense of a social and medico-scientific phenomenon involving the emergence of Western bourgeois identity and values. The chapter focuses on issues of 'hygiene', a term which comes from the French *hygiène* and is derived from the ancient Greek goddess of health, Hygeia. Hygiene became a shorthand term for the Greek natural science of preserving and extending life,[21] and the use of the word to refer to 'that department of knowledge or practice which relates to the maintenance of health'[22] continued into the nineteenth century. I use the term in this way when speaking of 'public hygiene', which was largely concerned with practices for preserving health. By the late nineteenth century, however, the triumphs of the sanitary reform movement made hygiene synonymous with 'cleanliness', and by the end of the century, hygiene held 'a considerably narrower meaning than [it] had held historically, reflective of the overriding significance cleanliness had acquired over the course of the nineteenth century'.[23] On the whole, this chapter uses the term 'hygiene' on its own in this narrower sense of purity or cleanliness, the meaning acquired by the end of the nineteenth century and still used today.

I will place the analysis in the context of new scientific understandings of bacteria that began to develop in the late nineteenth century. It was during this century that filth, and particularly human excrement, came to dominate discussions of health and disease: as waste removal became a major issue with the unprecedented growth of cities, diseases that were spread through contamination with excrement (such as typhus, typhoid fever, and cholera) became prevalent, and the volume of urban filth and efforts to remove it 'surpassed its previous dimensions'.[24] Within this context, France and Britain were leading nations in public hygiene, the founding of which has been noted by historians and sociologists as a significant factor in the emergence of modern Western societies.[25] The establishment of public hygiene as a distinct scientific discipline began in France in the 1820s with the formation of the first dedicated journal, the *Annales d'hygiène publique et de médecine légale*, in 1829, and the pioneering work of individuals calling themselves hygienists, especially Louis-René Villermé and Alexandre Parent-Duchâtelet.[26] In terms of practical public health measures, Britain soon took the lead, and by the second half of the century the British were largely regarded as the front runners in public health reform. On the level of theory and research, however, France continued to make major contributions to the field, and it was in France that the germ theory of disease was born in the last decades of the century with Pasteur's research on microorganisms.

Up until the second half of the nineteenth century the causes of infection remained in dispute,[27] and it was in the 1860s and 1870s that experimental work to link germs and diseases began to show marked signs of success.[28] The main contributions to the debate were made by Louis Pasteur and Robert Koch, who linked particular microorganisms to specific diseases. Up to this point, miasma theory had provided the predominant explanation of disease – the belief that disease developed through the spontaneous generation of harmful elements from putrefying matter – and a whole range of potential sources of disease had been identified, such as dampness, bad soil, and bad air.[29] Bacteriology, however, now posited that disease was the outcome of contagion by germs, specifically the transmission of germs through water-based means and through human contact.[30] The repugnance towards dirt was already present in miasma theory, with the fear towards bad smells emanating, in particular, from human excrement as a potential cause of disease. This fear now intensified into a more specific anxiety, since the seemingly clean could be harbouring a host of invisible microbes. Further, although the cause and nature of disease was now better understood, cures through antimicrobial drugs would not be discovered until the first half of the twentieth century, and thus the implications of early bacteriology on a practical level was a focus on prevention and a heightened preoccupation with cleanliness.[31]

One of the texts that most obviously exemplifies the obsession with hygiene in the late nineteenth century is Jules Verne's *Cinq cents millions de la Bégum* (1880). In this text, a French Napoleonic soldier settles in India and marries the widow (the begum) of a wealthy rajah. When he and the widow die, the fortune is divided between the two remaining heirs: Dr Sarrasin, a French hygienist, and Dr Schultz, professor of chemistry at Jena University. Both decide to use the money to set up their ideal city; the benevolent Sarrasin creates 'France-Ville', a society engineered to promote health and longevity in Oregon, USA, whereas the despotic Schultz forms Stahlstadt, a hierarchical city which produces firearms and aims to destroy or conquer all other communities. Those few critics who refer to Verne's novel highlight the contrast between the utopian France-Ville and the dystopian Stahlstadt and its 'evil scientist' creator.[32] Nadia Minerva has perceptively suggested that the portrayal of Stahlstadt is in fact more compelling than that of France-Ville.[33] Indeed, Verne himself wrote in a letter that he preferred Stahlstadt.[34] But this is precisely what makes France-Ville, an apparently ideal city of hygiene, such an arresting case.

Peter Schulman argues that docteur Sarrasin in *Bégum* is 'propelled by fear of microbial contamination' in his preoccupation with health and hygiene,[35] while historian Georges Vigarello refers to Verne's text as 'the first Utopia dominated by the war against the microbe'.[36] However, there are no references to microbes in *Bégum*, and neither Schulman nor Vigarello go any further in examining the medical context of the novel or in explaining what leads them to make these inferences. The term 'microbe' was first coined (in both French and English) when Verne was writing his novel, in 1878. *Bégum* refers instead to 'germs', a word that had long been used to denote the 'seed' of contagion.[37] Advocates of the new germ theory of disease in the 1870s adopted the term to refer to microscopic organisms capable of causing human or animal disease. The 'germ theory of disease' came into common use in medical literature around 1870 as a scientific shorthand for propositions associated with the work of Pasteur, Koch, Tyndall, and others.[38] *Bégum* does include a direct reference to Benjamin Richardson's *Hygeia*, an address delivered by the renowned public health activist in 1876. Richardson's understanding of disease was largely based on the earlier theory which posited that disease agents were chemical ferments produced by decaying filth, and could generate spontaneously.[39] Richardson's sanitarian ideal was based on the view that miasma emanating from filth, particularly from human excrement, caused disease. It would therefore seem that Verne's text draws on earlier, pre-bacteriological understandings of disease.

However, bacteriology and miasmatic theory initially existed in tandem until at least the beginning of the twentieth century, and in some senses the new science simply replaced the already existing emphasis on excrement in miasma theory.[40] The prominent French physician, Fonssagrives, for example, refers in his *La Maison. Étude d'hygiène et de bien-être* (1871), to 'putrid' or 'fetid' emanations and 'mephitis through putrid matter'[41] whilst also noting the work of Tyndall and the idea that 'many contagious illnesses or epidemics are due to the movement and dissemination of living germs'.[42] Initially, bacteriological theories were woven into earlier conceptions of filth, and strengthened and justified aspects of miasmatism.

We now know that when he was writing *Bégum*, Verne was reworking a manuscript by Paschal Grousset and it seems that it was Grousset who initially drew on Richardson. The manuscript by Grousset has not survived but we have Verne's letters outlining his response to the work, where he notes his intention of making quite considerable changes. Verne specialists, however, consider the novel as a thoroughly Vernian text[43] and it is known that Verne himself was exceptionally well read in contemporary science.[44] When writing the novel in the late 1870s he specifically showed strong respect for Pasteur, placing him alongside writer Victor Hugo as one of the greatest Frenchmen of the nineteenth century for his contributions to science.[45]

Verne was writing *Bégum* before Pasteur's theory was widely accepted and understood by the general public. Nevertheless, the new bacteriological view of disease was beginning to be introduced to both medical and popular audiences,[46] and Verne would certainly have been aware of the developments in the understanding of disease and the gradual adaptation of earlier sanitarian principles in the service of germ theory. The language used for hygiene and infection in *Bégum* presents a combination of miasma theory and the newer understanding of germs: carpets and wallpaper are referred to as 'veritable nests of miasma', and the government's main task is said to be 'cleaning, ceaseless cleaning, destroying and annihilating the miasma that constantly emanate from human agglomerations as soon as they are formed'.[47] But with regards to offensive materials such as carpets and wallpaper, 'not a single morbid *germ* can conceal itself' within them.[48] The laundrettes in the city feature 'disinfection rooms', and illnesses are said to be due to contagion transmitted either through air (adhering to earlier miasmatic theory) or through food – a more recent finding of bacteriology.[49] Rather than demonstrating a preoccupation with microbes, *Bégum* presents a transitioning moment between the earlier sanitarian model and the newer principles of bacteriology.

Moreover, in *Bégum*, Verne is less interested in disseminating new knowledge of disease and bacteriology than with exploring the implications of extreme hygiene for society. France-Ville, 'the city of Wellbeing',[50] is entirely devoted to hygiene: a journalist notes that 'we would never be done if we tried to enumerate the hygienic perfections which the founders of the new city have put into place,[51] and asserts that 'the question of individual and collective cleanliness is the central preoccupation of the founders of France-Ville.'[52] Its creator, Sarrasin, repeatedly highlights his desire to build a city 'based on rigorously scientific data'[53] in the name of Humanity and of Progress.[54] The city has no theft or murders, very few illnesses, and no epidemics. Whereas the annual mortality rate in affluent European cities is said to be at least 3%, in France-Ville the average is 1.5%.[55] All the inhabitants lead healthy, regular, hardworking lives in an egalitarian community run by a committee which rejects 'the tiring and insipid uniformity' of other cities.[56] *Bégum* thus seems to depict the perfect balance between public hygiene and individual freedom.

However, as Peter Schulman notes, France-Ville is 'somewhat frightful.'[57] The ambiguous nature of France-Ville is suggested through its unequal status in the text: only a very few pages are devoted exclusively to descriptions of France-Ville whereas Stahlstadt is the focus of several chapters. Further, the city of hygiene is presented indirectly: as a prospective project in Sarrasin's speech to the medical conference, in an article in a German review, and through other brief glimpses. Nadia Minerva suggests that this might be because 'perfection cannot be represented without falling into the stereotypes of a well-worn genre.'[58] But the refusal to offer direct descriptions of France-Ville might also be due to its problematic nature. Whereas the novel appears to offer a model city, the absence of dirt and disease entails the absence of passion, excitement, and independence of thought.

The regularity of the inhabitants' lifestyle or 'scientific regime' is repressive.[59] A set of ten rules, for example, is laid out for all households, including specific regulations for their construction: the walls will be made of 'tubular bricks conforming to the patented model,'[60] a model that is 'perfectly regular in form, weight and density, and pierced lengthways by a series of cylindrical and parallel holes.'[61] More specifically with regards to hygiene, certain materials are forbidden due to their threat to human health, and the streets and pavements are to be kept as clean as the tiles in a Dutch court: an extremely high standard.[62] Food markets are kept under strict surveillance by trained experts through 'sanitarian policing'[63] and the city is made up entirely of streets lined up 'at right angles, at equal distances, of uniform width, planted with trees and designated by ordering numbers.'[64] Dirt is immediately removed: a stain on a child's clothes, for example, is considered 'an absolute disgrace'.[65] All excrement is swiftly expelled from the city.[66]

The effect of this rigorous hygienic regime on the inhabitants is telling. The city has reached 'the highest degree of prosperity' in material and intellectual terms,[67] but when it comes to the citizens' psychological condition, it is the absence of emotion that is striking. During the peak crisis of the book, when the population is at risk of extermination, they remain perfectly composed, 'above all disorderly emotion of alarm or anger'.[68] They are steady, calm and silent, and, troublingly, 'in thrall'[69] to Sarrasin's words. The hygienic lifestyle leaves them incapable of experiencing strong emotions or of exhibiting independence of thought. Underneath the portrayal of this 'model city'[70] of health and well-being, then, is a covert criticism of extreme hygiene.

In this sense, *Bégum* can be read as an example of the 'utopian afterlife' as defined by Daniel Sipe. Scholars have argued that the yearning for utopia disappears from literature in France after the Enlightenment and is expressed instead through social experiments and technological projects.[71] Sipe, however, points to the 'utopian afterlife' as a literary form which both takes up and rejects aspects of the literary and scientific utopia.[72] J. J. Grandville's *Un autre monde* (1844), for example, which mockingly fictionalises Charles Fourier's utopian system, embarks on a utopian adventure whilst undertaking 'a critique of the manner in which utopian designers like Fourier intend to bring it about'.[73] *Bégum* draws on the literary tradition of utopian writing though its creation of a model city and the exploration of this space through a foreigner's gaze, that of a young Alsatian worker. It is also utopian in the socio-scientific sense in that its North American setting echoes the social experiments of Robert Owen or Étienne Cabet. However, whilst the novel does not offer the explicit critique that Grandville's text does, it rejects the utopian tradition by failing to demonstrate wider social happiness in France-Ville, by refusing to offer precise descriptions of the city, and through its distressing portrayal of a life 'regulated by science'.[74]

Camille Flammarion's *Uranie* (1889) goes one step further both in its setting and in its take on hygiene. Flammarion published several successful popular science books in the second half of the century, and he is perhaps best known for his defence of intelligent life on other planets. But Flammarion also wrote philosophical dialogues and fiction, and in *Uranie* he combines his interest in astronomical explanation with reflections on hygiene and the body. As one of the leading popularisers of science in the second half of the nineteenth century, Flammarion would have been familiar with the evolving understanding of disease. *Uranie* was written in the 1880s, by which point new understandings of infection were more widely disseminated beyond scientists and physicians.[75] It is important that the first disease convincingly linked to a specific microorganism (in a paper of 1876 by Koch) was anthrax, as this disease had hardy spores, which could survive even though the bacteria might have been killed. The resistant nature of anthrax had a particular effect on the preventative strategies developed against disease in the name of germ theory: it was widely believed that all pathogenic microorganisms were tenacious and needed to be addressed in aggressive terms, leading to a heightened emphasis on the removal of dirt.[76] Although filth had long been linked with disease and was central to miasmatic theory, the idea that everyday substances such as food, clothing, and even body parts might be teeming with pathogenic and highly resilient organisms, added a new urgency to the battle against dirt.

In the only commentary I have found on *Uranie*, Everett Bleiler criticises the work's lack of cohesion.[77] I would argue, however, that its three main sections are unified through a consistent attempt to transcend earthly reality. In the first section, for example, the narrator is taken on a journey to other planets inhabited by a range of creatures superior to human beings. On one planet he sees creatures that are translucent, androgynous, and blessed with superior intellectual and moral qualities. On another, he comes across individuals that have been reborn as superior beings through a process of 'transmigration'.[78] There is a yearning for the ideal in Section II also, as 'Uranie', a symbol for astronomy, is said to lead to infinity.[79] Throughout the text there is an attempt to move beyond material, earth-bound existence.

The most significant section from a hygienist standpoint is the final one, 'Ciel et Terre' (Earth and Sky), where the first-person narrator wakes up to find himself on Mars. Two aliens explain to him that life on Earth is 'a total failure'[80] due to humanity's reliance on the body. Tracing our planet's downfall to the moment when the first mollusc developed a stomach, the Martians criticise our practice of killing and consuming other creatures and explicitly identify 'the first digestive

A disease-free world

tube' as the cause of our baseness.[81] Human bodies are 'repugnant', 'base', and 'monstrous',[82] whereas the Martians nourish themselves simply through breathing and have never digested food: 'we do not eat, we have never eaten and we will never eat'.[83] They consider it impossible for human beings ('ignoble organisms') to have thoughts that are 'healthy, pure, elevated, ... clean'.[84] Cleanliness is thus identified as the basis for moral and intellectual superiority, achieved through detachment from the body. On Mars, for instance, there has never been religious intolerance, martyrs, torturers, war, or murder, and the Martians live in peace, liberated from all material needs and constantly engaged in intellectual activity.

Uranie combines fiction (utopia, fantasy, love story), popular astronomy, religion, and psychic research, fulfilling the generic diversity and multiplicity which Sipe insists characterises the utopian afterlife.[85] In its exploration of space, the text calls to mind the writings of Bergerac (*L'Autre monde: ou les états et empires de la lune*, 1657), Voltaire (*Micromégas*, 1752), and Verne (*De la terre à la lune*, 1865), and it draws on the tradition of literary utopianism by using the framework of a fictional account to consider an imagined world. Yet, like *Bégum*, *Uranie* also rejects the utopian tradition, as the novel offers little sense of any coherent form of society. Moreover, although the narrator is disappointed to find himself back on Earth and seems to idealise what he has seen on Mars, the portrayal of life on the other planet is ambiguous.

The Martians live an apparently ideal existence free from pain and all physical needs. The text repeatedly notes the immaterial nature of their existence: they live 'for the spirit and through the spirit' and 'material forces play only a secondary role' in their lives.[86] Bodily waste is not mentioned at all, presumably since, if the Martians do not eat, neither do they defecate. Excrement only appears in the earlier sections in the text. It is said, for example, that, without the awareness of the soul, the earth's entire history would be doomed to nothingness and become 'a disappointing absurdity, more miserable and more senseless than the excrement of an earthworm'.[87] A later tale involves the discovery of a corpse in a pile of manure. Excrement is thus posited as a worthless by-product or is associated with death.

Beyond the elimination of excrement from their lives, the Martians are also explicitly free from decay or disease: 'the heavy burdens of the earth and the suffering of pain are completely unknown. Everything [on

Mars] is more heavenly, more ethereal, more immaterial.'[88] But the release from the body comes at a price. The Martians' nervous systems are so advanced that they are compared with electrical appliances,[89] and their most sensual impressions are experienced 'more by the soul rather than by the body'.[90] They live without passion: their liberation from 'the crudeness of earthly needs'[91] means not only that they do not eat, but that they are also asexual. Conception takes place through a method similar to that of flowers. They feel no erotic pleasure, and all sensations are experienced on an intellectual level only. The novel presents a passionless existence.

Despite the constant denial of materiality in *Uranie*, however, the narrator does notice some physical activity being carried out on Mars by machines 'operated by perfected animal races, whose intelligence is similar to that of humans on earth'.[92] No more is said of the status or well-being of these creatures. Although they are referred to as animals, the comparison with human intelligence leads us as readers to make uncomfortable connections with them. This sinister reference to exploited entities in *Uranie* can be compared with the explicit subjugation of individuals in Verne's *Bégum*. Chinese workers are essential to the construction of France-Ville, for example, with 'an army of twenty thousand Chinese coolies' toiling under the direction of 'five hundred European supervisors and engineers'.[93] When the city is threatened by an attack from Schultz, it is these labourers who mobilise to protect it: 'armies of coolies moved the ground, dug trenches, raised ramparts and fortifications at all appropriate points'.[94] The list of verbs stresses the active contribution made by the workers. But, having supplied their labour, the 'coolies' are no longer welcome in the city: they can only access their earnings by promising not to return. This discriminatory policy is presented by the narrator as 'an indispensable precaution for getting rid of a yellow population, which would certainly have had an adverse effect on the character and genius of the new city'.[95] The workers are discarded to ensure the economic, ethnic, and intellectual stability of France-Ville. Hygiene is thus presented as a multilayered phenomenon in Verne's text, not only physical and mental, but also racial.

Laura Otis has shown that the germ theory of disease was crucially intertwined in the late nineteenth century with concepts of invasion and colonialism, especially in France and Britain: 'if one believes that

A disease-free world

invisible germs, spread by human contact, can make one sick, one becomes more and more anxious about penetration and about any connection with other people – the same anxieties inspired by imperialism'.[96] These comments are particularly pertinent to the context of *Bégum* and *Uranie*, written after France's bitter defeat in the Franco-Prussian war and at a point when France was acutely aware of its ailing position on the world stage, with falling birth rates, and a range of serious pathologies plaguing the nation.[97] Docteur Sarrasin in *Bégum*, for example, reads an article at the beginning of the novel, entitled 'Why are all Frenchmen suffering from varying degrees of hereditary degeneration?'[98] There is therefore a dark side to the relentless emphasis on health and strength in these texts which can be linked with France's contemporary desire for racial and national purity.

The portrayals of ideal hygienic societies in Verne and Flammarion and the unsettling consequences of dirt removal can be compared with William Morris's *News from Nowhere* (1890), a novel which Virginia Smith reads as 'a full account of [the] wonderful hygienic world to come'.[99] The new world in Morris's text is set in a fictional London of the future, removed of filth, and offering a vision of pastoral, ecological, and hygienic harmony. Society has been cleansed of literal dirt – industrial soot, grime, and urban squalor –and filthy lucre, crime, and disease are also absent. Morris's work focuses mainly on social organisation, and this is the main angle from which the text has been analysed by critics. Unlike Verne and Flammarion, who famously engaged with the new scientific developments of the day, Morris is primarily known for his contributions to socialist theory, aesthetics, and his ecological consciousness. There are no explicit references to germs or bacteria in the novel. Rather, it is on a more indirect level that the preoccupation with cleanliness and purity surfaces here.

There is a strong emphasis, for instance, on health, vigour, and longevity in Morris's text. The women that the narrator meets are 'well-knit of body, and thoroughly healthy-looking and strong' and he observes that beauty is now 'not so fleeting as it was in the days when we were burdened heavily by self-inflicted diseases'.[100] The fact that the diseases of earlier times were self-inflicted shows that they can be removed through effort of will. Indeed, almost all diseases have been eradicated from the new society, including the scourge which posed one of the greatest threats to nineteenth-century urban centres: cholera. The residents' youthfulness is highlighted in contrast with the nineteenth-century narrator's wizened appearance: he meets a lady who is forty-two, for example, but looks as though she were twenty.

In contrast with Flammarion's text and Verne's *Bégum*, Morris's *News from Nowhere* offers an apparently anxiety-free view of excrement. In Verne's and Flammarion's works, human waste is mentioned only to be denied. In *Bégum*, for example, the 'products of the sewers'[101] are immediately expelled and transported to the countryside, and in *Uranie*, the lack of digestion makes excrement non-existent; indeed, the Martians place strong emphasis on the digestive system as the epitome of human baseness. Although in *Bégum* human waste seems to be used as fertiliser, this is only briefly mentioned, whereas in *News from Nowhere*, England is said to be 'a garden where nothing is wasted' and dung is explicitly highlighted as a source of fertility.[102]

There is also a freedom and openness towards sexuality and the body in *News from Nowhere* that is absent in Verne's and Flammarion's novels. Morris's protagonist, William Guest, repeatedly responds to women on an erotic level, especially the central female figure, Ellen. Guest notices her scantily clad physique, for example, and comments on 'her face and hands and bare feet'.[103] His main interlocutor, Dick, also draws attention to women's physical attributes and the main object of these comments, Clara, responds by reddening with pleasure.[104] Morris's novel was in some ways a reaction against the highly regimented society presented in Edward Bellamy's *Looking Backward* (1888), and desire is a central and valorised force in *News from Nowhere*.[105]

The novel's emphasis on personal relations is not surprising given Morris's privileging of love and desire in his thinking about the socialist future.[106] The stronger utopian dimension of *News from Nowhere*, compared with the two French novels, might also be explained by the sense of disillusionment in France towards the possibility of social renewal following the failure of the 1848 Revolution.[107] Morris's less troubled approach to the body can further be situated in the context of developments in public health reform, which were in a much more advanced state in Britain by the 1880s. The linking of homes with sewers and the prohibition of cesspits, for example, had been achieved in London by the late 1840s whereas this did not happen in Paris until the early twentieth century. Britain passed its first Public Health Act in 1848, while France had to wait until 1902 for this to happen. Whatever the reasons, Morris's novel appears to offer one of the most viable visions of an alternative world, and the society in this text is often viewed as one of the most attractive literary utopias created.[108]

Yet the society in *News from Nowhere* continues to be haunted by the spectre of disease. Idleness and crime are pathologised, with the latter seen as a 'spasmodic disease' cured by society's many 'nurse[s] or doctor[s]'.[109] David Pike also argues that, even though Morris shows London as a purified space, 'not everything can be made useful and beautiful' in this novel, as 'the dust of the new city of London is symbolically disposed of in another filthy and irredeemable institution, the Houses of Parliament'.[110] Although the novel is offering political symbolism and not a hygienic blueprint, it is notable that whereas the value of manure is highlighted as a source of fruitfulness and fertility, there is no mention of what happens to the 'dust' placed in Westminster.

Moreover, in addition to the reference to Parliament as a dungheap, excrement is used in Morris's novel to refer back to nineteenth-century society as a place of dirt and depravity –'these people, whether they found the dung sweet or not, certainly lived in it' – and America is also described as 'a stinking dust-heap'.[111] In both examples, faeces are used to denigrate societies distanced from the speaker in space or time, exposing more unease towards bodily waste in Morris's text than at first seems apparent. Therefore, although both *Bégum* and *News from Nowhere* gesture towards a valorisation of excrement in the form of manure, at the same time, all three novels display a continuing level of anxiety towards the body and especially bodily waste.[112]

Some psychoanalytic theorists have argued that excrement disturbs us because it stands for a hostile residue of the past: Norman Brown, for example, argues that excrement represents the past in that it is 'the dead life of the body'.[113] Such interpretations of faeces as residues of the past are especially relevant to *News from Nowhere*, which engages so essentially with the question of time. Natalka Freeland has argued that the novel refuses the genealogical continuity and historical determination of realist narrative in favour of temporal 'rupture' which enables a new evaluation of waste as a bounteous resource to be reused.[114] A similar argument regarding the novel's release from conventional narrative is put forward by Patrick Parrinder, who asserts that the novel 'show[s] Morris subsuming and rejecting the tradition of Victorian fiction and historiography'.[115] Of more interest to this chapter is the link between the rejection of the past and the rejection of human waste.

Some thinkers suggest that the revulsion towards faeces as a remnant of the past is in fact a fear of death, as excrement highlights our bodily nature and reminds us of our own mortality. Such theories are put forward, for example, by Freud and more recent theoreticians of disgust, such as Paul Rozin.[116] But Colin McGinn points out that some forms of death, such as skeletons or frozen bodies, do not elicit the same degree of disgust as others. He therefore suggests that the greatest cause of disgust is in fact 'the interpenetration of life and death'.[117] The thinker who articulates this position most powerfully is Aurel Kolnai in his phenomenological study *On Disgust* (originally published in German in 1929). Kolnai argues that what causes disgust is the persistence of life in death: our inability to keep the two seemingly separate categories apart causes us distress, such as in a rotting corpse teeming with maggots.[118] This 'death-in-life theory' is clearly expressed in excrement: our digestive system is founded on death since it involves the consumption and excretion of other living things (animal, plants) and produces an inert object (faeces), but it is also this process that sustains life.[119]

In Morris's novel, the inhabitants notably know nothing of the past and are horrified by references to social history.[120] Clara, for example, refers with scorn to 'the dreadful times of the past' in contrast with 'our modern life', and feels a distinct unease towards the idea of 'talking of past miseries' – 'I don't like this: something or another troubles me'.[121] This refusal to confront the past suggests a deep psychological disturbance, and the erasure of history in this text can be linked with the novel's negative understanding of the dungheap. It is just at the point when old Hammond starts discussing the state of America as 'a stinking dust-heap', for instance, that Dick and Clara re-enter and Clara firmly breaks in with the retort: 'no more questions now before dinner'.[122] Shortly afterwards, Dick's comment on the stories of the past brings a cloud over her face.[123] Although *News from Nowhere* offers a more positive approach to the body than *Bégum* or *Uranie*, and even seems to valorise waste (with the 'dustman', for example, highly valued in society[124]), the denial of the past and use of excremental imagery to vilify others reveals underlying anxieties towards the body and its ephemerality.

Furthermore, an indirect upshot of our disgust towards life-in-death is a potential rejection of passion and desire. Psychoanalytic thinking is well known for connecting anal products with sexual pleasure,[125] but Freud also more broadly links disgust with the archaic libido.[126] Other thinkers have also developed an affirmative position on the disgusting as an erotic, energising force.[127] With specific reference to nineteenth-century France, for instance, historian Jonathan Strauss suggests that the fear of illness and dirt is, on a deep and dissimulated level, 'the attempt to manage a recurrent and unspeakable erotic desire'.[128] If hygienic concern regarding dirt and disease is permeated with a form of desire, then the suppression or elimination of dirt entails a rejection of this desire, as seen in Verne's and Flammarion's texts. France-Ville's inhabitants in Verne's *Bégum* show an alarming lack of emotion or passion, and Flammarion's *Uranie* demonstrates the passionless and sexless existence that results from extreme hygiene. Morris's novel, by contrast, is permeated by the erotic and seems to advocate the value of desire and sexuality.

There is little emotional depth to the characters in *News from Nowhere*, however; while the novel includes lengthy discussions on questions of political and social organisation, scant analysis is offered of the inhabitants' inner lives, undermining the sense that the emotional and libidinal dimensions of life are valorised in the community. Moreover, as argued by Norman Kelvin, by removing many of the legal and social constraints placed on love in the nineteenth century, Morris's society of Nowhere 'manages' the erotic and thus 'extinguishes' its power.[129] By ensuring that all inhabitants are healthy and attractive such that 'every Jack may have his Jill',[130] society makes fights over beautiful mates unnecessary. There is therefore a link between the management of desire in *News from Nowhere* and physical attractiveness, as the novel's focus on health, vigour, and longevity is a means of diminishing erotic desire's potentially dangerous and disruptive influence.

The attenuation of the erotic is also revealed in Guest's relationship with Ellen. In many analyses of desire in this novel there is a degree of slippage in the use of the term, as critics move from erotic desire to 'socialist desire' or 'utopian desire' – a much broader force, which might more accurately be defined as aspiration or ambition.[131] Such slippage is, however, faithful to the novel itself in that Guest's feelings for Ellen also shift into a tamer wish for solidarity and friendship. By the end, they become 'good friends' and Guest's erotic longings go unfulfilled.[132] He learns instead to appreciate Ellen's beauty as part of the wider attractiveness and happiness of the new society. This shift from the erotic and the personal to the social and the general is a further example of the way in which the society of Nowhere controls and neutralises the power of the erotic.

Like Verne and Flammarion, Morris creates a hygienic, disease-free society just at the moment when such a world was emerging as a possibility with the discovery of microbes as the cause of disease, and on one level, *News from Nowhere* does offer a 'glowing vision of an actualized utopia'.[133] At the same time, however, the novel reveals some of the more disturbing implications of moving away from dirt and the body.

Conclusion

This chapter has focused on utopian visions of alternative worlds as a way of considering the increasing attempts made in nineteenth-century society to overcome the dirty body. Such attempts are often regarded by scholars as central to the project of modernity. Helen Sullivan, for example, posits that 'the challenge of shaping dirt ... functions as a metaphor for the project of modernity'.[134] Scholars of history and sociology also point to increasing levels of disgust, and especially lowering tolerance of dirt and smell, as constitutive of the modern Western subject.[135] However, whilst the dissemination of germ theory from 1880s onwards certainly rendered fears of dirt and pollution particularly acute, a narrative of straightforward human advancement away from the lowly and animalistic towards an apparently sanitised, civilised Western society needs to be re-evaluated, as has been argued by Mark Jenner.[136] I would argue that looking at novels written in this period offers a starting point for this process.

As the texts examined here reveal, the outright rejection of dirt is problematic and at times paradoxical. Verne, Flammarion, and Morris all present positive images of a disease-free world and the benefits of a hygienic society. All three, however, also reveal the unintended consequences of extreme cleanliness and suggest that dirt cannot be straightforwardly removed. Bound up with the rejection of excrement, filth, and bodily processes is a rational rejection of disease, infirmity, and infection, but also an indirect rejection of passion, diversity, and desire.

Notes

1. D. P. Strachan, 'Hay fever, hygiene, and household size', *British Medical Journal*, 299 (1989), 1259–60.
2. G. A. W. Rook, '99th Dahlem Conference on infection, inflammation and chronic inflammatory disorders: Darwinian medicine and the "hygiene" or "old friends" hypothesis', *Clinical and Experimental Immunology*, 160 (2010), 70–9.
3. For example, M. Blaser, *Missing Microbes: How Killing Bacteria Creates Modern Plagues* (London: Oneworld, 2015).
4. L. Brookes, 'The hygiene hypothesis – redefine, rename, or just clean it up?', *Medscape*, 6 April 2015, www.medscape.com/viewarticle/842500. Accessed 9 August 2017.
5. T. S. Chen and P. S. Y. Chen, 'Intestinal autointoxication: a medical leitmotif', *Journal of Clinical Gastroenterology*, 11 (1989), 434–41 (pp. 434–6).
6. M. Sullivan-Fowler, 'Doubtful theories, drastic therapies: autointoxication and faddism in the late nineteenth and early twentieth centuries', *Journal of the History of Medicine and Allied Sciences*, 50 (July 1995), 364–90 (p. 364).
7. S. Signe Morrison, *Excrement in the Late Middle Ages* (New York: Palgrave Macmillan, 2008), 133.
8. For example, S. Greenblatt, 'Filthy rites', *Daedalus*, 111:3 (Summer 1982), 1–16. See also R. Ganim and J. Persels (eds), *Fecal Matters in Early Modern Literature and Art: Studies in Scatology* (Aldershot: Ashgate, 2004); W. Stockton, *Playing Dirty: Sexuality and Waste in Early Modern Comedy* (Minneapolis/London: University of Minnesota Press, 2011); P. J. Smith, *Between Two Stools: Scatology and its Representations in English Literature, Chaucer to Swift* (Manchester: Manchester University Press, 2012).
9. Rozin et al., 'Disgust', in L. Feldman Barrett, M. Lewis, and J. M. Haviland-Jones (eds), *Handbook of Emotions* (New York/London: Guildford Press, 2000), 637–53 (pp. 637–8).
10. D. Inglis, *A Sociological History of Excretory Experience* (Lewiston: Edwin Mellen Press, 2000), 18.
11. M. Douglas, *Purity and Danger* (Routledge: London, 1966), 2.
12. For example, S. Strasser, *Waste and Want: A Social History of Trash* (New York: Metropolitan Books, 1999); E. O'Connor, *Raw Material: Producing Pathology in Victorian Culture* (London/Durham, NC: Duke University

Press, 2000); W. Menninghaus, *Disgust: The Theory and History of a Strong Sensation*, trans. H. Eiland and J. Golb (New York: State University of New York Press, 2003); K. Forde (ed.), *Dirt: The Filthy Reality of Everyday Life* (London: Profile Books, 2011).

13 C. Hamlin, *Public Health and Social Justice*, 7–8; W. A. Cohen, 'Introduction: Locating Filth', in W. A. Cohen and R. Johnson (eds), *Filth: Dirt, Disgust, and Modern Life* (London: University of Minnesota Press, 2005), pp. vii–xxxvii (p. xviii).

14 D. S. Barnes, *The Great Stink of Paris and the Nineteenth-Century Struggle Against Filth and Germs* (Baltimore, MD: Johns Hopkins University Press, 2006).

15 For example, A. R. Aisenberg, who examines the prolonged debates surrounding the removal of human waste in Third Republic Paris. See *Contagion: Disease, Government, and the 'Social Question' in Nineteenth-Century France* (Stanford, CA: Stanford University Press, 1999), 105–112.

16 For example, N. Tomes, *The Gospel of Germs: Men, Women, and the Microbe in American Life* (Cambridge, MA: Harvard University Press, 1998), 62–3, 66–7.

17 Both texts have been translated into English: A. Corbin, *The Foul and the Fragrant: Odour and the Social Imagination* (London: Papermac, 1996); D. Laporte, *History of Shit* (Cambridge, MA: The MIT Press, 2002).

18 M. S. R. Jenner, 'Civilization and Deodorization? Smell in Early Modern English Culture', in P. Burke, B. Harrison, and P. Slack (eds), *Civil Histories: Essays Presented to Sir Keith Thomas* (Oxford: Oxford University Press, 2000), 127–44 (p. 129). Such a narrative is exemplified in Sigmund Freud's *Civilization and its Discontents* [1930], trans. J. Strachey (New York: Norton, 1961), 93–4; 97; 99 n. 1. Freud's linking of increasing cleanliness with the development of human civilisation has been highly influential. Corbin's *The Foul and the Fragrant*, for example, broadly conforms to this narrative.

19 G. Vigarello, *Concepts of Cleanliness: Changing Attitudes in France since the Middle Ages*, trans. J. Birrel (Cambridge: Cambridge University Press, 1988), 204.

20 Cohen, 'Introduction: Locating Filth', ix.

21 V. Smith, *Clean: A History of Personal Hygiene and Purity* (Oxford: Oxford University Press, 2007), 3.

22 *Oxford English Dictionary*, s.v. 'hygiene'. www.oed.com/view/Entry/90139?redirectedFrom=hygiene#eid. Accessed 15 August 2017.

23 J. C. Whorton, *Inner Hygiene: Constipation and the Pursuit of Health in Modern Society* (Oxford: Oxford University Press, 2000), 20.

24 Cohen, 'Introduction: Locating Filth', ix.

25 Corbin, *The Foul and the Fragrant*, 232; Inglis, *A Sociological History*, 11.
26 A. E. La Berge, *Mission and Method: The Early Nineteenth-Century French Public Health Movement* (Cambridge: Cambridge University Press, 1992), 99.
27 Hamlin, *Public Health*, 7.
28 N. Tomes, *The Gospel of Germs: Men, Women, and the Microbe in American Life* (Cambridge, MA: Harvard University Press, 1998), 28, 32.
29 Hamlin, *Public Health*, 110, 124, 126.
30 Inglis, *A Sociological History*, 213.
31 See R. Dubos, *Louis Pasteur: Free Lance of Science* (New York: DaCapo, 1960), 270; Tomes, *The Gospel of Germs*, 6.
32 A. B. Evans, *Jules Verne Rediscovered: Didacticism and the Scientific Novel* (New York: Greenwood Press, 1988), 83. See also N. Minerva, *Jules Verne aux confins de l'utopie* (Paris: L'Harmattan, 2001), 95; Christian Chelebourg, *Jules Verne. L'Oeil et le ventre* (Paris: Minard, 1999), 22.
33 Minerva, *Jules Verne aux confins de l'utopie*, 105.
34 Letter, 8 September 1878 (Olivier Dumas et al. (eds), *Correspondance inédite de Jules Verne et de Pierre-Jules Hetzel*, 3 vols (Geneva: Slatkine, 1999–2003), vol. 2 (2001), 294–5).
35 P. Schulman, 'Jules Verne's *Very* Far West: America as testing ground in *Les 500 millions de la Bégum*', *Dalhousie French Studies*, 76 (Autumn 2006), 63–71 (p. 63).
36 Vigarello, *Concepts of Cleanliness*, 208.
37 D. S. Barnes, *The Great Stink*, 45; L. Murard and P. Zylberman (eds), *L'Hygiène dans la république: la santé publique en France, ou l'utopie contrariée (1870–1918)* (Paris: Fayard, 1996), 98.
38 Tomes, *The Gospel of Germs*, 33.
39 *Ibid.*, 27.
40 Barnes, for example, refers to a 'sanitary-bacteriological synthesis' (*The Great Stink*, 2). See also Murard and Zylberman, *L'Hygiène dans la république*, 89 and B. Latour, *The Pasteurization of France* (Cambridge: Cambridge University Press, 1988), 22.
41 J.-B. Fonssagrives, *La Maison. Étude d'hygiène et de bien-être* (Montpellier: de Gras, 1871), 174, 186, 187: 'les émanations putrides', 'les émanations fétides', 'le méphitisme par les matières putrides'.
42 *Ibid.*, 191: 'des germes animés qui existent dans l'atmosphère'; 'beaucoup de maladies contagieuses ou épidémiques [sont] dues au transporte et à la dissémination de germes vivants'.
43 Y. Chevrel, 'Questions de méthodes et d'idéologies chez Verne et Zola. *Les Cinq cents millions de la Bégum* et *Travail*', in F. Raymond (ed.), *Jules*

Verne 2. *L'Ecriture vernienne* (Paris: Lettres Modernes, 1978), vol. 2, 69–96 (p. 73); Chelebourg, *Jules Verne*, 23.

44 Verne regularly read publications which reported on scientific discoveries such as *La Science illustrée, Le magasin pittoresque, Tour du monde*. See T. Unwin, *Jules Verne: Journeys in Writing* (Liverpool: Liverpool University Press, 2005), 56.

45 K. Allott, *Jules Verne* (London: Cresset Press, 1940), 145.

46 Barnes, *The Great Stink*, 24.

47 Verne, *Les Cinq cents millions de la Bégum* (Lyon: Editions Drôles de, 2013), 151, 153, 201: 'véritables nids à miasmes', 'nettoyer, nettoyer sans cesse, détruire et annuler aussitôt qu'ils sont formés les miasmes qui émanent constamment d'une agglomération humaine, telle est l'œuvre principale du gouvernement central'.

48 *Ibid.*, 151: 'Pas un germe morbide ne peut s'y mettre en embuscade'. Emphasis added.

49 *Ibid.*, 154, 156: '[les] blanchisseries ... [sont] pourvues de ... chambres désinfectantes'; 'neuf dixièmes des maladies sont dues à la contagion transmise par l'air ou les aliments'.

50 *Ibid.*, 39: 'la Cité du Bien-Être'.

51 *Ibid.*, 155: 'on ne finirait pas si l'on voulait énumérer tous les perfectionnements hygiéniques que les fondateurs de la ville nouvelle ont inaugurés'.

52 *Ibid.*, 153: 'La question de la propreté individuelle et collective est ... la préoccupation capitale des fondateurs de France-Ville'.

53 *Ibid.*, 37: 'une cité modelé sur des données rigoureusement scientifiques'. See also pp. 14, 35, 53.

54 *Ibid.*, 35: 'ce n'est pas à moi que ce capital appartient de droit, c'est à l'Humanité, c'est au Progrès!'.

55 *Ibid.*, 158.

56 *Ibid.*, 150: 'Le comité ... était plutôt l'adversaire de cette uniformité fatigante et insipide'.

57 Schulman, 'Jules Verne's *Very* Far West', 67. Schulman does not expand on this comment and focuses instead on Verne's criticism of American domination through capitalist exploitation.

58 Minerva, *Jules Verne aux confins de l'utopie*, 104.

59 Verne, *Bégum*, 158: 'un régime aussi scientifique'.

60 *Ibid.*, 150: 'les murs seront faits de briques tubulaires brevetées, conformes au modèle'.

61 *Ibid.*, 149: 'les maisons seraient faites ... de briques légères, parfaitement régulières de forme, de poids et de densité, transpercés dans le sens de leur longueur d'une série de trous cylindriques et parallèles'.

62 *Ibid.*, 151, 154.

63 *Ibid.*, 154: 'cette police sanitaire'.

64 *Ibid.*, 152: 'Les rues, croisées à angles droits, sont tracées à distances égales, de largeur uniformes, plantées d'arbres et désignées par des numéros d'ordre'.
65 *Ibid.*, 152: 'un déshonneur véritable'.
66 *Ibid.*, 154.
67 *Ibid.*, 65: 'France-Ville avait atteint le plus haut degré de prospérité, non seulement matérielle, mais intellectuelle'.
68 *Ibid.*, 173: 'chacun [était] au-dessus de toute émotion désordonnée d'alarme ou de colère'.
69 *Ibid.*, 173: 'subjugué'.
70 *Ibid.*, 144: 'cité modèle'.
71 See, for example, K. M. Roemer, 'Paradise Transformed: Varieties of Nineteenth-Century Utopias', in G. Claeys (ed.), *The Cambridge Companion to Utopian Literature* (Cambridge: Cambridge University Press, 2010), 79–106 (p. 79).
72 D. Sipe, *Text, Image, and the Problem with Perfection in Nineteenth-Century France: Utopia and its Afterlives* (Burlington, VT: Ashgate, 2013), 4.
73 *Ibid.*, 5.
74 Verne, *Bégum*, 131: 'une vie réglée selon la science'.
75 See Barnes, *The Great Stink*, 188.
76 Tomes, *The Gospel of Germs*, 37.
77 E. F. Bleiler, *Science Fiction: The Early Years* (Kent, OH: Kent State University Press, 1990), 248.
78 Camille Flammarion, *Uranie* (Paris: Librairie Spirite Francophone, 2011), 30.
79 *Ibid.*, 109: 'nous fait vivre dans l'infini'.
80 *Ibid.*, 175: 'votre planète est absolument manquée'.
81 *Ibid.*, 175–6: 'le premier tube digestif'.
82 *Ibid.*, 176, 178: '[des] corps grossiers et repoussants'; 'des monstres grossiers'.
83 *Ibid.*, 176: 'on ne mange pas, on n'a jamais mangé, on ne mangera jamais'.
84 *Ibid.*, 176: 'des organismes aussi grossiers'; 'des idées saines, pures, élevées, ... des idées propres'.
85 Sipe, *Text, Image*, 12.
86 Flammarion, *Uranie*, 180, 187: 'les habitants ne vivent que par l'esprit et pour l'esprit'; 'la force matérielle ne joue qu'un rôle secondaire'.
87 *Ibid.*, 92: 'une absurdité décevante, plus misérable et plus idiote que l'excrément d'un ver de terre'.
88 *Ibid.*, 192: 'On n'y connaît point les lourdes fardeaux terrestres ni les déchirements de la douleur. Tout y est plus aérien, plus éthéré, plus immatériel'.
89 *Ibid.*, 180: 'chacun de ces êtres ... semble un appareil électrique'.

90 *Ibid.*, 180: 'leurs impressions les plus sensuelles [sont] ressenties bien plus par leurs âmes que par leurs corps'.
91 *Ibid.*, 189: 'la grossièreté des besoins terrestres'.
92 *Ibid.*, 180: 'Tous les travaux matériels sont accomplis par des machines et dirigés par quelques races animales perfectionnées, dont l'intelligence est à peu près du même ordre que celle des humains de la Terre'.
93 Verne, *Bégum*, 146: 'une armée de vingt mille coolies chinois, sous la direction de cinq cents contremaîtres européens, était à l'œuvre'.
94 *Ibid.*, 187: 'des essaims de coolies remuaient la terre, creusaient des fosses, élevaient des retranchements et des redoutes sur tous les points favorables'.
95 *Ibid.*, 147: 'une précaution indispensable pour se débarrasser d'une population jaune, qui n'aurait pas manqué de modifier d'une manières assez fâcheuse le type et le génie de la cité nouvelle'.
96 L. Otis, *Membranes: Metaphors of Invasion in Nineteenth-Century Literature, Science, and Politics* (Baltimore, MD/London: Johns Hopkins University Press, 1999), 5.
97 See R. Nye, *Crime, Madness and Politics in Modern France: The Medical Concept of National Decline* (Princeton, NJ: Princeton University Press, 1984), 330.
98 Verne, *Bégum*, 41: 'Pourquoi tous les Français sont-ils atteints à des degrés différents de dégénérescence héréditaire?'.
99 Smith, *Clean*, 5.
100 W. Morris, *News from Nowhere* (Oxford: Oxford University Press, 2009), 13, 50.
101 Verne, *Bégum*, 154: 'les produits des égouts'.
102 Morris, *News*, 62, 65.
103 *Ibid.*, 128
104 *Ibid.*, 118.
105 N. Kelvin, 'The Erotic in *News from Nowhere* and *The Well at the World's End*', in C. Silver and J. R. Dunlap (eds), *Studies in the Late Romances of William Morris* (New York: William Morris Society, 1976), 97–114; J. Marsh, 'Concerning Love: *News from Nowhere* and Gender', in S. Coleman and P. O'Sullivan (eds), *William Morris & News from Nowhere: A Vision for our Time* (Bideford: Green Books, 1990), 107–27.
106 *Ibid.*
107 Sipe, *Text, Image*, 18.
108 Bleiler, *Science Fiction*, 524.
109 Morris, *News*, 72.
110 D. Pike, *Subterranean Cities: The World beneath Paris and London, 1800–1945* (Ithaca, NY: Cornell University Press, 2005), 204.

111 Morris, *News*, 85.
112 The recycling of excrement was popular in the mid-nineteenth century in both Britain and France. See, for example, N. Goddard, 'Nineteenth-century recycling: the Victorians and the agricultural utilisation of sewage', *History Today*, 31 (June 1981), 32–6; D. Simmons, 'Waste not, want not: excrement and economy in nineteenth-century France', *Representations*, 96 (Autumn 2006), 73–98. For an analysis of excremental recycling within the French novel, see Manon Mathias, 'Recycling excrement in Flaubert and Zola', *Forum for Modern Language Studies* (2017).
113 N. Brown, *Life against Death: The Psychoanalytic Meaning of History* (Middletown, CT: Wesleyan University Press, 1985), 295. See also J. Strauss, *Human Remains: Medicine, Death and Desire in Nineteenth-Century Paris* (New York: Fordham University Press, 2012), 151.
114 N. Freeland, 'The Dustbins of History: Waste Management in Late-Victorian Utopias', in Cohen and Johnson (eds), *Filth*, 225–49 (p. 231).
115 P. Parrinder, '*News from Nowhere*, *The Time Machine*, and the break-up of classical realism', *Science Fiction Studies*, 3:3 (November 1976), 265–74 (p. 269).
116 See Brown, *Life against Death*, 294–5; Rozin, 'Disgust', 642.
117 C. McGinn, *The Meaning of Disgust* (Oxford: Oxford University Press, 2011), 90.
118 A. Kolnai, *On Disgust* (Chicago: Open Court, 2004).
119 McGinn, *Meaning of Disgust*, 102.
120 Morris, *News*, 26, 47.
121 *Ibid.*, 88, 87–8, 117.
122 *Ibid.*, 85, 86.
123 *Ibid.*, 87.
124 *Ibid.*, 18.
125 S. Freud, 'Character and Anal Erotism' [1908], in A. Richards (ed.), *On Sexuality: Three Essays on the Theory of Sexuality and Other Works* (London: Penguin, 1977), 205–15.
126 Menninghaus, *Disgust*, 400.
127 G. Bataille, *Visions of Excess: Selected Writings, 1927–1939*, trans. Allan Stoekl (Minnesota: University of Minnesota Press, 1985), 77; M. Bakhtin, *Rabelais and his World* (Cambridge, MA: MIT Press, 1968), 147–9.
128 Strauss, *Human Remains*, 14.
129 Kelvin, 'The Erotic in *News from Nowhere*', 103, 99.
130 Morris, *News*, 31.
131 Marsh, 'Concerning Love', 124–5. See also Krishan Kumar, '*News from Nowhere*: the renewal of utopia', *History of Political Thought*, 14 (1993), 133–43 (p. 134).

132 Morris, *News*, 166, 170.
133 C. Hampton, 'The Feast's Beginning: *News from Nowhere* and the Utopian Tradition', in Coleman and O'Sullivan (eds), *William Morris & News from Nowhere*, 43–55 (p. 44).
134 H. I. Sullivan, 'Dirt theory and material ecocriticism', *Interdisciplinary Studies in Literature and Environment*, 19:3 (Summer 2012), 515–31 (p. 526).
135 Inglis, *A Sociological History*, 239, 290; D. Reid, *Paris Sewers and Sewermen: Realities and Representations* (Cambridge, MA: Harvard University Press, 1991), 2; D. Laporte, *History of Shit*, 119.
136 M. S. R. Jenner, 'Civilization and Deodorization', 136–8.

6

'Drooping with the century': fatigue and the *fin de siècle*[1]

Steffan Blayney

In the prologue to his 1892 short story, *Number Twenty*, the English satirist Henry Duff Traill personifies the nineteenth century as an exhausted, dying old man. Opening at 11.30 p.m. on 31 December 1900, Traill's story finds Old Seekleham – an ungainly pun on the Latin *saeculum* (century) – with just half an hour to live. Far from mourning his impending death, however, Seekleham greets it with a weary resignation, even relief: 'It was not that he had attained to a greater age than his ancestors, who, in fact, had all been centenarians like himself; it was that his life, as measured by exciting and consequently fatiguing experiences, had already far exceeded most of theirs.'[2]

From the violent wars and conflicts of his youth, through a middle age spent in energetic trade and travel, to yet further achievements in old age as a scientist and inventor, Seekleham's life is one that has been uniquely enervating. At the same time however – for all of its frenzied activity – it has also been singularly unsatisfying. While industry and empire have opened up the globe to an extent unknown to his ancestors, he feels more alone in the world than ever. For all of its promise, modern science has revealed 'almost everything except what he most wanted to discover.'[3] All the effort that Seekleham has spent on his own progress, has only advanced him closer to oblivion. With less than half an hour of his life remaining, he is left reclining limply on a couch, disillusioned, dissatisfied, and above all, exhausted.

As he reaches his final minutes, Seekleham is joined at his bedside by a choir of 'Decadents', who sing 'in praise of exhaustion, and disillusion, and failure, and emptiness, and weariness'. Individual singers explore themes of 'decay' and 'decline', with another reciting a 'sombre poem' on the subject of exhaustion. Finally, as the clock strikes midnight, they all join in an 'Ode to the Spirit of Decadence'.[4] Before the performance ends, however, Seekleham has already succumbed to his fatigue, disappearing to make way for the newborn Twentieth Century.

Traill, who fittingly died himself in 1900, was not alone in associating the end of the nineteenth century with exhaustion. Medical writers, as the physician Clifford Allbutt observed in 1895, were likewise concerned that the British population was 'drooping with the century'.[5] The final decades of the century saw a proliferation of attempts to define, describe, measure, and control physical and mental fatigue, a category that had been practically absent from medical or scientific discourse before the late 1860s. At the same time, the question of the conservation of bodily energies was discussed by commentators across disciplinary boundaries (including, not only physicians, but physicists, philosophers, and political economists), as one of the key problems of the modern age. By the close of the century, contemporaries were certain that they lived in an 'age of fatigue', with medical professionals concerned that their era would be remembered by posterity as 'the Tired Age'.[6]

Late nineteenth-century discourse on fatigue expressed a variety of concerns about modernity and its limits, and about social, political, and cultural decline. It did so in a language that drew on a range of scientific and cultural tropes. Crucially, this discourse relied on a new scientific understanding of the material world and of the body, grounded in the concepts of 'energy' and 'work'. As Anson Rabinbach has shown, this new paradigm, inaugurated by the 'discovery' of the laws of thermodynamics, exerted a pervasive influence across Europe in the second half of the nineteenth century.[7] At its centre was the metaphor of the 'human motor': the notion that the body operated in the same way as a thermodynamic engine, converting nature's 'energies' into productive 'work'. In this context, older moral proscriptions against sloth and idleness were superseded by materialist concerns about the limits of bodily efficiency. Fatigue – understood as the body's inbuilt resistance to continued productivity – emerged as 'the endemic disorder of industrial society', coming to embody a vast range of anxieties about social, economic, political, and cultural decline.[8]

While Rabinbach's account, focusing primarily on Continental Europe, barely mentions developments in Britain, for a number of British scientific writers and cultural commentators in the second half of the nineteenth century, energy and fatigue were central preoccupations. Particularly after 1870 – with Britain's dominant global status increasingly threatened by the rise of international competitors such as Germany and the United States – bodily exhaustion became a focus for a wide range of anxieties about economic and political decline, cultural stagnation, and the challenges of industrial civilisation. Fatigue took its place alongside those other richly overdetermined *fin-de-siècle* signifiers – decline, degeneration, and decadence – with which historians of late nineteenth-century Britain are familiar.

Fin-de-siècle discourse was characterised by a powerful homology between the biological and the social. Repeatedly, physical and mental exhaustion were characterised as symptoms of a much broader national deterioration. Across a range of texts, metaphors of fatigue were mobilised to signify political decline, social regression, and cultural deterioration. In an influential article of 1871, the historian James Froude painted a picture of an England overcome by 'lethargy', the political and racial 'vigor' of its people teetering on the brink of 'exhaustion'.[9] By the end of the century, in the words of Conservative politician Joseph Chamberlain, Britain had become a 'Weary Titan', overburdened by its vast colonial possessions and struggling to match the energy and dynamism of its international rivals.[10] In British cultural life the critic John Addington Symonds diagnosed a pervasive 'world-fatigue [which has] penetrated deep into our spirit'.[11]

Medical writers were likewise concerned that modern civilisation was taking its toll on the physical and mental constitution of the British population. The 'working powers of the community at large', it was argued, were undergoing depletion as a result of the vast and rapid social and technological changes that had characterised the nineteenth century.[12] The spread of industrialisation, urbanisation, education, and new technologies such as the railway and the telegraph had increased the pace and intensity of modern life to such a degree that the body was unable to muster the energy to withstand its constant pressures and demands.

While it is possible to emphasise the pessimistic overtones of these writers, the status of fatigue in medical discourse – and its relationship to modernity in particular – was always ambiguous. While the spectre of exhaustion produced anxieties about the detrimental consequences of civilisation, the limits to progress, and the inevitability of degeneration, scientific investigation of the body's energies at the same time held out the hope of revitalised and reinvigorated bodies, increased productivity, and social efficiency.[13]

Notions of energy and fatigue were shaped at the intersection of various nineteenth-century discourses, from physics and chemistry, to biology and medicine, to philosophy and literature. This chapter does not seek to identify direct lines of influence from a putatively discrete sphere of 'science' or 'medicine' to one of 'culture'. Instead, it examines the ways in which ideas from a variety of discursive arenas were adopted, modified, and reincorporated in a continual and reciprocal process. A number of historians and researchers in the medical humanities have drawn attention to the 'rich and complex interplay' between various scientific and cultural 'languages and systems of representation' operating in the late nineteenth century.[14] The *fin-de-siècle* preoccupation with fatigue is here treated in these terms: not simply as the consequence of certain scientific ideas or empirical findings, nor as an isolated cultural phenomenon, but as the result of a complex exchange of ideas, images, and concepts.

Energy, work, and waste

In broad terms, the two faces of the *fin-de-siècle* discourse on fatigue can be mapped onto the first and second laws of thermodynamics, which, in turn, formed the basis of a new scientific understanding of the human body in the second half of the nineteenth century. The first law – originally theorised by Hermann von Helmholtz in 1847 and variously developed and elaborated by a number of physicists from the mid-nineteenth century onwards – asserted that all of the different physical forces observable in the universe were in fact manifestations of a single and universal 'force' (or later 'energy'). This energy could be neither created nor destroyed, but was capable of infinite interconversion into its different forms. Most importantly, as the example of the steam engine showed, nature's energies could be converted – through the intercession of human agency – into useful mechanical work.

The 'law of the conservation of energy', as an article in the *British Medical Journal* asserted in 1870, was of 'immense importance in its bearing on the subject of physiology'. It was now possible to understand the 'vital energy' of animals and human beings to be 'merely a form of physical energy, and convertible with it'.[15] Furthermore, from the principle of the conservation of energy it followed that 'the total quantity of work of which a healthy man was capable ... [was] constant, no matter in what description of labour he was employed'.[16] The human body could now be seen – like the productive machines of the Victorian factory – as simply another arena for the conversion of an abstract and universal labour-power into useful 'work'. Increasingly, medical textbooks envisioned the human body as a 'physical machine': an 'engine furnace ... convert[ing] energy into work'.[17]

However, the reassuring picture of a constant supply of universal energy ripe for conversion into useful 'work' offered by the first law of thermodynamics was almost immediately undercut by the arrival of the second. As William Thomson explained in 1851, in any transfer of energy from a warm body to a cold one, only a small fraction of the heat generated could actually be harnessed for useful 'work', with 'the remainder being irrecoverably lost to man'.[18] In 1865, the German physicist Rudolf Clausius coined the term 'entropy' to describe the result of this irreversible loss of energy which accompanied any real-life process of energy conversion. Followed to its conclusion, the second law implied 'a universal tendency to the dissipation of mechanical energy': the universe was gradually tending towards an equilibrium at which point human life, let alone useful work, would, 'within a finite amount of time', be impossible.[19] In the *fin-de-siècle* imagination, the image of a universe slowly, but inexorably, running out of energy both reinforced and further fuelled contemporary notions of decline and cultural pessimism. If the principle of the conservation of energy opened a space for utopian dreams of a society engineered so as to best exploit the infinite productive potentials of nature, the notion of entropy brought shadows of 'deterioration, decay, and dissolution'.[20]

The upshot of the second law was that 'all work implies waste', and that 'the work of life' was no exception.[21] From the very beginning, discussion of 'energy' in British medical and scientific discourse was characterised by a preoccupation with its dissipation. Rather than being a boundless productive resource, 'the energy of a human body' was 'a definite and not inexhaustible quantity'.[22] It was in this context that fatigue – the body's inbuilt 'resistance to effort', or 'to the conversion of latent energy into active motion' – emerged as a distinct phenomenon and object of concern.[23] If degeneration, in the words of Stephen G. Brush, was the 'cultural counterpart of the second law of thermodynamics', then fatigue appeared as its bodily expression.[24]

In the mid-1870s, the question of 'overwork' became a locus for medical negotiations of energy and fatigue, and of the relationships between the body and modernity. An 1874 article in the *Contemporary Review* argued that the late nineteenth century was characterised by 'life at high pressure', with the 'severity of exertion' and 'incessant strain' demanded by modern industrial and commercial life leaving large numbers 'shattered, paralysed, reduced to premature inaction or senility'.[25] From 1875, a series of articles and letters in the *Lancet* and the *Journal of Mental Science* debated the extent to which 'society at large is really suffering from an amount of work, physical and mental, which is injurious to the individual, and therefore to the human race'.[26] Doctors mobilised the language of the physical sciences to argue that the natural 'energies' and 'nervous power' of patients were being depleted through overuse.[27]

While fatigue had rarely before been considered a medical issue, now it was increasingly associated with pain, disease, or even death. For the esteemed surgeon, Sir James Paget, writing in 1871, fatigue had 'a larger share in the promotion or permission of disease than any other single causal condition you can name'.[28] By 1875, the physician George Poore was able to elevate fatigue from a mere predisposing factor in illness to a medical condition in its own right, which he further subdivided into its 'general' and 'local', 'acute' and 'chronic' forms.[29] Increasingly, distinctions were drawn between normal and pathological states of fatigue, or 'between fatigue and over-fatigue'.[30] By the early twentieth century the 'pathology of fatigue' was also supplemented by a proliferation of related conditions, from 'fatigue dyspepsia' to 'exhaustion psychosis'.[31]

The particular discursive configuration of pathological exhaustion with which historians of medicine and *fin-de-siècle* culture are most familiar is neurasthenia. Introduced into the medical vocabulary by the American physician George Miller Beard in 1869, the diagnosis gained widespread currency internationally from the late 1870s.[32] Translated by Beard as 'nervous exhaustion', neurasthenia referred to a syndrome consisting of a wide range of symptoms, but defined most prominently and consistently by chronic fatigue. Characterised as a specifically modern (and for Beard, specifically American) disorder, neurasthenia is arguably the archetypal 'disease of modernity'. While the diagnosis was never as popular in Britain as elsewhere (notably in the United States, France, and Germany), a steady flow of publications on the subject began to emerge from the 1880s onwards, and neurasthenia, often in combination with earlier concepts of 'nervous exhaustion', became an increasingly common framework for interpreting the problems of life at high pressure.

Like fatigue from overwork, neurasthenia was interpreted as a special case of the second law of thermodynamics. Its explanation in terms of the dissipation of 'nervous energy' was ubiquitous. 'It is a general principle in physics that energy in performing work is expended and finally exhausted', wrote Thomas Stretch Dowse, one of the first British physicians to adopt the diagnosis. For Dowse, biologists and physicians could 'account for the exhaustion of nervous energy in very much the same way as the physicist'.[33] Neurasthenia was a pathology of energy conservation. In the healthy individual, fatigue was the 'natural consequence of some accomplished muscular or mental work', after which 'the store of our latent forces' could be 'readily and easily replenished'. For the neurasthenic, however, 'fatigue means that such a demand has been made upon the already inefficient reserve forces that they cannot be well repaired, and nervous exhaustion is thus increased'.[34] Or, as another expert on neurasthenia put it, 'instead of fatigue the result is exhaustion'.[35] While a certain amount of fatigue was the natural consequence of normal work, continued overexertion put body and mind at risk of severe, or even permanent, debility. Behind every discussion of fatigue lay the dark entropic spectre of 'total collapse' or 'irrecoverable degeneration'.[36]

Tiredness and civilisation

While some discussions of pathological exhaustion emphasised the dangers of pushing the body beyond its physiological limits, for other writers, the idea of fatigue as a naturally set limit on working capacity seemed to provide the key to a healthy accommodation between the body and modern civilisation. As the frenetic pace of late Victorian society placed increasing demands on bodies and minds it was argued, fatigue acted as a kind of biological safety mechanism, alerting the subject to the dangers of overexertion, and preventing any permanent damage to the body's tissues. Fatigue was a 'warning illness', ignored at one's peril.[37] The authority of nature was placed in opposition to the pressures of modernity: in contrast to a 'primitive life' in which humans lived in harmony with nature and with their bodies, the demands of modern life were 'opposed to all biological laws'.[38] It was the task of the physician 'to see that Nature is not thwarted'.[39]

Similar appeals to nature – and further claims of fatigue's beneficial qualities – can be found in medical and physiological discussions of the body's inbuilt 'rhythms', which were supposed to govern both voluntary movements and automatic biological functions. Like the idea of a single motive force behind the material universe, the unifying concept of natural rhythms had a pre-existing philosophical pedigree. For the philosopher Herbert Spencer, writing in 1862, rhythm was a law of nature: 'a necessary characteristic of all motion' uniting phenomena as diverse as the movement of the tides and the vibrations of a violin string.[40] Though perhaps nowhere, Spencer speculated, were 'the illustrations of rhythm so numerous and so manifest as among the phenomena of life'.[41] The beating of the heart, the rhythms of digestion, and the breathing cycle were all undeniable evidence of the body's innate periodicities.

For medical writers in the second half of the nineteenth century, the concept of rhythm was key to understanding how the body conserved its energies. Periods of action, in which work was done, alternated with periods of rest, when the body's energies could be restored. 'Every living structure', as one author claimed, 'passes through alternating conditions of repose and activity: when active, the tissue is consumed; when at rest, the tissue is nourished, and the waste repaired'.[42] Rest, it followed, was not truly inaction, but an active process of 're-creation'.[43] In this context, fatigue was seen to play a crucial role in regulating the body's rhythms of work and rest. In a state of nature, the physical and mental sensations of weariness had the protective function of compelling rest at regular intervals and so preventing the body's rhythms from becoming dangerously syncopated.

Here again, the problem of fatigue was understood less as the inevitable consequence of modern progress than as a failure of adaptation. Biological and social rhythms had fallen out of step. The natural synchronisation of human beings with their environment had been disrupted. The unnatural rhythms of economic and industrial life, of motors and machines, had not been designed with the natural tempos of body or society in mind, and fatigue was the price paid by bodies – both biological and social. As George Poore explained in his article on the subject, 'Fatigue occurs directly we attempt to alter the rhythm of our vital vibrations by prolonging the periods of tension at the expense of the periods of relaxation, or by demanding for any length of time a quickening of the normal rate of vibration.'[44]

For the physician Joseph Mortimer Granville, neurasthenia likewise consisted 'in the disturbance of the rhythm of the vibration of the nerve elements', caused, for example, by the body's exposure to the artificial and mechanically driven rhythms of a railway carriage.[45] Such malign rhythms, Granville and others proposed, could be corrected via the application of electronic vibrating instruments, specially designed – it was claimed – to 'control and rectify the disorderly vibrations'.[46] Thus the fatigue wrought on modern bodies as a result of technological changes could be palliated or prevented through technological means, reconfiguring the challenges of modernity as solutions.

Similarly, while modern civilisation was often placed in opposition to a supposedly 'natural' order governed by the rhythms of the body, at other times biological comparisons functioned to naturalise the rhythms of modernity. The metaphors used to describe energy and fatigue commonly aligned the body either with the technologies of industrial machinery (for example, the 'human motor'), or with the economic logic of the market. Susan Sontag is one of a number of theorists to observe that nineteenth-century anxieties about the waste of energy often 'echo[ed] the attitudes of early capitalist accumulation. One has a limited amount of energy, which must be properly spent ... Energy, like savings, can be depleted, can run out or be used up, through reckless expenditure.'[47]

For health to be maintained and exhaustion avoided, *fin-de-siècle* doctors argued, the 'economy of the body' needed to be properly balanced.[48] If the 'daily out-goings' of 'bodily expenditure' exceeded the 'body-income ... paid in daily from the food we eat', the inevitable result would be 'the exhaustion of the body-capital' and 'physiological bankruptcy'.[49] As Chandak Sengoopta has observed, neurasthenia, in particular, was often presented as a pathology of economic efficiency, striking down 'the most productive section of society in the most productive years of their life'.[50]

Anson Rabinbach attributes an intensified focus on 'the wasteful expenditure of energy' in 1870s Britain to concerns about rising costs of labour, and the accompanying recognition that 'the costs of reproducing labour power could be turned into profit' through the development of a lucrative working-class consumer market.[51] However – in contrast to much of the early discourse on fatigue in Continental Europe – the object of medical concern in Britain in the late nineteenth century was not, at least at first, the industrial working class. In almost every article on the subject, overwork, fatigue, and neurasthenia were problems said, for the most part, to affect 'the official, the professional, the commercial, and the literary classes'.[52] It was not the manual worker, but 'the eminent lawyer, the physician in full practice, the minister, and the politician who aspires to be a minister ... the literary workman, or the eager man of science' who were the archetypal subjects of fatigue.[53] In general, concerns about overwork focused on the 'excessive mental labour' that many saw as being increasingly demanded of a swelling class of so-called 'brain workers'.[54] As one article on neurasthenia categorially put it, 'it is not among the working classes that we meet with examples of nerve exhaustion'.[55]

For these writers, neurasthenic and fatigued patients were less the discontents of modern civilisation than they were its agents. While pathological fatigue was associated with weakness and degeneration, it was, at the same time, an affliction of success. If it could be called upon to explain Britain's decline, it could also be used as evidence of its social and cultural pre-eminence and imperial dominance; in a word, its modernity. 'The more advanced a nation becomes', wrote one physician, 'the more prevalent have nervous diseases been amongst its people'.[56] The tendency to exhaustion, wrote another, was 'characteristic of high states of civilisation'.[57]

Late Victorian doctors were thus faced with an uncomfortable paradox. Fatigue represented the failure of the human body to meet the demands of modern life, and yet, at the same time, its increasing incidence was the best possible evidence of a society's modernity.[58] An epidemic of pathological exhaustion, if alarming, at least proved that the British nation – and particularly its 'strenuous' middle classes – stood at the forefront of human progress.[59] The problem that preoccupied medical and scientific writers, therefore, was to reconcile immutable constraints on the powers of the body with continuing social and economic progress. Did fatigue represent the impassable boundary of modernity, or an obstacle which it was possible to overcome?

Re-energised bodies

As Catherine Oakley has argued, while scholarship on the Victorian *fin de siècle* has often stressed fears surrounding 'the dissipation or curtailment of human capacity', less attention has been paid to 'the ways in which these anxieties about biological, moral and racial decline were counterbalanced by a more optimistic interest in the physical potential of the human body'. While the spectres of physical and social degeneration provoked anxiety, Oakley argues, they also offered a rationale for new 'interventionist strategies of corporeal "*re*generation"', which aimed to recuperate, augment, or maximise bodily energy.[60] If concerns about overwork, exhaustion, and neurasthenia were frequently implicated in pessimistic narratives at the end of the nineteenth century, medical and physiological writing on human energy was, at the same time, often characterised by an optimistic – or even utopian – confidence that fatigue and inefficiency could be conquered. Through the discovery of the scientific 'laws' of human effort, it was argued, fatigue, the body's inbuilt resistance to work, could be understood, controlled, or even eliminated.

In his essay on 'metaphors of human biology', the medical historian Owsei Temkin argued that the elaboration of mechanical models of human physiology allowed the development of 'a more active attitude toward the body' than was previously possible. Whereas older notions of the body as a divine creation 'imagined the human organism to be so perfectly constructed that an improvement was not even thinkable', the idea of the body as a machine or motor implied that improvements were both possible and desirable.[61] While mechanical models of animal and human physiology had been articulated since at least the seventeenth century, the development of thermodynamics from the middle of the nineteenth century – for a number of thinkers – effectively closed the gap between animate and inanimate mechanisms. For dogmatic materialists, such as the biologist Thomas Huxley, 'the idea that the physical processes of life are capable of being explained in the same way as other physical phenomena' was no less than 'the expressed or implied fundamental proposition of the whole doctrine of scientific Physiology'.[62] The concept of 'Life' itself, the chemist H. A. Huntley went so far as to suggest, should, 'scientifically speaking', be referred to under the term 'Thermo Dynamical Phenomena'.[63] For those who insisted on the 'physical doctrine of life', the 'human motor' was more than just a metaphor: the human body was, in its essential properties, *no different* from any other heat engine, motor, or industrial machine converting energy (or 'force') into useful work.[64] Increasingly, physiologists and physicians viewed themselves as engineers, tasked with maintaining and increasing the efficiency of the body, optimising its potentials and expanding its capacity to convert energy into work.

In this context, fatigue – the body's inbuilt resistance to continued effort – was viewed less as an absolute barrier to the expansion of the body's productive powers, than a contingent and surmountable inefficiency. '[T]he power, and hence the usefulness, of the machine we call the human body is limited by two shortcomings prominent among others', the physiologist Michael Foster proclaimed in 1893: 'by the inertia, the sluggishness which makes it so hard to set agoing, and the readiness with which it wearies, so that its work is stopped before its task is done'. For Foster, the scientific study of fatigue would indicate how both the individual, and society as a whole, might 'extend [the] limits' of working capacity and productivity.[65] While fatigue might be the 'inevitable' consequence of work, others argued, the 'suitable management' of the body would make it possible 'to secure the maximum efficiency for the human machine'.[66]

As concerns mounted about the dissipation of the nation's energetic resources towards the end of the nineteenth century, scientific research into the physiology of fatigue gained social significance. As Richard Gillespie has argued, the problem of fatigue enabled physiology, as a distinct branch of medical science and as a profession, to forge itself a 'social role' in the application of laboratory research to questions of supposedly national importance: systematic knowledge of the body's mechanisms, physiologists argued, could provide the key to industrial and social efficiency.[67] This was a period which saw the creation of Britain's first professional association for physiologists, the Physiological Society, in 1876, and the early issues of the society's journal carried numerous articles on the origins and nature of the body's energies, the biochemical mechanisms of fatigue, the optimal rhythms of muscular contractions, the effects of different foods and drugs on bodily efficiency, and different means to measure the extent of fatigue.

In the last decades of the nineteenth century, social, industrial, and economic problems were increasingly framed in terms of the efficient deployment of human energy. Through scientific research into the 'maximum efficiency' of the body, the economist William Stanley Jevons argued in 1870, 'definiteness might possibly be given by degrees to some of the principles and laws which form the basis of our science of political economy'.[68] Physiological research into the 'laws of fatigue' focused increasingly on the rate and quantity of 'useful work' which the human body was capable of giving out.[69]

For psychology, too, questions of fatigue and efficiency provided a means by which researchers could assert the practical utility of their methods. In the rush of late nineteenth-century industrial modernity, psychologists argued, mental fatigue was becoming an increasingly important problem, and its objective measurement was seen as an essential step in combating its effects. For William McDougall – a key figure in the development of a new, self-consciously scientific psychology at the turn of the twentieth century – 'the general speeding up of life' was 'the most striking characteristic of modern civilisation', and was 'rendering the study of the problems of fatigue a matter of the most urgent practical importance'. The study of fatigue, McDougall argued, 'must always be of the deepest interest from the point of view of pure science, because in studying fatigue we are studying the source of human energies, the modes and conditions of their operations, and, above all, their limitations'.[70]

For McDougall, psychological fatigue had nothing to do with the subjective feelings of the individual, but was an entirely *objective* phenomenon measurable in terms of declining capacity for work. While acknowledging that of 'all the manifestations of fatigue the most familiar are the *subjective*', McDougall maintained that feelings of tiredness bore no direct relation to the capacity of the body or mind for exertion.[71] As his close associate and former tutor W. H. R. Rivers put it, in 1908:

> In the performance of mental work especially, decided sensations of fatigue may be experienced when the objective record shows that

increasing and not decreasing amounts of work are being done; and there may be complete absence of any sensations of fatigue when the objective record shows that the work is falling off in quantity, or in quality, or in both.[72]

In order to measure 'objective' fatigue, the subjective elements of tiredness had to be ruthlessly dispensed with. Instead of seeking to understand the psychology of fatigue from the internal perspective of the individual, mental fatigue was externalised and objectified. It could be measured without reference to any feelings of tiredness, purely in terms of the amount of 'work' which a subject was able to produce. In the psychology of McDougall and Rivers, the brain, as well as the body, became just another site of the transformation of potential energy into useful, productive work.

If the image of the body-machine paved the way to a more interventionist attitude towards the physiological engineering of the individual, its combination with social Darwinism and eugenics at the end of the nineteenth century introduced the prospect of improving the efficiency of the race *en masse*. While Geoffrey Searle long ago associated the eugenics movement in Britain with the 'quest for national efficiency', ideas of energy and human productivity have been underexamined in histories of eugenic discourse.[73] In Francis Galton's project of racial regeneration, the category of 'energy' was central. In the work in which he introduced the term 'eugenics', in 1883, Galton proclaimed that energy – 'the capacity for labour' – was 'an attribute of the higher races'. 'In any scheme of eugenics', he argued, 'energy is *the most important quality* to favour'.[74] While some human beings were born with 'large powers of endurance', others were naturally 'quickly fatigued'.[75] Particularly, under 'the strain and exhausting calls of modern civilised life', Galton argued, the need for a 'measure of fatigue' was essential to ensuring the progressive evolution of a re-energised human race.[76]

Conclusion: fatigue and the *fin de siècle*

In their introduction to *fin-de-siècle* culture, written at the turn of the twenty-first century, Sally Ledger and Roger Luckhurst stress the ambivalence of end-of-the-century thinking. Too great an emphasis on degeneration in accounts of the Victorian *fin de siècle*, they argue, risks 'forgetting a host of other voices that contested visions of collapse with dreams of regeneration.'[77] Likewise, any history of fatigue and its scientists at the end of the nineteenth and beginning of the twentieth century needs to accommodate both deep anxieties about the dissipation of the body's powers *and* optimistic projects for the restoration and expansion of human energies.

In Oscar Wilde's *The Picture of Dorian Gray* – perhaps the text (and author) most readily associated with the *fin de siècle* and its paradoxes – the phrase itself is immediately associated with exhaustion:

> '*Fin de siècle*,' murmured Lord Henry.
>
> '*Fin du globe*,' answered his hostess.
>
> 'I wish it were *fin du globe*,' said Dorian, with a sigh. 'Life is a great disappointment.'
>
> 'Ah, my dear,' cried Lady Narborough, putting on her gloves, 'don't tell me that you have exhausted Life. When a man says that one knows that Life has exhausted him.'[78]

Like Old Seekleham in Traill's *Number Twenty*, Dorian finds fatigue to be the inevitable consequence of modern life. In both cases, however, decline is only one side of the story. If Dorian fantasises about the end of the world, he is at the same time hopelessly enchanted with the idea of his own rejuvenation; degeneration and regeneration are two sides of the same coin. Likewise, in Traill's story, the moment of death is coextensive with that of rebirth: in the same instant that Seekleham succumbs to his accumulated exhaustion, the infant Twentieth Century is born.

In *fin-de-siècle* Britain, fantasies of fatigue spawned visions of efficiency. Far from resigning themselves to the march of entropy, or relapsing into a gloomy therapeutic pessimism, a significant number of doctors, scientists, and social thinkers expressed – implicitly or explicitly – the confident conviction that, if fatigue could not be eliminated altogether, the accumulation of scientific knowledge of the body's energies would create the potential for an unparalleled increase in the efficiency and productivity of bodies both biological and social. In the first decades of the twentieth century – as concerns mounted about the physical deterioration of the working population – these convictions would form the basis of a new scientific approach to industrial work. Fatigue research turned its attention explicitly to the working class, with the British government and employers sponsoring large-scale scientific investigations into factories and workplaces aimed at the optimisation of the working body, and the physiological and psychological rationalisation of work.[79] If fatigue had seemed to some late nineteenth-century observers to be a pathology caused by modern life, for others, as Rabinbach has argued, the science of fatigue itself became 'part of a broader strategy of social modernity', in which social problems would be overcome through technical knowledge, empirical investigation, and scientific and industrial progress.[80]

Notes

1 This research was funded by a Wellcome Trust Medical Humanities doctoral grant. Thanks are due to my PhD supervisor Joanna Bourke, whose advice and guidance on this project have been invaluable, and to Violeta Ruiz and Cat Oakley, whose comments on drafts of this chapter improved it immeasurably. Any errors of fact or judgement which remain are, of course, my own.
2 H. D. Traill, *Number Twenty: Fables and Fantasies* (London: Henry & Co., 1892), 1.
3 *Ibid.*, 2.
4 *Ibid.*, 11–12.
5 T. Clifford Allbutt, 'Nervous diseases and modern life', *Contemporary Review*, 67 (February 1895), 210.
6 M. Caird, 'The evolution of compassion', *Westminster Review*, 145 (1896), 643; 'A physician', 'Fatigue', *Quiver*, 429 (1908), 1012.
7 A. Rabinbach, *The Human Motor: Energy, Fatigue, and the Origins of Modernity* (New York: Basic Books, 1990).
8 *Ibid.*, 2.
9 J. A. Froude, 'England's war', *Fraser's Magazine*, 3 (February 1871), 135, 144.
10 J. Chamberlain (1902), quoted in J. Amery, *The Life of Joseph Chamberlain* (London: Macmillan & Co., 1951), vol. 4, p. 421.
11 J. A. Symonds, 'A comparison of Elizabethan with Victorian poetry', *Fortnightly Review*, 45 (January 1889), 60.
12 S. Wilks, 'On overwork', *Lancet*, 105 (26 June 1875), 886.
13 For further reading on scientific and cultural reflections on the possibilities for revitalising the human body in this time period, see 'Knocking Some Sense Into Them: Overpressure Debates and the Education of Mind and

Body', in A. Bonea, M. Dickson, S. Shuttleworth, and J. Wallis, *Anxious Times* (Pittsburgh, PA: University of Pittsburgh Press, 2019).
14 M. S. Micale, 'Two Cultures Revisited: The Case of the Fin de Siècle', in R. Bivins and J. V. Pickstone (eds), *Medicine, Madness and Social History: Essays in Honour of Roy Porter* (Basingstoke: Palgrave Macmillan, 2007), 210–23 (pp. 211–12); R. B. Yeazell, 'Introduction', in R. B. Yeazell (ed.), *Sex, Politics, and Science in the Nineteenth-Century Novel* (Baltimore, MD: Johns Hopkins University Press, 1986), p. vii.
15 D. Ferrier, 'Introductory lecture on life and vital energy considered in relation to physiology and medicine', *British Medical Journal*, 2:512 (22 October 1870), 430.
16 S. Haughton, *On the Natural Constants of the Healthy Urine of Man, and a Theory of Work Founded Thereon* (Dublin: Trinity College Dublin Press, 1860), 1.
17 E. H. Starling, *Elements of Human Physiology* (London: J. & A. Churchill, 1892), 3.
18 W. Thomson, *Mathematical and Physical Papers* (Cambridge: Cambridge University Press, 1882), vol. 1, pp. 188–9.
19 Thomson, *Mathematical and Physical Papers*, 511–14; W. Thomson, 'On the age of the sun's heat', *Macmillan's Magazine*, 5 (1862), 388–9.
20 S. G. Brush, *The Temperature of History: Phases of Science and Culture in the Nineteenth Century* (New York: Burt Franklin & Co., 1978), 14.
21 T. H. Huxley, 'On the physical basis of life', *Fortnightly Review*, 5 (February 1869), 136–7.
22 H. Maudsley, 'Sex in mind and in education', *Fortnightly Review*, 15 (April 1874), 67.
23 T. H. Huxley, *Lessons in Elementary Physiology* (London: Macmillan & Co., 1866), 194; H. B. Jones, *Croonian Lectures on Matter and Force* (London: John Churchill & Sons, 1868), 76.
24 Brush, *Temperature of History*, 14.
25 W. R. Greg, 'Life at high pressure', *Contemporary Review*, 25 (December 1874), 623–38 (pp. 629–30).
26 S. Wilks, 'On overwork', *Lancet*, 105 (26 June 1875), 886–7.
27 F. G. Stanley-Wilde, *Sleeplessness: Its Treatment by Homoeopathy, Hydropathy, and Other Accessory Means* (London: E. Gould & Son, 1879), 1–2.
28 J. Paget, 'Notes for a clinical lecture on dissection poisons', *Lancet*, 97 (3 June 1871), 736.
29 G. V. Poore, 'On fatigue', *Lancet*, 106 (31 July 1875), 163–4.
30 J. Adams, 'Mental fatigue', *The Practical Teacher*, 22 (April 1902), 503.
31 A. Haig, *Diet and Food* (London: J. & A. Churchill, 1898), 26–40; G. Rankin, 'Fatigue dyspepsia', *British Medical Journal*, 1:2842 (19 June 1915),

1033–6; W. H. B. Stoddart, 'A theory of the toxic and exhaustion psychoses', *Journal of Mental Science*, 56:234 (July 1910), 418–22.
32 G. M. Beard, 'Neurasthenia, or nervous exhaustion', *The Boston Medical and Surgical Journal*, 80:13 (29 April 1869), 217–21; M. Gijswijt-Hofstra and R. Porter (eds), *Cultures of Neurasthenia from Beard to the First World War* (Amsterdam: Rodopi, 2001).
33 T. S. Dowse, *On Brain and Nerve Exhaustion* (London: Baillière, Tindall and Cox, 1880), 5–7.
34 *Ibid.*, 66–7.
35 D. de Berdt Hovell, *On Some Conditions of Neurasthenia* (London: J. & A. Churchill, 1886), 14.
36 R. Farquharson, 'On overwork', *Lancet*, 107 (1 January 1876), 10; J. Mortimer Granville, *Nerve-Vibration and Excitation as Agents in the Treatment of Functional Disorder and Organic Disease* (London: J. & A. Churchill, 1883), 11.
37 G. Beddoes, *Habit and Health: A Book of Golden Hints for Middle Age* (London: Swan, Sonnenschein & Co, 1890), pp. xv–xvi
38 B. Ward Richardson, *Diseases of Modern Life* (London: Macmillan & Co., 1876), 173; Dowse, *On Brain and Nerve Exhaustion*, 42–3.
39 Beddoes, *Habit and Health*, p. xvi
40 H. Spencer, *First Principles* (London: Williams & Norgate, 1862), 334.
41 *Ibid.*, 324.
42 A. E. Durham, 'The physiology of sleep', *Guy's Hospital Reports*, 3rd series, 6 (1860), 150.
43 W. R. Gowers, 'Fatigue', *The Quarterly Review*, 200 (October 1904), 575.
44 Poore, 'On fatigue', 163.
45 Granville, *Nerve-Vibration*, 112.
46 H. Campbell, *The Anatomy of Nervousness and Nervous Exhaustion* (London: Henry Renshaw, 1886), 61.
47 S. Sontag, *Illness as Metaphor and AIDS and Its Metaphors* (London: Penguin, 2002), 64.
48 M. Foster, 'Weariness', *The Nineteenth Century*, 34 (September 1893), 339–41, 350.
49 J. Milner Fothergill, 'Work and overwork', *Good Words*, 23 (December 1882), 571.
50 C. Sengoopta, '"A Mess of Incoherent Symptoms"? Neurasthenia in British Medical Discourse, 1860–1920', in Gijswijt-Hofstra and Porter (eds), *Cultures of Neurasthenia*, 97–116 (p. 98). See also J. Oppenheim, *'Shattered Nerves': Doctors, Patients, and Depression in Victorian England* (New York: Oxford University Press, 1991), 144–5.

'Drooping with the century' 171

51 A. Rabinbach, 'The body without fatigue: a nineteenth-century utopia', in S. Drescher, D. Sabean, and A. Sharlin (eds), *Political Symbolism in Modern Europe: Essays in Honor of George L. Mosse* (New Brunswick: Transaction Books, 1982), 42–62 (p. 50).
52 F. MacCabe, 'On mental strain and overwork', *Journal of Mental Science*, 21:95 (1 October 1875), 394.
53 Greg, 'Life at high pressure', 629.
54 G. V. Poore, 'Exhaustion', in R. Quain (ed.), *A Dictionary of Medicine: Including General Pathology, General Therapeutics, Hygiene, and the Diseases Peculiar to Women and Children* (London: Longmans, Green, & Co, 1882), 469.
55 A. S. Myrtle, 'Neurasthenia – true and false', *Provincial Medical Journal*, 8:86 (1 February 1889), 86.
56 H. Campbell, *Nervous Exhaustion and the Diseases Induced by It, with Observations on the Origin and Nature of Nerve Force* (London: Longmans, Green, Reader, and Dyer, 1873), 1.
57 MacCabe, 'On mental strain and overwork', 398.
58 A similar model is apparent in arguments about the modern body and cancer, discussed by Arnold-Forster in Chapter 7 of this volume.
59 'A physician', 'Fatigue', 1012.
60 C. Oakley, 'Vital Forms: Bodily Energy in Medicine and Culture, 1870–1925' (PhD dissertation, University of York, 2016), 14. Emphasis added.
61 O. Temkin, 'Metaphors of Human Biology', in R. C. Stauffer (ed.), *Science and Civilisation* (Madison: University of Wisconsin Press, 1949), 178–82.
62 T. H. Huxley, *Collected Essays* (London: Macmillan & Co., 1904), vol. 1, pp. 199–200.
63 H. A. Huntley, *Thermo Dynamical Phenomena, or the Origin and Physical Doctrine of 'Life'* (Madras: Foster & Co., 1875), 23.
64 See, for example, H. B. Jones, *Lectures on Some of the Applications of Chemistry and Mechanics to Pathology and Therapeutics* (London: John Churchill & Sons, 1867), 1–2.
65 Foster, 'Weariness', 337, 352.
66 'A physician', 'Fatigue', 1013.
67 R. Gillespie, 'Industrial fatigue and the discipline of physiology', in J. C. Wood and M. C. Wood (eds), *George Elton Mayo: Critical Evaluations in Business Management* (London: Routledge, 2004), 429–57.
68 W. Stanley Jevons, 'On the natural laws of muscular exertion', *Nature*, 2 (30 June 1870), 158–60.
69 'On the law of fatigue in the work done by men or animals', *Nature*, 22 (10 June 1880), 128–9.

70 W. McDougall, 'Fatigue', in *Report of the British Association for the Advancement of Science 1908* (London: John Murray, 1909), 479.
71 *Ibid.* Emphasis in original.
72 W. H. R. Rivers, *The Influence of Alcohol and Other Drugs on Fatigue* (London: Edward Arnold, 1908), 2.
73 G. R. Searle, *Eugenics and Politics in Britain, 1900–1914* (Leyden: Noordhoff International Publishing, 1976), 34.
74 F. Galton, *Inquiries into Human Faculty and its Development* (London: Macmillan & Co., 1883), 25–7. (Emphasis added.)
75 F. Galton, *Essays on Eugenics* (London: The Eugenics Education Society, 1909), 2.
76 F. Galton, 'Remarks on replies by teachers to questions respecting mental fatigue', *Journal of the Anthropological Institute*, 18 (1889), 165.
77 S. Ledger and R. Luckhurst (eds), 'Introduction: reading the "fin de siècle"', in *The Fin de Siècle: A Reader in Cultural History, c. 1880–1900* (Oxford: Oxford University Press, 2000), p. xxiii.
78 O. Wilde, *The Picture of Dorian Gray* (London: Penguin Classics, 2003 [1891]), 171.
79 See A. McIvor, 'Employers, the government, and industrial fatigue in Britain, 1890–1918', *British Journal of Industrial Medicine* 44:11 (1987), 724–32; A. McIvor, 'Manual work, technology, and industrial health, 1918–39', *Medical History*, 31 (1987), 160–89.
80 Rabinbach, *Human Motor*, 8.

7

'A rebellion of the cells': cancer, modernity, and decline in *fin-de-siècle* Britain

Agnes Arnold-Forster

In 1899, the *Contemporary Review* published an article by the English physician Woods Hutchinson (1862–1930) entitled 'The cancer problem: or, treason in the republic of the body'.[1] In this article, thick with metaphorical allusions and polemic, Hutchinson condensed to thirteen pages the diverse and fraught anxieties that attended cancer in late nineteenth-century Britain. He wrote about how, over the past thirty years, the 'deaths per thousand living from this malady' had doubled in England, and 'nearly trebled' in the United States. Writing in the *fin de siècle*, Hutchinson argued that cancer was among 'our oldest, deadliest, and most-studied diseases', while at the same time positioning it as an unintended consequence of Victorian civilisation and progress. He presciently posed cancer as 'the riddle of the Sphinx for the twentieth century'.[2]

It is a well-known and often rehashed trope that cancer today constitutes an unintended consequence of modernity. Or, as Charles Rosenberg so eloquently puts it, 'the notion that the incidence of much late twentieth-century chronic disease reflects a poor fit between modern styles of life and humankind's genetic heritage'.[3] However, while Roy Porter called cancer 'the modern disease *par excellence*' and Siddhartha Mukherjee described it as 'the quintessential product of modernity', they locate that modernity firmly in the twentieth century.[4] Thus, while cancer is widely recognised today as a problem of progress, it is strangely absent from histories of this idea. This chapter goes some way towards filling this lacuna by exploring the construction of cancer as a 'disease of civilisation' in Victorian Britain. Cancer in the nineteenth century remains understudied, and work that has been done has predominantly focused on the twentieth century.[5] This asymmetry can be partly explained by the ways in which cancer and chronic disease have been conceptualised. There is an internalised understanding of the history of health as aligning with the epidemiological transition model, which posits era-specific diseases: from the age of pandemics in the medieval and early modern periods, to the age of infectious diseases in the nineteenth century, to the age of degenerative or man-made maladies in the twentieth.[6] All this works to obscure cancer from our view of the nineteenth century.

Yet, and as exemplified by Woods Hutchinson's anxieties, this posited relationship between civilised life and the incidence of cancer is not confined to the present day. Rather, similar debates about the impact of modern life on the integrity of our cells can be found circulating at the end of the nineteenth century. This chapter owes much to recent historiography on the *fin de siècle*. Such scholarship has focused on microhistories and examined the period through 'kaleidoscopic edited collections'.[7] Cancer is one such micro-history, and allows us not only to trace the metanarratives of progress and decline, but also to interrogate what, if anything, was specific to the conceptualisation of the disease at the turn of the nineteenth into the twentieth century. In what follows, I will outline the ways in which this perceived 'cancer epidemic' captured the medical and lay imagination, and promoted fierce debate in the pages of medical journals, general-interest periodicals, and in parliament. Drawing from literature on medical metaphors by scholars such as Laura Otis, Michael Stolberg, and Susan Sontag, I argue that cancer was easily incorporated into contemporary anxieties about degeneration and decline, and constructed as a malady of modern life using long-standing and flexible disease metaphors.[8] In this way, the disease was used to interrogate those facets of society and culture that appeared new and 'modern' to nineteenth-century medical men.

Cancer in the nineteenth century

From the late eighteenth century, cancer was increasingly addressed in both medical practice and culture, corresponding with rising popular and professional anxiety about the disease. Cancer appeared regularly in print and periodical material: alternative and itinerant practitioners hawked their wares, philanthropists lamented the cancerous pauper, and obituaries recorded it as cause of death among the wealthy and notable. It was also etched on the urban landscape – from the late eighteenth and early nineteenth centuries, cancer-specific institutions were constructed in London and later in other towns and cities across the British Isles. In 1792, the Middlesex Hospital established a ward devoted to the care of cancer patients, and in 1802 a close-knit circle of medical and surgical elites founded a cancer hospital just off Tottenham Court Road.[9] Both institutions served the local, urban, plebeian population, but people also travelled in from the surrounding countryside.

These two hospitals provided clinical evidence for a flurry of publications, and various familiar figures – urban surgical elites like John Abernethy, Everard Home, Charles Bell, and Thomas Denman – wrote tracts and treatises on the disease, derived from their new encounters with cancer on the hospital wards.[10] Thus, both institutions contributed to the codification of cancer, by which various incidental features of the disease were transformed into essential, identifying characteristics. For both doctor and patient, cancer was first indicated by the presence of a mass or growth. When someone arrived at the hospital they were subjected to physical examination – the surgeon on the ward poked, prodded, felt, smelt, and tasted the tumour. However, cancer could not be diagnosed by the senses alone; it was also defined by its long duration, its irreversible capacity for growth and spread, and ultimately its incurability. The clinical context made the disease more visible to the practitioner by enabling them to witness the entire 'life course' of the disease, from diagnosis through to death and beyond.

These cancer-specific institutions were explicit in allowing patients to remain 'until either relieved by Art, or released by Death.'[11] Consequently, people could be housed for months or even years, and frequently made repeat visits to the hospital for increasingly lengthy stretches of time. Most people who sought medical care at the hospitals did so while suffering under tumours of considerable magnitude. A patient treated by the surgeon John Pearson had a 'cancer in her right breast the bulk of a man's head.'[12] These extreme scales confirmed cancer as a disease with a monstrous capacity for growth and expansion. The Irish physician and pioneer in the study of cancer, Walter Hayle Walshe wrote in 1842, 'One of the most essential attributes of cancerous substance is an unswerving tendency to grow'.[13] This growth potential was not just about the tumours' ability to expand, but also about cancer's tendency to metastasise. Practitioners were well aware that masses on the surface of the skin might have ancestors or descendants buried deep within internal flesh. Finally, with depressing regularity, the patients on the cancer ward died. Thus, cancer in the nineteenth century was defined as an intractable malady, unassailable by medical intervention and nature alike.

However, cancerous growth and spread was not confined to the textures of the human body. In the middle of the nineteenth century, the disease was increasingly conceptualised as extending through the populations of the British Isles. This new anxiety depended on the increasing use and authority of vital statistics. The 1840s and 1850s saw the British populace increasingly quantified on a local, regional, and national scale. This practice derived in part from the development of statistical methods and epidemiology, and grew alongside a quantitative study of people and their activities more generally.[14] These intellectual movements were increasingly institutionalised and professionalised, and by the 1860s the government was systematically undertaking a large quantity of official, numerical inquiries into the health of the nation. The main source of disease statistics was the *Annual Report of the Registrar-General on Births, Deaths and Marriages in England*, first presented to Parliament in 1838.[15] In 1839, the statistician William Farr joined the General Registry Office (GRO), and proceeded to tabulate regional and national vital statistics – births, marriages, and deaths – for each of the country's divisions. The GRO also calculated the annual mortality by each cause and the proportion of deaths in 100,000 effected by each class of disease in each region. Parallel reports were later produced for Scotland, Wales, and Ireland.[16] Cancer was integrated into this practice from the outset.[17] The Medical Officers of Health (MOH) reports, first produced in 1848, ran parallel to the GRO's output. They, too, provided vital data on birth and death rates, infant mortality, incidence of infectious and other diseases, and a general statement on the condition of the population. The MOHs tabulated causes of death according to disease and stratified by age. From 1856, the reports included cancer in their nosology. Narrative prefaces to each annual report situated individual investigations within a broad chronology, and enabled doctors and public health professionals to comment on yearly shifts in the disease profile of the nation.[18]

As the quantity of data on cancer accumulated, observers began to draw conclusions about the changing incidence of the disease over time. Cancer appeared to be increasing. The *Forty-Second Annual Report*, published in 1879, recorded that among men of all ages, cancer was the cause of 4,121 deaths, the same order as diseases such as diarrhoea (5,712), whooping cough (5,804), scarlet fever (9,148), and measles (4,678). It also caused many more deaths than cholera, the quintessential Victorian malady (122). Among women the figures were even more dramatic, accounting for 8,508 deaths, more than any other disease.[19] The preface elaborated on these high numbers, and expressed concern over the increased mortality from cancer, which had 'maintained the increase to which it has been gradually mounting for many years'.[20]

Responses to this observed increase became progressively fretful. In 1883, the *British Medical Journal* published an article which lamented that, 'a cursory examination only is sufficient to divulge that the Fell disease claims year by year a higher ratio of victims'.[21] Commenters made use of an emotive vocabulary to express their concern: 'Unhappily ... a strict examination of the facts and figures bearing upon it, must lead to the painful and disquieting conviction that cancerous disease is, year by year, becoming more fatal in this country.'[22] This bleak prognosis – both for individuals afflicted with cancer, and for the population as a whole – filtered through multiple strata of nineteenth-century society. Concern over the new 'cancer epidemic' was not confined to professional discourse; rather evidence for, and debates about, the increase in cancer appeared in a variety of publications. Writers frequently invoked melodramatic language to impress upon the public the gravity of the cancer epidemic. In 1895, the English physician and inventor of the clinical thermometer, Clifford Allbutt, commented in the *Contemporary Review*: 'There is a bitter cry that cancer is on the increase.'[23] In 1907, the *New York Times* wrote, 'The cancer problem is assuming more and more menacing proportions ... we are doing nothing to hold cancer in check as a cause of mortality.'[24] Even the fashion magazine *Vogue* despaired: 'It is sad news indeed that cancer is increasing at such a rate that it begins to rival the white plague – as tuberculosis is called – in the number of its victims.'[25] Comparing cancer to consumption – the archetypal romantic tragedy of the *fin de siècle* – would have had a powerful impact on readers and cemented the supposed increase in the incidence of cancer in the imaginations of the middle classes.[26]

Why, then, was cancer increasing at such a rate? Writers at the end of the nineteenth century drew on an eclectic range of theories, all grounded in the intellectual, cultural, and political climate of the *fin de siècle*. Some argued that diet and lifestyle were key to the shifting epidemiological profile of the disease. The medical officer of Freetown, Sierra Leone, W. Renner suggested that 'preserved and imported foreign [European] food' was responsible for cancer's spread and increase amongst indigenous populations.[27] Similarly, the Surgical Registrar to the Middlesex Hospital, W. Roger Williams proposed that a simpler, less decadent diet was likely to protect against the disease.[28] Cancer – then as now – was conceptualised as a disease of civilisation, an unintended consequence of progress. Anxiety over the perceived increase of cancer was provoked in part by research that seemed to suggest the epidemic was not confined to Western or so-called 'developed' nations. Doctors across the British Empire were, at the end of the nineteenth century, engaged in a large-scale evidence-gathering mission. Data and anecdotal evidence was compiled to create cancer maps of the globe. Commenters plotted populations on a gradient – from immune to cancer-riddled – at one end Sub-Saharan African communities, at the other Anglo-Saxon or Teutonic races: 'Observation has shown that cancer has a certain geographical distribution. It prevails extensively in some parts of the globe, and is scarcely known in others.'[29] This mapping was marshalled as evidence for cancer as a 'disease of civilisation'. Not only was the disease on the increase, the epidemic was confined to nations that were understood as biologically, culturally, and economically superior.

If Britain was particularly susceptible, its colonies were at the other end of the spectrum. The *British Medical Journal* acted as a nexus of cancer evidence, sent in from across the empire. Medical men reported back from their respective colonies with quantified and narrative assessments. In 1906, the *British Medical Journal* commented: 'There can be no doubt that cancer in natives of British Central Africa is of the utmost rarity. Repeated efforts made by Government medical officers throughout the country for some time past have so far resulted in the discovery of but a single case.'[30] The situation in Sierra Leone was similar: 'Cancer as a disease is very rare among the aborigines ... I would rather not say that the aborigines are immune from the disease, but that the disease is rare among them.'[31] Dr A. J. Craigen, writing from Port Moresby in New Guinea in 1905, reported 'that during his stay of nearly four years in the Possession he has not yet seen a single case of cancer among the native population.'[32] The disease was also rare in Ceylon.[33] Cancer rates were slightly higher in Hong Kong: 'The returns made to the Registrar-General show that the total number of deaths among the Chinese in the period 1895–1904 was eleven, giving an annual death rate from cancer of 4.45 per 100, 000 of population.'[34] However, as Dr Francis Clark, Acting Principal Civil Medical Officer pointed out, this compared 'very favourably with the death rate from the same cause in England'.[35]

Cancer was also used to subdivide the 'advanced' races. William Hill-Climo, a fringe clinician articulating mainstream views, wrote in 1903:

> During the past forty years the death-rate from cancerous diseases in all European countries, and in the United States of America has steadily risen ... So widespread and so continuous is this increase, that it cannot be ascribed to local or accidental causes, but it must be sought for in the growth of new conditions, to a greater or less extent, common to all the affected countries, which the people themselves have produced.[36]

According to Hill-Climo, the 'cancer epidemic' was man-made, and produced by some shared element of civilised society. England appeared to suffer the greatest burden: 'Englishmen may be regarded as unfortunate; for within the geographical area of these islands cancer asserts largely its malignant and fatal influence'.[37] The *British Medical Journal* wrote in 1903, 'In considering countries as a whole it appears that the disease is more common in rich countries such as England, France, Holland, and Bavaria, while the lowest rates are among the poorer nations, Italy and Ireland'.[38]

It was in this period in Britain that meditations on national decline and biological degeneration reached their zenith. Thus, this pathological asymmetry was explained through then current notions of racial hierarchy.[39] In 1880, E. Ray Lankester wrote, 'We are subject to the general laws of evolution, and are as likely to degenerate as to progress'.[40] He was one of many writers negotiating theories of decline at the turn of the nineteenth into the twentieth century. This body of literature dealt with the 'apparent paradox' that civilisation itself 'might be the catalyst of, as much as the defence against, physical and social pathology'.[41] *Fin-de-siècle* commenters were anxious that neither the 'natural' triumph of the 'civilising' imperial Western powers, nor the stability of the racial order, was guaranteed. Such a socio-cultural evolutionary viewpoint was characteristic of British anthropology after *c.* 1860 and infiltrated a range of academic pursuits and public conversations.[42] Scholarship in this area is extensive and the historical narratives are complex; cancer theorists, however, were drawing on a variety of overlapping concepts that formed the vocabulary of the late Victorian bourgeoisie. These concepts included ideas about the diversity of humankind and its maintained relationship with biblically determined hierarchies; the positivistic and naturalistic study of the progress of civilisation; a tradition of Anglo-Saxon racialism and ideas about inherent Teutonic superiority; and broader notions of biological and racial determinism.[43] These intellectual movements were taking place in a context of increasingly punitive and violent imperialism, intra-European competition, rising nationalism, and anxieties about demographic realities within the United States of America, Britain, France, and the rest of Europe.[44]

Animal health was used as a proxy for human diversity in disease incidence and the shape of the debate confirmed the causal relationship between cancer and civilisation. Wild animals were discursively connected to 'wild' or 'uncivilised' peoples. And, parallels were drawn between 'civilised' man and domesticated creatures: 'Cancer is by no means an uncommon disease among the domesticated animals, while in wild animals and uncivilized man it is rare'.[45] This comparative exercise rested on the assumption that cancer was the same disease in both humans and animals.[46] W. Roger Williams claimed: 'I have never met with a single instance of cancer in any wild animal in a state of nature … It is, of course, well known that wild animals that have been kept long in confinement may be thus affected'.[47] This caveat tapped into a key question for late nineteenth-century cancer theorists: was the differential between civilised and uncivilised cancer rates (in both animals and humans) caused by body or lifestyle? If you brought a wild creature into a domestic context – a menagerie for example – would its propensity to cancer increase? Or, did the inherent bodily structure of each dictate its vulnerability?

Thus, various commenters sought to explain why 'civilised' races might be more prone to cancer than their 'barbarous' counterparts. Some argued that a propensity towards cancer was created by inherent racial distinctions between home and abroad, whereas others suggested the uneven epidemic was a product of correlating styles of life. This opposition (although not an explicit one) was in part a product of chronology, and can be mapped on to a broader shift from environmental determinism to biological determinism in *fin-de-siècle* science and medicine. It is a hallmark of late nineteenth-century anthropology that race was believed to rest on material facts – 'it is no arbitrary idea, no abstraction.'[48] Moreover, that certain races were inherently more or less vulnerable to certain diseases was a common concept in Victorian medicine. In his 1883 'Address in Pathology', the parasitologist Charles Creighton wrote that smallpox was 'peculiarly an African disease'. This particularity was a biological one – 'the loathsomeness, the peculiar odour, and the no less peculiar scars of small-pox, might of themselves suggest another skin than ours.'[49] In contrast, cancer was a disease of white skin. However, for most *fin-de-siècle* commenters, cancer was less a product of the civilised *body*, and more of the civilised *way of living*.

The impact of the civilised experience was, for nineteenth-century writers, clearest in Creole or mixed-race populations. W. Renner wrote about the Creole populations of Sierra Leone – 'the descendants of the liberated Africans'. He claimed that there was an increase in cancer among them, in contrast with its, 'apparent rarity among the aborigines in the colony and in the hinterland of Sierra Leone.'[50] Renner's argument was that this was due to the influences of European civilisation and the adoption of the 'European mode of living': 'the existence of cancer and other malignant growths among the creoles, and its absence or rarity among the aborigines, are due in my opinion to the civilised habits of, and the civilising influences operating upon, the former, and to the primitive mode of living of the latter.'[51]

Renner was concerned that changes in lifestyle were making Creoles more prone to cancer – that through adopting the 'mode of living, the food and dress, of the Europeans', creoles had discarded their 'natural' African environment and styles of life, and substituted instead an inappropriate decadence. In their 'eager pursuit for wealth and luxury', they had brought about premature degeneration and decline.[52] This sentiment was echoed by Sir William MacGregor, Lieutenant-Governor of

British New Guinea, in the *Lancet*. During his nine-and-a-half-year tenure, the only example of cancer he ever saw was, 'in the person of a Papuan who had for seven or eight years lived practically a European life'.[53] Renner framed his analysis as concern for the well-being of the Creole population. However, it can equally be read as an invective against populations deviating from their 'proper' and 'natural' state of existence. In 'their eager pursuit for wealth and luxury', the Creoles were subverting the hierarchy inherent in the British Empire's system of rulers and ruled, and suffering increased rates of cancer as a result. Renner was reflecting commonly held views at the end of the nineteenth and beginning of the twentieth centuries. His concerns manifested widespread beliefs about the dangers of transgressing natural racial divisions. Many Victorian commentators saw Nature as aristocratic, mercilessly punishing impure blood.[54]

W. Roger Williams made parallel arguments about Africans. While they remained in Africa, 'negroes' appeared to be 'almost exempt' from cancer. Similarly, living in slavery in the United States – 'with hard work and frugal diet' – cancer remained uncommon. However, since the abolition of slavery, 'and the altered habits thus entailed', the 'United States negroes have become almost as prone to cancer as their white neighbours'. According to Williams, there was nothing inherent in the bodies of black Africans, rather their susceptibility to malignancy was conditioned by the way they lived.[55]

Metaphors of degeneration and decline

Why did *fin-de-siècle* citizens construct cancer as a disease of civilisation?[56] Why did they discursively connect it to social degeneration and decline? I argue that this phenomenon was dependent on the metaphorical fluidity of cancer's identity in the nineteenth century and before. Scholars such as Laura Otis have argued that metaphors and analogies are not just rhetorical techniques, but express actual scientific and medical understanding.[57] The extent to which cancer, in particular, has been understood through metaphors and analogies is well documented.[58] In her seminal work, *Illness as Metaphor*, Susan Sontag wrote, 'I want to describe, not what it is really like to emigrate to the kingdom of the ill and live there, but the punitive or sentimental fantasies concocted about that situation: not real geography, but stereotypes of national character.'[59] She navigates various diseases, but returns to cancer time and again: 'Cancer remains the most radical of disease metaphors.'[60]

There was a confluence between imaginings of society and biological understandings of cancer in this period – a relationship made possible by the well-established 'essential congruity between medicine and culture.'[61] Crucial to this connection was language that linked the body biological to the body politic. This relationship was not specific to cancer, but common to cultural and medical discourse throughout the nineteenth century and before. In Hutchinson's text, the body is described through analogy to the state; he speaks of 'cell-citizens', 'lymph-roads', and 'the body-fortresses.'[62] Similarly, Rudolf Virchow repeatedly described the cell through analogy to the individual person: 'A cell … yes, that is really a person and in truth a busy, and active person.'[63] Thus, the 'cancer epidemic' was read through this metaphorical body–nation connection, and its narration was particularly dependent on prevalent assumptions about the disease's specific causes and cures.

Various aspects of cancer's identity in this period shaped the disease's discursive relationship to civilisation and its decline. Cellular pathology – introduced into Britain in the late 1850s – played a significant role. As applied to cancer, the idea was that normal human cells were converted to malignant cells – that these diseased units arose spontaneously in the body and were derived from healthy tissue. As one observer wrote in 1858, 'there appears, then, no reason to regard the cells found in cancerous growths other than as the ordinary ones formed for the development of healthy tissue, which have taken on an abnormal character.'[64] This 'abnormal character' was primarily their capacity for growth: 'the primordial cell divides and divides again, till the whole has become converted, by the process of segmentation, into a mass of nucleated cells.'[65] Frequently, this process was described in 'unnatural' terms. In his 1874 Goulstonian Lectures, J. F. Payne wrote that 'the tumour … has no very definite limit, and shows no conformity to rule in its shape.'[66] Unlike 'natural' bodily processes, cancer was not governed by discernible laws; cancerous tumours instead demonstrated a 'monstrous exaggeration of growth.'[67]

Such narratives found easy parallels with *fin-de-siècle* discourses about the civilised nation and its supposed inevitable decline. There were clear parallels to be drawn between a healthy body ultimately succumbing to disorder, and a prosperous nation or empire suffering necessary deterioration. The new 'cancer epidemic' emerged in a climate of widespread anxiety about the vigour of empire, concerns about imperial overstretch, and worries that Britain might be vulnerable to the destructive effects of the unruly, ungovernable, and the newly enfranchised 'crowd'.[68] This latter anxiety tracked contemporary bourgeois fears over the threat of social revolution, political anarchy, and urban proliferation. The idea that these 'advanced' societies (or bodies) – marked in every other way by order and design – could be particularly susceptible to cancerous growth resonated with the metaphorical language used to describe the disease's physiology and pathology, and only cemented the connections between cancer and these worrying aspects of late nineteenth-century Western civilisation.

In line with the links drawn between cells and citizens, Hutchinson described cancer as 'a rebellion of the cells'.[69] He went on to describe how, 'in the body-republic, where we have come to regard harmony and loyalty as the almost invariable rule, we suddenly find ourselves confronted by anarchy and revolt'.[70] Another writer outlined the cancer process: 'one day, from an unknown cause, these microcosms are thrown into disorder. A cell or a group of cells commences to multiply and proliferate in an unusual manner, and the mass thus formed forces back the healthy tissue around it'.[71] When a cancer is discovered in the body, 'anarchy may have been said to have arisen in the community, and everything is in confusion'.[72] This is a declinist narrative of the body – hitherto governed by order and progress, now entropy takes over, and it descends into chaos. Drawing on cellular pathology, these evocative descriptions personify the cancer cell: 'In a cancer we have cells and nothing but cells, which refuse to explain why they have left their places, and have much less the air of policemen than the suspicious demeanour of vagabonds.'[73]

This declinist narrative of cells and nation was not without its discontents. While cancer might have been tied to the late stages of civilisation, the same metaphors that linked the body biological to the body politic also provided evidence of social advance and prosperity. In 1893, George King and Arthur Newsholme published a thirty-three-page article entitled 'On the Alleged Increase of Cancer' in the *Proceedings of the Royal Society of London*.[74] The introduction sculpted the shape and profile of the debate at the *fin de siècle*: 'During the last few years the minds of medical men and of the general public has been exercised over the rapid and striking increase in the mortality from cancer, as shown by the statistics contained in the Registrar-General's Annual Reports.'[75] However, they then went on to offer a rebuttal to the dominant narrative of increasing cancer rates. They presented a careful consideration of the GRO data and summarised many of the key critiques of the supposed increase in the incidence of cancer. King and Newsholme were not alone. For every commenter insisting on the epic proportions of the cancer epidemic there was a countervailing argument suggesting that the panic was baseless.

Anthropologist Erin O'Connor has argued that the metaphors used by nineteenth-century doctors allowed them to 'contemplate breast cancer as a surgical rather than sexual problem'. The discursive connections they drew between cancer and civilisation, so she argues, separated the breast from 'questions of sexuality, identity, and womanhood' and so enabled surgeons to develop effective operative techniques: 'objectifying, yes: but only as a saving grace'.[76] O'Connor suggests that these processes were intimately associated with, and led up to, the development of the radical mastectomy in the 1890s. I argue instead that these rhetorical devices not only continued into the new century, but they also served a slightly different purpose. Rather than just enabling increasingly radical surgical intervention, metaphorical allusions to progress and decline in cancer discourse allowed medical men to invert the distressing conclusions of social commentators. Cancer was articulated not as an indicator of collective failure, but as a barometer for the quality of a nation's social medicine and public health. This helped to redefine cancers as a *disease of health*. This was both explicit and implicit in the writings of medical men and their lay counterparts. Hugh P. Dunn wrote, 'cancer is said to abound in the healthiest districts and amongst the people who are most robust'.[77] This claim was supported by close statistical analysis, undertaken by the Scottish statistician and later president of the Royal Statistical Society (1947–49), David Heron. He wrote in 1906, 'the conditions of prosperity and culture which lead to a low birth rate also conduce to a high cancer death-rate. In other words, cancer cannot, like phthisis, be taken as a measure of that unhealthy environment with which a high birth-rate seems to be associated'.[78] Here, Heron inverted contemporary speculation that falling birth rates were the result of national decline and degeneration.[79] For Dunn and Heron the relationship between cancer and civilisation was *unlike* the conceptualisation of various diseases of poverty such as cholera, rickets, and typhoid. Cancer may have been a pathology of progress, but it was not caused by industrialisation and its well-known pathological corollaries: filth, overcrowding, lack of sunlight, and moral depravity. But rather, and somewhat paradoxically, the disease was an unintended consequence of civilisation and its attendant health, wealth, and social improvement.

Even publications sceptical of Heron's analysis had to begrudgingly admit their research revealed that the cancer death rate tended to rise with increasing social status.[80] This inverse relationship worked on a national level as well. Dunn emphasised a correlation between an entire population's ill health and infrequent cancer incidence, 'a high general mortality would be associated with a low cancer one'.[81] Hutchinson was succinct in his analysis of the question of cancer and national health, 'Paradoxical as it may sound, [cancer's] greater prevalence is a symptom of increasing longevity and vigour on the part of the community. Cancer is the price paid for longer life'.[82] Dunn went even further, 'a disease such as cancer, which is characteristic of the healthy, may be expected to abound amid conditions of health'.[83]

Key to this conceptualisation of cancer as a disease of individual or national health was the increasingly prevalent understanding that this was a malady that particularly affected the elderly. Hutchinson described cancer as 'emphatically a disease of senility, of age'.[84] This tendency was used to explain the increase in the incidence of the disease as the nineteenth century progressed. Commenters criticised statistics that failed to correct for error due to the survival of an increasing number of persons to higher ages. The age-incidence of cancer was also brought to bear on discussions of the disease's geographical variations. Head of the Imperial Cancer Research Fund, E. F. Bashford observed:

> Civilised man's responsibility for the occurrence of cancer among native races brought into contact with civilisation, and in domesticated mammals, may merely be limited to providing them with opportunities for reaching their respective cancer ages.[85]

Civilisation was indeed bringing cancer to colonised territories, but only, he suggests, in that it was improving the life expectancy of their inhabitants. The cancer incidence of various nations and regions was now tied up with their demographic profiles. Shifting birth rates, death rates, and infant mortality were responsible for variations in cancer rates, further cementing the association between cancer, the population, and national health.

Cancer was, therefore, constructed as a disease of late nineteenth-century modernity. For some it was a product of social and biological progress, and for others, a consequence of national and imperial decline. In the minds of nineteenth-century writers, the nation-state mirrored the processes of the natural body. It grew, advanced, and improved, before beginning an inevitable and irreversible decline, only for life to be ended by a catastrophic rebellion of cells, or rather population. This trajectory was only available to those nations/individuals who achieved both longevity and modernity. Thus, societies and communities that were situated on lower rungs of the Victorian racial hierarchy were vulnerable to neither cancer nor collapse.

However, the age incidence of cancer, and discourse that used it to explain away the epidemic, was not without its paradoxes and complications. There are clear parallels to be drawn between a healthy body ultimately succumbing to disorder, and a prosperous nation or empire suffering inevitable decline. Cancer was understood to affect organs that had begun to 'atrophy' (breasts after the menopause, for example), and to flourish in countries and empires that had diminished in influence (as many interpreted Britain to be). High cancer incidence was, therefore, both an indicator of civilisation, and the mechanism by which that civilisation would fall apart. This metaphorical coating around the age-incidence of cancer gestures towards the paradoxes inherent in late nineteenth-century disease discourse. A greater proportion of your population living to old age was in many ways a positive indication of the 'quality' of your people and the 'quality' of your governance and ways of living. However, if that 'old age' was also a 'cancer age' there were certain implications – practical and theoretical – for the nature and trajectory of individual bodies and societies at large. Anxieties about social and national decline were particularly fraught in the *fin de siècle* – the '*end* of the century'. What did it say about the logic of the human body if at a certain point its internal order broke down? And what might that suggest about the logic of the body politic? And what was the role of public health and the medical profession in this unstable climate?

Perhaps the late-Victorian faith in progress buttressed a belief in these professionals' ability to tackle the new array of challenges presented by a healthier, and yet more cancerous, population. Cancer at the beginning of the twentieth century was simultaneously the 'dread disease' – a malady synonymous with death and disorder, which found easy metaphorical parallels in debates concerning the health and wealth of the nation and empire –and a disease of health. Accordingly, it came to be conceptualised in ways that reflected the complexities and ambiguities of 'civilisation' as a concept in *fin-de-siècle* Britain.

Roy Porter and Mikulas Teich's edited collection, *Fin de Siècle and its Legacy*, argues that this period was both a turning point and an enduring influence.[86] Various contributors trace the after-effects of the period through the twentieth century, and seek to show the ramifications of fundamental changes from before 1900. My micro-history of ideas around cancer slots into this approach, and provides an example of how the meta-narratives of progress, degeneration, and decline were themselves contextualised. While understandings of cancer at the *fin de siècle* owed much to their ancestors in the eighteenth century and before, they nonetheless acquired a unique character during the nineteenth century. This character persists into the twentieth century, and continues to shape our troubled relationship with the disease today. Cancer remains both the archetypal modern malady – tied to Western civilisation and necessitating the full technical arsenal of biomedical science – and an intractable and untameable foe, one that draws out our basest fears and anxieties about suffering and death. The most deadly of diseases is paradoxically a consequence of an increasingly healthy society. There is, therefore, an initimate and interdependent relationship between cancer and civilisation, which should cause us to rethink the nature of modern life and its capacity to incorporate death and disease.

Notes

1 W. Hutchinson, 'The cancer problem: or, treason in the republic of the body', *Contemporary Review* (July 1899), 105–17.
2 *Ibid.*, 105.
3 C. E. Rosenberg, 'Pathologies of progress: the idea of civilization as risk', *Bulletin of the History of Medicine*, 72:4 (1998), 714–30 (p. 714).

4 R. Porter, *The Greatest Benefit to Mankind: A Medical History of Humanity from Antiquity to the Present* (Fontana Press: London, 1999), 574; S. Mukherjee, *The Emperor of All Maladies: A Biography of Cancer* (Scribner: New York, 2011), 241.
5 There are, of course, exceptions. Frances Burney's 1811 mastectomy has received detailed scrutiny from feminist scholars such as J. Epstein and S. Mediratta: J. E. Epstein, 'Writing the unspeakable: Fanny Burney's mastectomy and the fictive body', *Representations*, 16 (1986), 131–66; S. Mediratta, 'Beauty and the breast: the poetics of physical absence and narrative presence in Frances Burney's mastectomy letter (1811)', *Women: A Cultural Review*, 19:2 (2008), 188–207. Cancer and gender in the nineteenth century has also been studied: I. Löwy, '"Because of their praiseworthy modesty, they consult too late": regimes of hope and cancer of the womb, 1800–1910', *Bulletin of the History of Medicine*, 85 (2001), 356–83; O. Moscucci, 'Gender and cancer in Britain, 1860–1910', *American Journal of Public Health*, 95:8 (2005), 1312–21; *Gender and Cancer in England, 1860–1948* (Basingstoke: Palgrave Macmillan, 2016). Finally, cancer in nineteenth-century America has received more attention than in the UK: R. A. Aronowitz, *Unnatural History: Breast Cancer and American Society* (Cambridge: Cambridge University Press, 2007).
6 See A. Omran, 'The epidemiological transition: a theory of the epidemiology of population change', *The Milbank Quarterly*, 83:4 (1971), 731–57.
7 M. Teich and R. Porter (eds), *Fin de Siècle and its Legacy* (Cambridge: Cambridge University Press, 1990); S. Ledger and S. McCracken (eds), *Cultural Politics at the Fin de Siècle* (Cambridge: Cambridge University Press, 1990); S. Ledger and R. Luckhurst (eds), *The Fin-de-Siècle: A Reader in Cultural History, c. 1880–1900* (Oxford: Oxford University Press, 2000); M. Saler (ed.), *The Fin-de-Siècle World* (London: Routledge, 2015).
8 L. Otis, *Membranes: Metaphors of Invasion in Nineteenth-Century Literature, Science, and Politics* (Baltimore, MD/London: Johns Hopkins University Press, 1999); S. Sontag, *Illness as Metaphor and AIDS and its Metaphors* (London: Penguin, 2013); M. Stolberg, 'Metaphors and images of cancer in early modern Europe', *Bulletin of the History of Medicine*, 88:1 (2014), 48–74.
9 J. Howard, *The Plan Adopted by the Governors of the Middlesex-Hospital for the Relief of Persons Afflicted with Cancer: With Notes and Observations* (London: H. L. Galabin, 1792); B. Schoenberg, 'A program for the conquest of cancer: 1802', *Journal of the History of Medicine and Allied Sciences*, 30:1 (1975), 3–22; V. A. Triolo, 'The institution for investigating the nature and cure of cancer: a study of four excerpts', *Medical History*, 13:1 (1969), 11–28.

10 J. Abernethy, *Surgical Observations on Tumours* (London: Longman, Hurst, Rees, Orme, and Brown, Paternoster Row, 1811); C. Bell, *Surgical Observations; Being a Quarterly Report of Cases in Surgery; Treated in the Middlesex Hospital, in the Cancer Establishment, and in Private Practice* (London: Longman, Hurst, Rees, Orme, and Brown, Paternoster Row, 1816); T. Denman, *Observations on the Cure of Cancer* (London: J. Johnson and Co., 1810); E. Home, *Observations on Cancer: Connected with Histories of the Disease* (London: W. Bulmer and Co., 1805).

11 UCLH Archive, London, 'Weekly Board Meeting', Middlesex Hospital Minutes, 10 January 1792.

12 J. Pearson, *Practical Observations on Cancerous Complaints: With an Account of Some Diseases Which Have Been Confounded with the Cancer* (London: J. Johnson, 1792), 38.

13 W. H. Walshe, *The Anatomy, Physiology, Pathology and Treatment of Cancer* (Boston: William D. Ticknor & Company, 1854), 146.

14 I. Hacking, *The Taming of Chance* (Cambridge: Cambridge University Press, 1990).

15 E. Higgs, 'Registrar General's Reports for England and Wales, 1838–1858', *Online Historical Population Reports* http://histpop.org/. Accessed 13 October 2016.

16 J. M. Eyler, 'The Conceptual Origins of William Farr's Epidemiology: Numerical Methods and Social Thought in the 1830s', in A. M. Lilienfeld (ed.), *Times, Places, and Persons* (Baltimore, MD: Johns Hopkins University Press, 1980), 1–27 (p. 1).

17 B. P. Henniker, 'Deaths from several zymotic and other causes, and inquest cases, in the divisions, counties, and districts of England', *Forty-Second Annual Report of the Registrar-General* (1879), 186–97.

18 E. Higgs, 'The Annual Report of the Registrar-General, 1839–1920: A Textual History', in E. Magnello and A. Hardy (eds), *The Road to Medical Statistics* (Leiden: Brill, 2002), 55–76 (p. 55).

19 Henniker, *Forty-Second Annual Report*, 186–97.

20 *Ibid.*, xxx.

21 H. P. Dunn, 'An inquiry into the causes of the increase of cancer', *British Medical Journal*, 1:1163 (1883), 708.

22 *Ibid.*

23 C. Allbutt, 'Nervous diseases and modern life', *Contemporary Review* (1 January 1895), 215.

24 'Cancer Deaths Increasing: Porter Says the Malady is Assuming Menacing Proportions', *New York Times* (5 November 1907), 1.

25 'Cancer Increasing at an Alarming Rate', *Vogue* (15 April 1909), 726.

26 See C. Lawler, *Consumption and Literature: The Making of the Romantic Disease* (Basingstoke: Palgrave Macmillan, 2006).

27 W. Renner, 'The spread of cancer among the descendants of the liberated Africans or Creoles of Sierra Leone', *British Medical Journal*, 2:2592 (1910), 588.
28 W. R. Williams, 'Cancer in Egypt and the causation of cancer', *British Medical Journal*, 2:2177 (1902), 917.
29 H. P. Dunn, 'English experience with cancer', *The Popular Science Monthly* (March 1885), 689.
30 'Cancer in the colonies', *British Medical Journal*, 1:2362 (1906), 812.
31 W. Renner, 'The spread of cancer', 588.
32 'Cancer in the colonies', 812.
33 *Ibid.*
34 *Ibid.*
35 *Ibid.*
36 W. Hill-Climo, 'Cancer in Ireland: an economic question', *Empire Review*, 6:34 (November 1903), 410.
37 *Ibid.*
38 'A comparative statistical study of cancer mortality. V. General summary (concluded), *British Medical Journal*, 1:2211 (1903), 1154.
39 A key text in this discourse is Max Nordau's *Degeneration*, first published in German in 1892 (New York: Howard Fertig, 1968).
40 E. R. Lankester, *Degeneration: A Chapter in Darwinism* (London: Macmillan and Co., 1880), 60.
41 D. Pick, *Faces of Degeneration: A European Disorder, c. 1848–c. 1918* (Cambridge: Cambridge University Press, 1989), 11. See, too, J. E. Chamberlin and S. Gilman (eds), *Degeneration: The Dark Side of Progress* (New York: Columbia University Press, 1985).
42 G. Stocking, *Victorian Anthropology* (London: Simon and Schuster, 1991).
43 *Ibid.*
44 *Ibid.*
45 Dunn, 'English experience with cancer', 689.
46 Professor Olt Giesson wrote in the *Journal of Comparative Pathology and Therapeutics*: 'Cancer in domestic animals exactly corresponds histogenetically with that of man.' O. Giessen, 'Cancer in domestic animals', *Journal of Comparative Pathology and Therapeutics*, 18 (1905), 278.
47 W. R. Williams, 'Cancer in the lower animals', *British Medical Journal*, 2:2021 (1899), 815.
48 H. S. Chamberlain, *Foundations of the Nineteenth Century*, trans. John Lees (New York: John Lane, 1913), 261.
49 C. Creighton, 'Address in pathology', *British Medical Journal*, 2:1179 (1883), 221.
50 W. Renner, 'The spread of cancer', 588.
51 *Ibid.*

52 Ibid.
53 W. MacGregor, 'Some problems of tropical medicine', *Lancet*, 2:13 (1900), 1059.
54 See Chamberlain, *Foundations*, 261; and A. de Gobineau, 'The Inequality of Human Races', in R. Bernasconi and T. L. Lott (eds), *The Idea of Race* (Indianapolis: Hackett Publishing Company, 2000), 45–53 (p. 48).
55 Williams, 'Cancer in Egypt', 917.
56 Anthropologist Erin O'Connor has argued that in the mid-nineteenth century, British medical men discursively connected breast cancer to the industrial city and 'forged strong linguistic associations between breast cancer and urban culture'. E. O'Connor, *Raw Material: Producing Pathology in Victorian Culture* (Durham, NC: Duke University Press, 2000), 61. However, elsewhere I have shown that Victorian practitioners were equally, if not more intensely, preoccupied by the relationship between cancer and rural space: A. Arnold-Forster, 'Mapmaking and mapthinking: cancer as a problem of place in nineteenth-century England', *Social History of Medicine*, 32:1 (2019).
57 L. Otis, 'The metaphoric circuit: organic and technological communication in the nineteenth century', *Journal of the History of Ideas*, 63:1 (2002), 105–28 (p. 127).
58 Metaphorical conceptualisations of the human body also took place in other medical and cultural contexts of the time. See Mukharji on the metaphors pertaining to the Ayurvedic body in Chapter 9 of this volume.
59 Sontag, *Illness as Metaphor*, 3.
60 Ibid.
61 As argued by Michael Brown and Mary Poovey, medical knowledge was a driver of social and conceptual change in the nineteenth century. M. Brown, 'Medicine, reform, and the "end" of charity in early nineteenth-century England', *English Historical Review* 124:511 (2009), 1353–88 (p. 1358); M. Poovey, *Making a Social Body: British Cultural Formation, 1830–1864* (Chicago: Chicago University Press, 1995).
62 Ibid.
63 R. Virchow quoted in Otis, *Membranes*, 18.
64 G. Southam, 'The nature and treatment of cancer: being the address in surgery', *British Medical Journal*, 1:53 (1858), 6.
65 J. F. Payne, 'The Goulstonian Lectures on the origin and relations of new growths', *British Medical Journal*, 1:688 (1874), 294.
66 Ibid., 293.
67 Ibid., 294.
68 Gustav le Bon argued that individuals as well as crowds often showed the survival of traits that characterised previous stages in the development of

society, or in the natural history of man. G. le Bon, *The Crowd. A Study of the Popular Mind* (London: Penguin, 1977), 13–23.
69 Hutchinson, 'The cancer problem', 106.
70 *Ibid.*
71 E. Burnet, *The Campaign Against Microbes*, trans. E. E. Austen (London: J. Bale & Sons and Danielsson Ltd, 1909), 2.
72 *Ibid.*, 2–3.
73 *Ibid.*, 4.
74 G. King and A. Newsholme, 'On the alleged increase of cancer', *Proceedings of the Royal Society of London*, 54 (1893), 209–42.
75 *Ibid.*, 209.
76 O'Connor, *Raw Material*, 99.
77 H. P. Dunn, 'An inquiry into the causes of the increase of cancer (continued)', *British Medical Journal*, 1:1164 (1883), 762.
78 D. Heron, *On the relation of fertility in man to social status etc.* (London: Dulau and Co., 1906).
79 The period between 1860 and 1914 witnessed a dramatic fall in fertility in Britain and awareness of these developments prompted widespread anxiety and introspection. See S. Szreter, *Fertility, Class and Gender in Britain, 1860–1940* (Cambridge: Cambridge University Press, 1996).
80 J. W. Brown and M. Lal, 'An inquiry into the relation between social status and cancer mortality', *Journal of Hygiene*, 14:2 (1914), 19.
81 Dunn, 'An inquiry into the causes of the increase of cancer', 762.
82 Hutchinson, 'The cancer problem', 115.
83 Dunn, 'An inquiry into the causes of the increase of cancer', 710.
84 Hutchinson, 'The cancer problem', 112.
85 E. F. Bashford, 'An address entitled are the problems of cancer insoluble?', *British Medical Journal*, 2:2345 (1905), 1509.
86 Teich and Porter (eds), *Fin de Siècle and its Legacy*.

8

The curse and the gift of modernity in late nineteenth-century suicide discourse in Finland

Mikko Myllykangas

'In greater nations, where large numbers of people create complicated social situations, where one can find plenty of riches, a lot of suffering, and high intelligence but also many degenerated individuals, the battle against self-murder can at times seem hopeless, and the onlooker is lead to believe it's all caused by grim determinism.'[1] This is how the Finnish physician Fredrik Wilhelm Westerlund (1844–1921) summarised the late nineteenth-century suicide discourse in April 1897. Observing the European debate on suicide from the north-eastern corner of Europe, the geographical distance and especially socio-economic remoteness between Finland and the leading countries of modernisation presented Westerlund with a bird's eye view of the burning question of the connection between suicide and industrialisation, urbanisation, and modern society. Westerlund, like his contemporaries, acknowledged that suicide – the most repugnant of sins for over a thousand years – was a disease brought about by progress, a dark stain that signified a modern society. In this chapter, I explore how suicide as a sign of modernity was interpreted in a country where the material side of modernity – big cities and railroads – were rarely seen by the majority of the population.

The relationship between suicide discourse and modernisation has been a recurring subject in the historiography of suicide since at least the 1980s. The historian Howard Kusher has described in his book *Self-Destruction in the Promised Land* and subsequent articles how 'the fear of modernity' was reflected in how suicide was conceptualised in the nineteenth century.[2] Yet, however frightening modernisation might have seemed, it was still worth pursuing. For many contemporaries, high suicide rates represented a sign of modernity, an undesirable but at the same time unavoidable price that a society had to pay on its path to the higher reaches of civilisation. While disturbing, the suicide phenomenon was often positioned as something to be proud of; the higher suicide rates in the West were seen as a proof of racial superiority. As Evelyne Leuf notes in her article on Scandinavian suicide statistics, some suicide researchers presented the local suicide figures with often barely disguised pride.[3] However, this rather widespread conception was not shared by all those who studied the suicide phenomenon in European countries. Towards the end of the century, suicide began to be seen more and more as a symptom of degeneration instead of a sign of increasing mental or cultural sophistication.

In this chapter, I analyse the conflicting views of nineteenth-century suicide researchers as they were faced with the increasing numbers of suicides in societies experiencing modernisation. I point out how local circumstances influenced the way concepts such as modernisation and progress were understood by those who studied suicide. As a historical case, I discuss a suicide study by F. W. Westerlund from 1897, published in 1900. Westerlund's essay 'Själfmorden i Finland' ('Suicide in Finland'), over 150 pages long, shows that suicide research in Finland followed closely in the footsteps of European authors in many ways. In this regard, Finnish suicide researchers viewed (or at least wished to view) their own nation as being part of the modern, civilised world, in which the increasing rates of suicide had become something of a yardstick of progress. However, the local idiosyncrasies of Finnish society also offered Westerlund an outside perspective from which to critically evaluate the established 'truths' about suicide and its connection with the modernisation process. Before examining the suicide discourse of the late nineteenth century, I look at the formation of what could be called 'a modern concept of suicide'.

The shaping of modern suicide

The difference between the modern conception of suicide and the pre-modern understanding of suicide is very clear. 'From Satan to Serotonin' and 'From Sin to Insanity': these are just two examples of how the historians of suicide (in this case Kushner and Jeffrey R. Watt, respectively[4]) have summarised this transition. The two millennia of premodern discourse of suicide were characterised by suicide being understood within the frameworks of philosophy and theology, both of which aimed at answering the question 'is it right or wrong to commit suicide?' In ancient Greek and Roman texts, we can find mythological accounts of suicide followed by both condemnation and apologies for suicide by the philosophers. Whether suicide was regarded as a crime depended on the social status of the actor and the circumstances of the act.[5] During 'the Middle Age of suicide', beginning around the dawn of the early medieval period, European culture became generally hostile towards suicide, and its criminalisation was backed by theological condemnation. The only escape from criminal sanctions, which were suffered by the relatives, was the verdict of madness.[6] During a transitional period of approximately three hundred years, starting around the 1500s and lasting until the dawn of the modern era, universal condemnation of suicide was contested gradually with the culmination of Enlightenment philosophers openly challenging the practices of legal prosecution of suicides.[7] The resulting contrast between the medieval suicide discourse firmly built on moral codes based on religious authority and the modern concept of suicide formed by the processes of medicalisation, secularisation, and decriminalisation is sharp. Suicide was removed from the realm of metaphysics and both religious and earthly condemnation and set on the field of scientific enquiry, rooted in modern medicine and the social sciences.

As the modern concept of suicide emerged during the long nineteenth century, phenomena such as industrialisation, urbanisation, institutions of democracy, nationalism, and capitalism and the free-market economy were spreading throughout the Western world and were already seeping into societies on the fringes of Europe, including Finland. Those who studied suicide in the nineteenth century pointed their fingers frequently at the very features that constituted what was understood as modernisation. After all, it was the new institutions of modern nation-states that raised awareness of the occurrence of suicide in the population. One of these new enterprises was the collecting of social statistics, as the gathering of data became part of the nation-building process.[8] For example, in the 1840s, the Finnish philosopher and statesman Johan Wilhelm Snellman (1806–81) urged Finnish officials to collect statistical data to get a better understanding of the Finnish people. Statistics, he believed, offered an in-depth view, not only of the material qualities of a society, but also of the psychological and moral character of its people.[9] It appears that Snellman was calling for more systematic and in-depth statistical inquiries to supplement the existing mortality statistics, the likes of which, including causes of death, had been collected in Finland since the 1740s. In fact, the Finnish and Swedish birth and mortality statistics are the oldest continuously collected population statistics in the world.[10] Gathered under the heading of 'moral statistics', the series of numbers representing crimes, suicide, and other forms of deviance consolidated a new way of regarding human behaviour, as just another measurable part of the world. Because of its moral, medical, and juridical aspects, suicide became the focal point of statistical investigations.[11]

In addition to statistics, the emergence of modern, secular, decriminalised suicide was closely linked to the formation and development of the psychiatric profession in the early years of the nineteenth century. Ian Marsh has gone as far as to claim that 'alienists' – the early French psychiatrists – and especially the renowned Jean-Étienne Dominique Esquirol (1772–1840) used the connection between suicide and madness to bolster their professional claims on the domain of mental health. Traditionally, the provision of 'spiritual counselling' (as a form of psychotherapy), as well as broader care for the mentally ill, had been the duty of the religious establishment.[12] The emerging psychiatric profession, through their contributions to medical and social debates, played an essential part in the formation of the modern conception of suicide, which can be characterised as 'medicalised suicide'.

The discussion of suicide among medical professionals began in France and Britain, and soon spread to other European countries and the rest of the Western world during the first two decades of the nineteenth century. The first scientific enquiries of suicide in Finland were published in the second half of the century (at the time Finland was a Grand Duchy of the Russian Empire, and remained so until independence in 1917). In 1864, psychiatrist Thiodolf Saelan (1834–1921) published his doctoral thesis *Om sjelfmordet I Finland I statistiskt och rättsmedicinskt afseende* (*On Suicide in Finland: A Study in Statistics and Medical Jurisprudence*), in which he examined the suicide phenomenon in Finland using statistical data from the past thirty years. Saelan's thesis introduced the international methodology of suicide research to Finnish academia. Based on official statistical data, edited by a private statistical enthusiast,[13] and illustrated by a handful of case descriptions, Saelan's study was in line with its European counterparts. By presenting several sets of statistics, Saelan endeavoured to shed light on various environmental and temporal circumstances as context for the reported causes of suicides. Saelan's study, like the majority of the suicide research written during the nineteenth century, followed a trend of 'cataloguing of causes',[14] a prominent feature of mid-nineteenth-century French psychiatry.[15] This was no wonder, as most of Saelan's quotations came from French authors, such as the psychiatrists Esquirol, Jean Pierre Falret (1794–1870), and Alexandre-Jacques-Francois Brierre de Boismont (1797–1881).[16]

As Saelan employed moral statistics as his chief instrument of enquiry, he also embraced mid-nineteenth-century determinism as a way to explain the rising suicide rates. Echoing one of the founding fathers of moral statistical research, the Belgian astronomer Adolph Quetelet (1796–1874), Saelan stated that suicide rates were governed by social laws, comparable to the laws of physics.[17] Quetelet and other early moral statisticians, such as André-Michel Guerry (1802–66), had been impressed by the regularities in statistical data that illustrated forms of behaviour traditionally attributed to free will, for example murder and suicide. Their conclusion was that there had to be something larger than individual volition at work.[18] These findings contributed to the rise of deterministic social theories, which became an integral part of late nineteenth-century suicide discourse. In Le suicide (1897), today the most famous work on suicide produced during the nineteenth century, the French sociologist Émile Durkheim (1858–1917) presented his own concept of suicide based on environmental determinism as he formulated his theory of 'suicidogenic currents'.[19]

The application of statistical data and statistical analysis in suicide research also contributed to the transformation of the meaning of suicide from an act defined by the individual's immorality (in premodern suicide discourse) and insanity (in modern suicide discourse), to a phenomenon with large-scale social significance. The primary concern for the early and the mid-nineteenth-century suicide researchers had been to establish whether or not suicide was to be regarded as a form of madness, or at least as a direct result of psychological morbidity. For example, in the 1860s, Saelan had underlined the importance of not assuming that all suicides were committed by the mentally ill, and of distinguishing mad and sane self-killers as separate categories to establish best possible ways to prevent suicides.[20] In the latter part of the century, the focus shifted towards the social aetiology of suicide. This change was facilitated by the creation of a mass of statistical suicide data. Another major reason for the shift towards epistemology grounded on moral statistical data was the rise of Darwinism in biology, and the introduction of evolutionary thinking into the social and human sciences.

In psychiatry, which had a tremendous significance in the shaping of understandings of modern suicide, Darwin's theory and other evolutionary ideas paved the way for conceptions of mental illness based on biological predisposition.[21] Simultaneously, the theory of evolution was being taken up by social scientists. Especially through the works of Herbert Spencer (1820–1903), evolutionary thinking was introduced into the emerging sociological perspective of understanding complex systems such as social organisation, and how various characteristics of a society, such as suicide rate, could be understood in terms of natural selection.[22] The theory of evolution and its applications in the nascent social sciences helped to undermine the conviction that human societies would be remain somewhat unchanged through time. Following social evolutionary thinking, it seemed that human societies were in constant change and that, by analysing the statistics, outcomes could be predicted. In some cases, the outcome could be undesirable if left unchecked. In the eyes of some contemporaries, modernity was seen as a catalyst for various new and harmful behaviours, such as a capitalistic, egocentric way of life, or urban idleness. These changes were thought to be injurious for individual and society alike, and if not addressed, they would spread in the society causing, for example, neurasthenia, mental illness, and suicide at increasing rate.[23]

Anxiety about the course of the evolution of a given society became more pronounced towards the end of the century, as the dark side of evolution – degeneration – entered the discourses of social sciences, medicine, and suicide.[24] Degeneration provided a theoretical framework in which to express fears of modernity using the language of science. The perceived increases in the incidence of suicide, mental illness, prostitution, alcoholism, and crime were explained within the parameters of theories of degeneration,[25] and, following a circular logic, degenerated individuals were typified by low morality, low intelligence, madness, and devious behaviour.[26] International competition fanned the fears of degeneration, which, in turn, created social programmes such as psychological testing of children in France and calls for policies to advance birth rates among people of 'good stock' in the UK and other Western countries.[27] The concern over the future of a nation was directed towards certain parts of the society as the poor and uneducated working classes began to be seen as threats to civilised society.[28]

Due to its political, social scientific, and biological connotations, it is little wonder that the theories of degeneration swept over academia in the wake of evolutionary thinking. According to Ian Dowbigging, for psychiatrists, in particular, the allure of theories of degeneration and evolutionary thinking in general was that they seemed to provide a conceptual framework for explaining the very nature of madness (and suicide) in seemingly empirical and scientific terms by pointing to heredity as the physical cause of insanity.[29] There were rather obvious reasons for psychiatrists to embrace the theory of degeneration. By the end of the nineteenth century, psychiatrists could not present any meaningful scientific breakthroughs in diagnosing and even less in curing madness, unlike their colleagues in bacteriology, for example. Degeneration theory offered a double-edged sword to psychiatrists, who wanted to be regarded as scientists.[30]

Following the increasingly mechanistic view of many social phenomena, the philosophical implications of presumed social laws became an integral part of explaining why suicide happened. For centuries, suicide had been understood as something that an individual chooses to commit. The perceived statistical regularities in people's behaviour raised doubts over whether such acts as suicide and homicide were in fact voluntary, or were somehow predetermined by social and cultural forces. The mounting statistical data on rising suicide rates provided groundwork for the idea that suicide was an illness of society rather than an outcome of voluntary human behaviour or, in a more modern view, a specific and individualised pathology.[31] Towards the end of the century, suicide together with madness was increasingly interpreted as a symptom of harmful aspects of modernity, but also as a sign of civilisation that separated modern nations from those who were regarded as barbaric races living outside of the Western cultural sphere.

The sickness of civilisation

The scientific and philosophical debates surrounding the use of social statistics produced a major transformation that restructured the discourse of suicide. These changes became visible in Fredrik Wilhelm Westerlund's 1897 study, as he fine-tuned the statistical analysis of Finnish suicides. Psychiatric considerations played a lesser part in Westerlund's study in comparison to the previous study by Saelan as he attempted to establish a social aetiology of suicide. Westerlund enriched his arguments by employing statistical data from abroad, and by quoting the international authors on suicide, moral statistics, and determinism, such as German moral statistician Adolph Wagner (1836–1917) and philosopher Moritz Wilhelm Drobisch (1802–96), as well as British author Thomas Henry Buckle (1821–62), whose deterministic *History of Civilization in England* was published in three volumes between 1857 and 1868.[32] By historically contextualising the changes in suicide statistics, Westerlund sought means for suicide prevention on a national scale. All of these features distanced Westerlund's work from Saelan's research of thirty years earlier. To understand the shift in focus of Finnish suicide research by the end of the nineteenth century, we need to look at one particular author on suicide, who was a major influence on Westerlund's study.

When it comes to late nineteenth-century suicide research, one work stands out for its major influence on subsequent research: the pan-European moral statistical analysis of suicide, *Il Suicidio. Saggio di statistica morale comparata* by the Italian psychiatrist Enrico Morselli (1852–1929), originally published in 1878. As Maria Teresa Brancaccio points out, what made Morselli's work so important and also so typical for the era was the way that he fused together some of the most popular topics in the human sciences of the late nineteenth century.[33] Statistics and statistical analysis formed the empirical foundation of Morselli's enquiry. He embraced statistics in general and moral statistics, in particular, as a way of uncovering the social laws that govern human behaviour. Statistics provided a supposedly objective view of the present state and historical development of a society. Furthermore, statistical analysis would provide answers to profound questions on the nature of human agency that philosophy had struggled to solve for centuries. For Morselli, the absolute independence of human actions had been refuted by observed statistical regularities in many forms of human behaviour.[34] He embraced the notion of determinism wholeheartedly, as he argued that the seemingly most arbitrary deeds, such as suicide, were, in fact, results of social laws that govern the behaviour of each individual.[35] Morselli's conclusion was a rather typical example of how the increasing interest in collecting and analysing moral statistics fed the debate over freedom of will and determinism intensified by the end of the nineteenth century.[36]

To come up with a universal explanation to interpret and explain his statistical findings on suicide, Morselli turned to evolutionary theories. He argued that psychologists and sociologists should seek the origins of social and psychological phenomena alike from the laws governing the evolution of life, and therefore they should base their arguments on natural laws instead of on idealistic rhetoric or sentimentalism.[37] From this premise, Morselli formulated an extremely deterministic definition of suicide: 'suicide is an effect of the struggle for existence and of human selection, which works according to the laws of evolution among civilized people.'[38] Those who did not come out of the struggle as victorious suffered from 'some morbid aberration' in their brains and were removed from the survival contest by voluntary death.[39] As we can see here, Morselli's definition of suicide was not meant to be a universal definition. Instead, his focus was on the suicide phenomenon in modern, 'civilised', societies, where the main source of misfortune and suffering causing suicides (and other individual and social maladies such as madness and prostitution) was the psychologically taxing struggle for existence.

The mechanism of suicide that Morselli outlined was rooted in a psychiatric understanding of nervous illnesses. Morselli argued, echoing the psychiatric and neurological conception of the causes of hysteria and neurasthenia, that in civilised societies the struggle for life manifested itself intellectually instead of through physical violence.[40] 'The struggle', as Morselli wrote, 'between civilized peoples tends to become still more a struggle of intelligence.'[41] Therefore, suicide was more common in civilised and secular societies, as intellectual aspirations were thought to cause strain and damage to the brain and nervous system, which then might lead to insanity. The connection between mental illness and suicide had already been made by early nineteenth-century psychiatrists, especially by Esquirol, although not all agreed with him on this point, and therefore high mental activity was seen as a possible risk factor that could lead to suicide.[42]

According to Morselli, as modern societies became more complex, if the suicide phenomenon were to be left unchecked, suicide rates would continue to increase at the same pace as cultural advancement. This hypothesis was shared by many late nineteenth-century suicide researchers, including the coroner William Wynn Westcott (1848–1925) in England, who had noted in 1885 how it was beyond dispute that 'a preponderant rate of suicide, and a high rate of madness exist in countries the farthest advanced in our modern ideas of civilization.'[43] In the German-speaking world, Alexander von Oettingen argued that materialism of modern civilisation made people weary of life, and his pupil in moral statistical research, Adolph Wagner, argued that Protestantism as a more 'modern' form of Christianity produced more suicides.[44] On the other side of the Atlantic, William Mathews (1818–1909) came to a similar conclusion in his essay 'Civilization and suicide', published in 1891. Praising Morselli as one of the most brilliant students of suicide, Mathews confirmed that modern civilisation was to blame for the increasing numbers of suicides.[45] A fast pace of living, excitement, and competition were at the centre of nineteenth-century life. 'Express-railway stock wears out far more rapidly … and man's nervous system is subject to the same law', Mathews wrote, conjuring images of a speeding mechanised lifestyle.[46] And finally, writing in 1897 – the same year that Westerlund completed his suicide study – Emile Durkheim described 'the hypercivilization which … refines nervous systems, making them excessively delicate … [and] more accessible both to violent irritation and to exaggerated depression.'[47] What we can gather from the aforementioned authors is that changes in the way people lived, as well as changes in their spatial and social environments – brought about by railroads, electricity, and urbanisation – were regarded as explanations for the modern prevalence of suicide. Here suicide is seen as a sign of modernity, and as a disease born out of progress. But how did this perception translate to societies where 'express-railway' and fast-paced urban life were only a rumour heard from those travelling abroad?

Death followed hunger and disease

As the quotation at the beginning of this chapter illustrates, Westerlund was well aware of the dissimilarities between his native country and the 'greater nations' of Central and Western Europe, conditions of which had been the subject of the existing literature on suicide. However, as any scholar who strives to create dialogue, he picked up the central concepts of the transnational discourse of suicide and employed them in his analysis of the Finnish suicide data. A logical starting point was to compare rural and urban suicide rates and to see how Finnish statistics answered their international counterparts.

For contemporary observers, the growth of urban centres was one of the most visible signs of modernisation. Unsurprisingly, urbanisation was often one of the prime explanations when the causes of suicide were sought. Urban life, it seemed, was especially plagued by the danger of suicide, while, as one American observer stated. People living in rural areas had no time to think mischievous thoughts of suicidal nature while they were engaged with agrarian activities.[48] The traditional agrarian way of life was regarded as morally superior to the busier character of urban life, which was generally considered to put a strain on the nerves due to its busier character.[49] Westerlund, like his international colleagues, considered the comparatively high suicide rates in Helsinki to be caused by an intensified struggle for existence in urban areas.[50] However, as Finland was quite far behind many of the Western European countries in its level of urbanisation, he thought generally lower Finnish suicide rates to be a result of a less intense struggle for existence. He stated that Finland was spared from the overtly strong influence of degeneration due to the agrarian and less urbanised structure of the society.[51] Despite this acknowledgement, Westerlund did consider suicide to be a problem for Finnish society, and one that was related to the country's level of modernisation. By looking at the measures that he proposed to prevent Finnish suicides, we get a clearer picture of exactly how suicide and modernisation were connected to each other in Westerlund's reasoning.

In the list of preventative measures, Westerlund placed a strong emphasis on the battle against famine, caused by failure of crops, as a measure to prevent suicides. He made a rather peculiar comparison between the 'struggle for existence' in other more developed nations and the impact of crop failures in Finland, arguing that they had a comparable influence on the suicide rates.[52] Westerlund's Western European colleagues generally viewed 'struggle for existence' in relation to the effects that modernisation had on society, usually targeting urban lifestyle as a way of life that was seen as harmful to moral and even physical well-being. In Finland, however, the 'struggle for existence' was interpreted through a more practical lens. Born in 1844, Fredrik Wilhelm Westerlund had been in his mid-twenties when consecutive failures of crops in Finland caused the famine of 1866–68. The winter of 1866–67 had been unusually cold and the spring of 1867 had come late, as the median temperature in May had been only +1.8°C in Helsinki, almost ten degrees below the average. On top of that, freezing weather in September had destroyed the crops in many parts of the country. Partially due to the slow reaction by the Senate of Finland, international food aid did not reach the country in time, and as a result Finland and especially the Finnish countryside was plunged into a food catastrophe. During these great hunger years, around 150,000 people died from hunger, diseases, and – for a small part – suicide, equating to almost 10% of the population of c. 1.7 million. In the worst-hit areas, the death rate reached 20% of the population.[53] The experience was engraved on people's imagination, and it was echoed in art and literature for decades after.

Looking at the suicide statistics of the 1860s, there was in fact an increase of over 40% in the suicide rate in 1868, the worst year of famine (see Table 8.1). A growth of similar magnitude in suicide numbers had been experienced in 1848, when in the aftermath of the 1846 crop failure, a cholera epidemic reached Finland.[54] During the famine, in addition to 'normal' suicides, it was fairly common for an individual who committed suicide to kill one or several family members before killing themselves. Westerlund described several cases of such 'extended' suicides, which he explained were caused by delirium due to typhoid fever and hunger.[55] Looking at the Finnish statistics, Westerlund saw a very different statistical reality from his European and American colleagues, who were mostly worried about the fast-paced progress of society and the nervous strain it caused.

After the great famine years of the late 1860s, Finland went through a rapid period of industrialisation. The experience of catastrophe partially speeded up the economic progress of the country; the government

TABLE 8.1 Suicide per 1 million inhabitants in Finland, 1841–90

1841: 36.2	1851: 44.3	1861: 44.05	1871: 31.05	1881: 34.57
1842: 36.4	1852: 44.6	1862: 40.87	1872: 29.98	1882: 34.54
1843: 49.2	1853: 41.4	1863: 38.39	1873: 30.11	1883: 44.73
1844: 37.4	1854: 42.3	1864: 42.12	1874: 36.05	1884: 38.53
1845: 29.1	1855: 49.0	1865: 47.20	1875: 40.78	1885: 40.30
1846: 40.4	1856: 52.0	1866: 47.34	1876: 33.97	1886: 46.01
1847: 43.7	1857: 52.0	1867: 42.76	1877: 36.52	1887: 37.75
1848: 60.7	1858: 46.9	**1868: 60.78**	1878: 38.10	1888: 40.62
1849: 43.3	1859: 40.6	1869: 46.57	1879: 32.47	1889: 32.80
1850: 45.2	1860: 48.7	1870: 39.58	1880: 27.18	1890: 39.92

Source: F. W. Westerlund, 'Själfmorden i Finland 1861–1895', *Bidrag till kännedom af Finlands natur och folk* (Helsingfors: Finska Vetenskaps-Societeten, 1900), p. 125.

instigated the development of the railroad network to ensure food aid would reach the periphery in cases of future famine, for example.[56] Between 1870 and 1910, the urban industrial labour force increased from 150,000 to over 600,000. However, when we look at the structure of the Finnish economy, only 4% of the population earned their livelihood in industrial occupations in 1870, and even by 1910 the figure had only increased to 14.7% of the population.[57] It is fair to say that the Grand Duchy of Finland was distinctly an agrarian society at the dawn of the twentieth century, around the time when Westerlund conducted his suicide study. Wide-scale urbanisation and the curses of the modern lifestyle that were thought to follow in its wake had not yet arrived in Finland. Social and economic circumstances that Westerlund considered as central points of focus of suicide prevention were very different in Finland from, for example, in France or the UK. But, as he noted that suicide and intensified struggle for existence were products of 'laws of nature' that gained their force from social circumstances, by manipulating these very same circumstances humankind could also work to decrease the number of suicides and other social ills. As 'progress gone too far' could hardly have been the cause of suicides in Finland, the development and modernisation of the society on a very basic level, such as food production and distribution, was the remedy that Westerlund recommended to combat suicides.[58] As Finland was still suffering from such societal problems as famine, it becomes understandable why a Finnish suicide researcher asked for more modernity rather than denouncing modernity and progress as the sources of suicide. The situation was almost an exact opposite of other Western nations, where the faster pace of modernisation and the moral debates surrounding various aspects of modern life had directed the attention of suicide researchers to see modernity as something that causes suicides rather than preventing them.

Free-willed progress and its benefits

While Westerlund agreed with Morselli's conclusion that there was indeed a connection between modernisation and suicide, he disagreed with Morselli's rather strict deterministic outlook on the progress of civilisation and its effects on individual behaviour. He pointed out how the causes of suicide varied between social classes, intellectual causes being typical for the upper echelons of society. More importantly, he argued that the power of determinism varied between the social classes. Committed by intellectually advanced and well-educated individuals (typically doctors, businessmen, scholars, and artisans), suicide could be regarded as a premeditated act, as the higher reaches of society exercised stronger moral freedom. The lower classes, due to generations of manual labour, alcoholism, poor education, and so on, were slaves to environmental determinism. In effect, Westerlund defined two different kinds of suicides: the more common kind was committed by morally inferior people, and it was determined by environment and inherited degeneration. The other kind of suicide was an act of self-sacrifice, to which free individuals sometimes had to resort. A wife caring for her sick husband knowing that she might also get ill and die in the process was one rather ambiguous example given by Westerlund.[59]

Westerlund was far from being alone as he distanced himself from the excessively deterministic interpretation of statistics. Although Westerlund was mainly influenced by Morselli's work, which exhibited a deterministic combination of materialism and Darwinism, he also studied the works of Oettingen and Wagner. Both German statisticians, especially after the former had convinced the latter, distanced themselves from rigid determinism and advocated social reforms as preventative measures to combat suicide.[60] A similar stance had been voiced in the early 1890s by Westerlund's compatriot, a Member of Parliament, and the founding father of the cooperative movement in Finland, Hannes Gebhardt (1864–1933). In his article 'Siveellisyystilastot ja ihmistahdon vapaus' ('Moral statistics and free will'), published in 1891, Gebhardt strongly rejected fatalistic implications of deterministic thinking. By pointing out correlations between suicide, mental illness, and other misfortunes, Gebhardt argued that with further social progress the freedom of individuals would increase and it would become possible to fix societal deficiencies that drove people into madness and suicide.[61] The only way to improve society was through the use of reason and rational planning of society; this was the approach taken by Westerlund and Gebhardt. Without freedom of will, deliberate societal development was considered impossible.[62] For those who distanced themselves from determinism, deliberate development of society was possible and also necessary to decrease the number of suicides.[63] Statistics would provide insight into the past and the present state of society, but they did not predict the future, and said nothing about ever-present laws that would govern human behaviour, as yet another Finnish statistician, Anders Boxtröm (1846–1906) had noted in 1891.[64]

Conclusion

It was clear that the lack of modernisation and progress – as in the case of the nation's inability to provide food aid in the case of crop failure – could also be considered as a cause of suicides, especially among the lowest classes of the society. Writing from a less developed country such as Finland, which had social problems due to lack of progress, Westerlund perceived suicide as a tragic outcome of vastly different scenarios, many of which had nothing to do with high levels of social progress, sophisticated brain development, or modern civilisation.[65] Consequently, Westerlund, with a critical attitude towards tying suicide and modernisation together, contested one of the most repeated statements of nineteenth-century suicide discourse, according to which only civilised people would commit suicide. By pointing out that even societies that had only just begun to go through modernisation produced suicides, Westerlund outlined suicide as an act universal to all humankind. He illustrated the argument by describing how many authors regarded suicide exclusively as a sign of modernity, as a privilege of culturally refined people, and therefore unheard of among the 'barbaric races'. Rather laconically, he pointed out that it was not uncommon for women in India to follow their husbands to death, or for a Chinese official to 'cut his stomach open at the slightest occasion of dishonour'.[66] It seems that Westerlund was here conflating Chinese customs with the Japanese practice of *harakiri*, but it is noteworthy that he saw suicide as a part of all cultures instead of as a phenomenon typical of a certain developmental stage of human society.

As we have seen, the introduction of modern suicide research presented the idea of suicide as a sickness of modernity. Statistical data and evolutionary theories provided suicide researchers with a theoretical framework with which to explain the increasing rates of suicide in civilised countries, and the bond between suicide and modernity was forged even more strongly by the end of the nineteenth century. But even as the fear of modernity and urban degeneration ruled suicide discourse in the most materially advanced nations, the fact remained that suicides were also committed in less-developed societies, and even outside of the Western cultural sphere. In fact, Westerlund attributed the Finnish suicide epidemics of the 1860s to the material underdevelopment of Finland. As mentioned in the Introduction of the present volume, one of the great theorists of the 'disease of modernity', George Miller Beard, attributed mental exhaustion, a typical cause of suicide, to such elements of progress as steam power and telegraphy. Ironically, the poor means of communication between coastal and inland regions was seen as one of the primary causes of the great famine and increase in suicide in Finland in the 1860s by contemporaries. Modernity, when it was regarded in the light of suicide statistics, became an ambiguous concept, which had to be interpreted in the local context.

For an observer like Westerlund, writing outside of the heart of modernisation, to see suicide as a universal human behaviour gave him an opportunity to critically evaluate dominant perceptions of suicide. As it turned out, the widely popular concept of the intimate connection between suicide and modernity was itself a product of modernisation. It was partially based on statistical findings as to what was happening in societies experiencing urbanisation, industrialisation, and other aspects of modernity. But the way these findings were interpreted was to aggrandise the material and cultural development of 'civilised' nations and to emphasise the gap between them and those which were regarded as cultures without modern civilisation.

Notes

1 'I större länder, där den stora mängder individer skapar mera invecklade förhållanden och flere sociala motsatser, större rikedomar och mera elände, högt stående intelligens och högre antal degenerade individer, kan väl kampen mot själfmorden ... stundom förefalla hopplös, ock låta betraktaren anse dem som oundvikliga följder af en grym determinism.' F. W. Westerlund, 'Själfmorden i Finland 1861–1895', *Bidrag till kännedom af Finlands natur och folk* (Helsingfors: Finska Vetenskaps-Societeten, 1900), 274.
2 H. Kushner, *Self-Destruction in the Promised Land: A Psychocultural Biology of American Suicide* (New Brunswick: Rutgers University Press, 1989); H. Kushner, 'Suicide, gender, and the fear of modernity in nineteenth-century medical and social thought', *Journal of Social History*, 26:3 (1993), 461–90; H. Kushner, 'Suicide, Gender and the Fear of Modernity', in J. Weaver and D. Wright (eds), *Histories of Suicide* (Toronto: University of Toronto Press, 2009), 19–52.
3 E. Leuf, 'Low morals at a high latitude? Suicide in nineteenth-century Scandinavia', *Journal of Social History*, 46:3 (2013), 1–16 (p. 10).
4 Kushner, *Self-Destruction in the Promised Land*, 11; J. Watt (ed.), *From Sin to Insanity: Suicide in Early Modern Europe* (Ithaca, NY: Cornell University Press, 2004).
5 G. Minois, *History of Suicide: Voluntary Death in Western Culture* (Baltimore, MD: Johns Hopkins University Press, 1999), 45–9. See also A. Hooff, *From Autothanasia to Suicide: Self-Killing in Classical Antiquity* (London: Routledge, 1990).
6 A. Murray, *Suicide in the Middle Ages* (Oxford: Oxford University Press, 1999), vol. 1, p. 170; H. Klemettilä, *Keskiajan julmuus* (Jyväskylä: Atena Kustannus, 2008), 181–5.
7 Minois, *History of Suicide*, 228–36, 250–3.
8 Leuf, 'Low morals', 1.
9 J. V. Snellman, 'Om Finsk Statistik', in *J. V. Snellman Samlade Arbeten IV 1844–1845* (Helsingfors: Statsrådets Kansli, 1994), 544.
10 G. Luther, *Suomen tilastotoimen historia vuoteen 1970* (Helsinki: WSOY, 1993), 22–3.

11 U. Baumann, *Vom Recht auf den eigenen Tod* (Weimar: Verl. Hermann Böhlaus Nachf., 2001), 220; D. Lederer, 'Sociology's "One Law": moral statistics, modernity, religion, and German nationalism in the suicide studies of Adolf Wagner and Alexander von Oettingen', *Journal of Social History*, 46:3 (2013), 688–9.
12 I. Marsh, *Suicide: Foucault, History and Truth* (Cambridge: Cambridge University Press, 2010), 100–2, 115–16.
13 In Finland, as in many other countries, publication of statistics was initially in the hands of private enthusiasts before public authorities began to produce official regularly appearing statistical publications. The Central Statistical Office of Finland was founded in 1865, one year after Saelan published his dissertation. Luther, *Suomen tilastotoimen historia*, 38–41.
14 See M. Myllykangas, *Rappeutuminen, tiedostamaton vai yhteiskunta? Lääketieteellinen itsemurhatutkimus Suomessa vuoteen 1985* [*Degeneration, unconscious, or society? Medical suicide research in Finland until 1985*, doctoral thesis] (Oulu: Universitatis Ouluensis, B 120, 2014), 45–6.
15 I. Dowbiggin, *Inheriting Madness: Professionalization and Psychiatric Knowledge in Nineteenth-Century France* (Berkeley: University of California Press, 1991), 29–30.
16 M. Myllykangas, 'The History of Suicide Prevention in Finland, 1860s–2010s', in D. Kritsotaki, V. Long, and M. Smith (eds), *Preventing Mental Illness: Past, Present, Future* (London: Palgrave Macmillan, 2019), 151–70 (p. 153).
17 T. Saelan, *Om sjelfmordet I Finland I statistiskt och rättsmedicinskt afseende* (Helsingfors: J. C. Frenckell & Son, 1864), 5.
18 J. Kivivuori, *Discovery of Hidden Crime* (Oxford: Oxford University Press, 2011), 31, 40; T. Porter, *The Rise of Statistical Thinking 1820–1900* (Princeton, NJ: Princeton University Press, 1986), 49.
19 J. Weaver, *A Sadly Troubled History: The Meanings of Suicide in the Modern Age* (Montreal: McGill-Queen's University Press, 2009), 47. According to Jack D. Douglas, Durkheim's 'suicidogenetic currents' that produced suicides were, in turn, caused by imbalance 'between the two sets of opposing forces' (egoism/altruism and anomie/fatalism). J. Douglas, *The Social Meaning of Suicide* (Princeton, NJ: Princeton University Press, 1967), 57.
20 Saelan, *Om sjelfmordet*, 63.
21 P. Pietikäinen, *Madness: A History* (London: Routledge, 2015), 125.
22 R. Smith, *Between Mind and Nature: A History of Psychology* (London: Reaktion Books, 2013), 59–60.
23 M. Jackson, *The Age of Stress: Science and the Search for Stability* (Oxford: Oxford University Press, 2013), 24–36.

24 On degeneration theory in nineteenth-century psychiatry, see Pietikäinen, *Madness*, 126–9; A. Scull, *Madness in Civilization: A Cultural History of Insanity from the Bible to Freud, from the Madhouse to Modern Medicine* (Princeton, NJ: Princeton University Press, 2015), 243–6.
25 Daniel Pick has argued that degeneration doctrine was never formalised as a single, coherent theory, but instead was redefined and restructured multiple times by different authors. It is therefore more accurate to talk about degeneration theories in the plural or of more general 'degeneration thinking'. D. Pick, *Faces of Degeneration: A European Disorder, c. 1848–c. 1918* (Cambridge: Cambridge University Press, 1989), 7.
26 H. Rimke and A. Hunt, 'From sinners to degenerates: the medicalization of morality in the 19th century', *History of the Human Sciences*, 15:1 (2002), 59–88 (p. 73).
27 Smith, *Between Mind and Nature*, 107, 112.
28 A. Herman, *The Idea of Decline in Western History* (New York: Free Press, 1997), 110–11.
29 Dowbiggin, *Inheriting Madness*, 5–6.
30 Even though degeneration theory offered tools to conceptualise madness, the concept of inherited mental illness left little room for therapeutic measures. P. Pietikäinen, *Neurosis and Modernity: The Age of Nervousness in Sweden* (Leiden: Brill, 2007), 78–81.
31 See e.g. E. Morselli, *Suicide: An Essay on Comparative Moral Statistics* (New York: D. Appleton and Company, 1882), 15–16.
32 See Myllykangas, *Rappeutuminen*, 69, 77.
33 M. Brancaccio, '"The fatal tendency of civilized society": Enrico Morselli's suicide, moral statistics, and positivism in Italy', *Journal of Social History*, 46:3 (2013), 700–15 (p. 700).
34 E. Morselli, *Suicide*, 16.
35 Brancaccio, 'Fatal Tendency', 700–1.
36 Weaver, *A Sadly Troubled History*, 61.
37 Morselli, *Suicide*, 355.
38 *Ibid.*, 354.
39 *Ibid.*, 361–2.
40 The diagnosis of 'neurasthenia' was introduced in 1880 by American neurologist George Beard (1839–1883). The disease was thought to plague the upper-middle-class businessmen and others who strained their mental capacity to the extreme. D. Schuster, *Neurasthenic Nation: America's Search for Health, Happiness, and Comfort, 1869–1920* (New Brunswick: Rutgers University Press, 2011).
41 *Ibid.*, 358.

The curse and the gift of modernity   213

42 Esquirol's countryman, for example, psychiatrist Pierre-Egiste Lisle disagreed with Esquirol completely and argued that suicide was never solely caused by madness. I. Hacking, *The Taming of Chance* (Cambridge: Cambridge University Press, 1990), 71. Saelan agreed with Lisle and stated that there were many instances, historical and present, where suicide could not be attributed to mental illness. Myllykangas, *Rappeutuminen*, 50–1.
43 W. Westcott, *Suicide: Its History, Literature, Jurisprudence, Causation, and Prevention* (London: H. K. Lewis, 1885), 81.
44 Lederer, 'Sociology's "One Law"', 690–3.
45 W. Mathews, 'Civilization and suicide', *The North American Review*, 152:413 (1891), 470–1, 477.
46 *Ibid.*, 482–3.
47 E. Durkheim, *Suicide: A Study in Sociology* (London: Routledge & Kegan Paul, 1970), 323.
48 Kushner, *Self-Destruction*, 42–3.
49 The debate over the effects of urbanisation on suicide rates continued among suicide researchers and psychiatrists in general well into the twentieth century. For example, as Finland went through yet another phase of modernisation in the 1960s, psychiatrists were worried about whether population moving into urban areas would experience more mental disorders and commit more suicides. M. Myllykangas, 'The social engineering of suicide: psychiatric epidemiology and suicide research in Finland in the 1960s and 1970s', *Medizinhistorisches Journal*, 54:2 (2019), 145–68.
50 Westerlund, 'Själfmorden', 195.
51 *Ibid.*, 274
52 *Ibid.*, 273.
53 O. Turpeinen, *Nälkä vai tauti tappoi? Kauhunvuodet 1866–1868* (Helsinki: Suomen historiallinen seura, 1986), 22; M. Klinge, *Keisarin Suomi* (Espoo: Schildts Miktor, 1997), 239.
54 Westerlund, 'Själfmorden', 127; H. Vuorinen, *Tautinen historia* (Tampere: Vastapaino, 2002), 124–6.
55 Westerlund, 'Själfmorden', 128–9.
56 Klinge, *Keisarin Suomi*, 240–2.
57 V. Rasila, *Torpparikysymyksen ratkaisuvaihe* (Helsinki: Suomen Historiallinen Seura, 1970), 18.
58 Westerlund, 'Själfmorden', 273–4.
59 *Ibid.*, 271.
60 Baumann, *Vom Recht*, 222.

61 H. Gebhardt, 'Siveellisyystilastot ja ihmistahdon vapaus', *Valvoja* 21 (1891), 152–3, 160–1.
62 Adolph Quetelet had already argued that by uncovering social laws by the use of statistics humanity could improve, instead being forced to obey the social laws as if they were as universal as the laws of physics. C. Emsley, *Crime, Police, and Penal Policy: European Experiences 1750–1940* (Oxford: Oxford University Press, 2007), 120.
63 Westerlund, 'Själfmorden', 273–4.
64 A. Boxtröm, *Jemförande befolknings-statistik: med särskildt afseende å förhållandena I Finland* (Helsingfors: G. W. Edlund, 1891), 11.
65 Myllykangas, 'Suicide Prevention', 156–7.
66 'eller i Kina, hvarest höga embetsmaän ej sällan rista upp sin mage, då deras ära fått någon flack'. Westerlund, 'Själfmorden', 227.

III
Negotiating global modernities

9

From physiograms to cosmograms: Daktar Binodbihari Ray Kabiraj and the metaphorics of the nineteenth-century Ayurvedic body

Projit Bihari Mukharji

To be modern, in its most fundamental sense, is to be distinct from the past (if not actually opposed to it) and to be an inalienable part of the present. To call something 'traditional' is therefore to deny it a rightful place in the present: to reduce it to an exotic anachronism. Johannes Fabian has described the anthropological trope of 'primitiveness' as a 'denial of coevalness' by which people and institutions – the anthropologist and her subject who are very obviously contemporary to each other – are split up and rendered within their own discrete temporal envelopes.[1] This is largely the case when we speak of 'traditional medicine'. Therapeutic practices that are labelled 'traditional' are marked off as leftovers from a bygone era.

A 2012 report by the World Health Organization, however, confirmed that over 115 countries in the world, including such demographic giants as China, India, South Africa, and Nigeria – to name but four – now have official policies for 'traditional medicine'.[2] To varying extents, all these countries have carved out officially recognised spaces for various so-called 'traditional medicines' within their state health systems, albeit often at a level subordinate to biomedicine. The nomenclature notwithstanding, these allegedly 'traditional medicines' do share the contemporary present with biomedicine and have done so for some time now. Yet it is partly by their continued framing as 'traditional' that their official subordination to biomedicine and their frequent erasure from scholarly overviews of the medical present is ensured.

Nowhere is this refusal of coevalness more conspicuous today than in overviews of the history of medicine. A 2008 work entitled *Medicine and Modernism*, for instance, has this to say about the conundrum of the modern: '"Modernity" and "modernization" are terms that historians use to refer to the interrelated series of economic, social, and political transformations that occurred in western societies during the period of the long nineteenth century. Urbanization, industrialization, and the spread of market capitalism were among the most salient features of these changes'.[3] Both modernity and modernisation are thus made synonymous with 'western societies'. A place like South Asia, though intimately connected to the developments in Britain and thus equally implicated in the dynamics of urbanisation, industrialisation, and the spread of market capitalism (though in different ways and at distinct rates), is yet expunged from the ambit of nineteenth-century modernity. In the same year that L. S. Jacyna wrote the above lines, William Bynum published *The History of Medicine: A Very Short Introduction*. Despite having deployed the definitive article in the title, and thus foreclosing any possibility of there being *Other Histories of Medicines*, Bynum's account remained firmly focused on the story of biomedicine. Even in his final chapter, entitled 'Medicine in the Modern World', the possibility of the 'modern world' being inhabited by anything but biomedicine is never allowed to interrupt the narrative.[4] A few years later, in 2011, Roger Cooter contributed a fascinating chapter entitled 'Medicine and Modernity' in an *Oxford Handbook of the History of Medicine*. Once again, notwithstanding Cooter's careful attention to how actors themselves used the notion of modernity and his just insistence that 'not only the history of medicine, but the history of modern thought depends upon an understanding of modernity in medicine and medicine in modernity', he completely eschews the possibility of their being *other modernities and other medicines*.[5]

I cite these authors not to single them out as somehow exceptionally blameworthy. Rather, I cite them for the exact opposite reasons. They are all eminent historians of medicine – amongst the very best in the field in fact – known for their archival rigour and their theoretical sophistication. Yet, and here's the rub, they seem entirely unaware of the debate over multiple modernities. The latter debate is now close to two decades old and in many circles it is already a fait accompli; but alas, not in medical history circles.

The watershed moment for the debate over multiple modernities came in 2000 when S. N. Eisenstadt edited a special issue of the journal *Daedalus* on the subject.[6] The contributors to the *Daedalus* volume described many different types of modernity ranging through Israeli, Turkish, Confucian, Islamic, Indian, Diasporic, Communist, and many more. Even before the *Daedalus* issue, however, postcolonial scholars such as Partha Chatterjee had made a powerful case about the fractured and plural nature of modernity.[7] In fact, Chatterjee's entry point into the question had been precisely through the actor's category of '*adhunikata*' or 'modernity' amongst nineteenth-century Bengali intellectuals. Along similar lines and more recently, Dipesh Chakrabarty has called for the 'provincializing' of European modernity.[8]

The argument I want to pursue here, however, is not merely that there are many medical modernities. Of course there are and the introduction to this volume does a splendid job in underlining that modernity is 'a constantly changing accretion of history, social context, and material conditions'. What I want to add here in this chapter is a recognition that just as there are many modernities, so too are there many medicines. Western, or biomedicine, is not the only form of 'medicine' that confronted, negotiated, or developed its own figure of modernity. Neither did all non-Western forms of medicine simply oppose modernity. Yet these *parallel medical modernities* continue unfortunately to be largely ignored within mainstream histories of medicine.

My ambition in this chapter, therefore, is to pursue the history of a specifically Ayurvedic medical modernity.[9] I do not wish to claim that Ayurvedic modernity was the only South Asian medical modernity. There were certainly both Western-style biomedical forms of modernity and vernacularised South Asian versions.[10] There were also other medical modernities engendered in and organised around other medical traditions such as Unani Tibb, Siddha, and Sowa Rigpa, to name only the most prominent ones.[11] Each of these medical modernities had their own specific accents, politics, and, above all, their distinctive body imaginaries. They were each shaped by their own historically specific trysts with what the practitioners themselves conceptualised as modernity. Each of these merits a devoted historical exploration. But in the present chapter, I shall focus exclusively on the Ayurvedic tradition, which has today emerged as not only the largest and best funded non-biomedical tradition in South Asia, but also as a global therapeutic option available in each of the major continents.[12] Moreover, my window into this Ayurvedic modernity will be the nineteenth-century Ayurvedic body.

In the interests of space, I have developed my account of Ayurvedic modernity through a discussion of the writings of one particular Ayurvedic author, Binodbihari Ray (1862–?). After a brief review of the extant literature on Asian medicines and modernity, I demonstrate how Ray developed an explicit and self-conscious discourse about Ayurvedic modernity. I follow this up with a more detailed interrogation of his descriptions of the Ayurvedic body and show how, through the use of metaphors, he radically refigured the Ayurvedic body. Finally, after another brief excursus contextualising the metaphors themselves, I conclude with a section on Ray's later cosmological writings and their relationship with his medical writings.

Binodbihari Ray and Ayurvedic modernity

Not a whole lot is known about Binodbihari Ray. He was born around 1862 and in his youth, he trained in Western-style medicine and eventually earned a VLMS (Vernacular Licentiate of Medicine & Surgery) diploma. Unfortunately, there is no record of his subsequent professional life. In January 1890, he launched a short-lived medical journal. At the time he was based in Talanda, Rajshahi, in present-day north Bangladesh. He also claimed to have run into huge debt to finance the publication. Very few issues of this journal have survived, suggesting that it probably did not last very long (though we cannot be sure of this). We next hear of him in 1908 when he published a lengthy book on Ayurveda written entirely in verse titled *Podyo Ayurbbed Siksha* ('Medical Educational Verses'). Also interestingly, while in 1890 he had described himself simply as a *Daktar*, that is, the vernacularised form of address for a Western-style physician, in 1908 he styled himself as 'Daktar Binodbihari Ray Kabiraj' (Kabiraj being the designation used to refer to Ayurvedic physicians).

In 1908, the same year that he published his last medical writing, Ray published his first cosmological work. In the years to come he went on to publish three more erudite cosmological works devoted to the theme of 'creation-existence-apocalypse' (*srishti-sthiti-pralay*). In none of the books did he refer to his life as a doctor, nor use addresses like *daktar* and *kabiraj*. Had it not been for his penchant for publishing photographs of himself in his books along with his birth year and his address in Rajshahi, there would be no way of knowing that the medical author and the cosmological author were one and the same person. Why he made such a clean and absolute break with his medical identity – at least in print – remains a mystery, as do the precise connections between his medical and his cosmological writings. These scant details are sadly the sum total of our knowledge about Ray's life.

We can add a little more to this by contextualising the sparse information we do possess. For instance, the VLMS diploma was a special qualification introduced in 1851 to cater to the colonial state's growing medical needs. The course followed for this diploma was shorter than the five years necessary for both the Bachelor of Medicine (MB) and the Licentiate of Medicine & Surgery (LMS) qualifications. Moreover, knowledge of English was unnecessary for the VLMS. Two separate classes of VLMS students were taught respectively in Hindustani and Bengali. Ray almost certainly read in the Bengali class. After a three-year truncated course, this would have rendered him eligible for appointment as either a Hospital Assistant or in one of the growing number of dispensaries under full or partial state funding. If Ray attended medical school in Calcutta, he would have attended classes at the Campbell Medical School in Sealdah where the Bengali class used to be held. There is, however, also a chance that he may have attended classes at the Dhaka Medical School that also offered VLMS diplomas from 1874 onwards.[13]

What we lack in circumstantial details for Ray is compensated by his own powerful voice. In explaining his decision to launch his short-lived medical journal, *Chikitshak* ('Physician'), Ray explained that 'Ayurveda, our national therapeutics' (*amader deshiya chikitsha byabostha*) had fallen on very bad times. 'Leave alone foreigners', he lamented, 'even our countrymen detest it and demean it by labelling it unscientific (*abaigyanik*)'.[14] Many 'great souls', he admitted, had already taken up the cudgels for Ayurveda and many Kabirajes too were making strenuous efforts to reverse the situation, but given the dire situation it was in, according to Ray, the 'help of locals trained as *daktars* was indispensible'. The likelihood of this happening, however, was remote. Many a local, Ray accused, began to hate Ayurveda the moment they entered through the gates of the Medical College. Yet he insisted that it was the 'beholden duty' of every *daktar* to labour for the revival of Ayurveda.[15]

Not one to be satisfied with abstract statements, Ray also had a clear plan for what needed to be done. He insisted that one of the foremost tasks was to publish more Ayurvedic journals. He lamented that one of the earliest journals, *Ayurveda Sanjeevani*, had proved short-lived and another, *Chikitsha Sammilani*, while faring better was often irregular and dependent on the magnanimity of a single generous aristocratic patron. The bigger aim, however, was 'to explain the complexities of Ayurveda and make it easily accessible, to elaborate on those issues that are only briefly mentioned in Ayurveda, to search for and to incorporate from other therapeutic traditions what is missing in Ayurveda.'[16]

In explaining this further, Ray mentioned that medicine is 'improving day by day' (*din din unnati hoitechhe*) and newer things are being discovered. None of this was there in the 'olden days that is in the days of the Aryans' (*purbakale arthat Arjyaganer samay*).[17] This is clearly a framing in terms of modernity by positing a clear break with an 'older time' of tradition. Ray's espousal of a classical time identified with ancestral 'Aryans', was fairly widespread amongst late nineteenth-century Indian, especially high-caste Hindu, intellectuals.[18] But unlike many others, Ray did not see the present as merely a degeneration of that classical, Aryan antiquity. Rather, the contemporary moment was for him marked by 'improvements' (*unnati*) and new discoveries (*abishkar*) that necessitated new efforts within the specific realm of Ayurvedic medicine.

Ray further suggested that some of the things that were being discovered were already there in Ayurveda but perhaps in complex, difficult-to-comprehend forms or indeed too briefly. He would elaborate on these and demonstrate that what appeared new was after all not so new, and already there in Ayurveda. But there were also things that were simply absent in Ayurveda. Ray confessed, for instance, that biomedical diagnosis (*nidan*) was much superior to Ayurveda, just as anatomy (*shaarir*) and physiology (*sharirkriya*) were weak in Ayurveda. Though he hastened to add that this was not a grievous fault since Ayurvedic diagnosis and therapeutics were not as heavily dependent on a thorough knowledge of anatomy and physiology as biomedicine was, the confession of a lack was telling.[19] It was particularly significant because he followed up this particular discussion with an entire serialised essay on physiology. Clearly, he was seeking to fill the gap here as he had promised to do in setting up the goals of his project.[20]

Ray's attitude towards modernity was further clarified when he intervened in a debate that had been taking place on the pages of another Ayurvedic journal, the *Chikitsha Sammilani* ('Meeting of Medicines'). The debate had originally involved a Bengali *daktar*, Pulinbihari Sanyal, and a Kabiraj, Prasannachandra Maitreya, and their respective definitions of the Ayurvedic notion of '*dhatu*'. Maitreya was opposed to Sanyal's attempts to interpret Ayurvedic concepts along biomedical lines and at one point had asserted that *pitta* (one of the key pathogenic principles in Ayurveda) was actually the 'Lord Brahma himself'. Ray summarised the debate in the *Chikitshak* and retorted that, 'if there is no other way of describing *pitta*, then Mr Maitreya's utterances are like the hollow boast of a child, for in the nineteenth century if we were to simply call *pitta* the god Brahma and left it at that, no one would accept it.'[21] Once more, in this exchange, we are given a clear sense in which Ray was thinking of his project as a modern project. His argument was a temporal one based on the attitudes of people in 'the nineteenth century'. People would not accept Maitreya's statement because it was incompatible with nineteenth-century horizons of belief and plausibility.

This horizon of plausibility seemed to be firmly linked, at least for Ray, to the idea of demonstrability. In every issue of his journal, he explained anatomical and physiological concepts by describing simple, do-it-yourself experiments or giving directions about the dissection of goats. One series of do-at-home experiments, for instance, was aimed at explaining to readers the chemical composition of the air and involved simple tools like candles, glasses, etc.[22] In another similar series of experiments, he demonstrated the chemical explanation for combustion.[23] Likewise, he advised readers to dissect a goat and conduct an experiment by blowing into the dead goat's trachea through a rubber tube and following the movements of the air.[24] Another similar demonstration involved dissecting the goat's stomach and examining the flexibility of the diaphragm by various simple experiments.[25]

As Steven Shapin and Simon Schaffer point out in their classical history of 'experimental life', there emerged towards the end of the seventeenth century in Britain a new paradigm of experimental knowledge, which generated 'moral certainty' around 'matters of fact'. The production of such experimental knowledge 'commenced with individuals' acts of seeing and believing, and was completed when all individuals voluntarily agreed with one another about what had been seen and ought to be believed'.[26] There were, therefore, two key moves involved in the production of such experimental knowledge. First, a faith that 'seeing is believing' and second, a consensus that everyone is seeing the same thing. The generation of this consensus, in turn, was premised upon the disciplining of the experimental community, that is the standardisation of the experiment itself as well as the ways of seeing. When 'Western' science and its oculo-centric ways of knowing were disseminated, therefore, it was not simply visual demonstration that was privileged. The eye of the seeing subject or experimentalist was also carefully trained and guided. Shigehisa Kuriyama's fascinating account of anatomical viewing amongst Japanese doctors amply illustrates that what distinguished older and new forms of anatomical knowledge in Japan was not so much cadaveric dissections per se, but rather what the dissector observed.[27] I would argue that Ray's detailed descriptions of do-at-home experiments were, in essence, attempts to disseminate a culture of visually anchored knowledge based upon standardised ways of seeing.

This experimental imperative, not to mention the actual experiments and demonstrations being recommended, was utterly new to Ayurveda but it seemed to be at the heart of the attitude that Ray thought necessary for the nineteenth century.[28] Ray was attempting not only to establish a novel, experimental basis of Ayurvedic knowledge, but also to create a community of experimentalists in the process. In an interesting early essay, Ray framed his new curiosity and quest for visual proof in terms of a generational difference in orientation. Structured as a dialogue between Ray and his aged grandfather around the chemical explanation of combustion, Ray repeatedly depicted his grandfather as lacking the curiosity to ask further questions. The grandfather seemed happy with the simple fact that the lamp stops burning when the oil runs dry, but deemed it foolish to ask why this should happen. Ray, on the other hand, urged his grandfather to ask more questions, while the latter feared that Ray was losing his mind. At one point in the exchange, the eponymous grandfather asked how Ray proposed to answer such absurd questions. Ray replied, 'We will ask nature (*prakriti*)'. Suitably taken aback, the grandfather asked again, 'And where will you find her?' 'I shall bring her here, into this room', explained Ray.[29]

There were a series of assumptions here about 'nature' as a discrete, rule-bound entity, about the ability to probe this 'nature' by way of experimentation, and of course, the alleged transparency of the meaning of these experiments. Carolyn Merchant argues that though the European idea of 'nature' as a discrete, frequently feminised, entity had roots in classical antiquity, it underwent one of the several crucial mutations at the end of the nineteenth century. An idea of 'nature' based on pure, idealised Forms, at this time, began to give way to a more 'materialist, process-oriented perspective'.[30] Whereas the idealised Forms derived their perfection from the Supreme Deity, the new natural laws were immanent in the regularity of the materialist world of nature. Rather than being plainly visible, they had to be made visible. Ray's dialogues sought to import this new, process-oriented, materialist nature into Ayurvedic thinking. By deploying the word *prakriti*, however, he also sought to braid this new idea of 'nature' with older notions of the cosmos available in Indic philosophies.

Being sensitive to this explicit recalibration of 'nature' by Ray is particularly important in view of Eduardo Viveiros de Castro's recent call to replace 'multi-culturalist' analysis – where nature remains ahistorical and universal and yet defined exclusively by the modern West – with a robust 'multi-naturalism' that acknowledges the different, historically specific ways in which people across the globe mobilised a sense of 'nature'.[31] As Ray made it clear through his trope of generational conflict, his 'nature' was a new one. It was this new 'nature' and its practical enactment that was constitutive of the modern present of the nineteenth century. Ray and his grandfather were clearly reified tropes standing in for 'tradition' and 'modernity', which, in turn, were themselves undergirded by distinct notions of the natural.

These themes were further elaborated in an essay Ray wrote in the third year of his journal *Chikitshak* on the scientificity of Ayurveda.[32] He mocked those who declared that Ayurveda was unscientific by saying that, when the ancient Aryan seers had composed the fundamentals of Ayurveda, those who now boast of science and claim to teach it to others (i.e. the British) had not even learnt to build the foundations of houses. The wisdom of such antiquity, he urged, ought not to be thrown away without some consideration. Notwithstanding the rhetorical broadside against the British, Ray's plea for the respect of tradition seemed almost to be in the vein of asking for some consideration for an aged grandfather.

This was not all. Having thus pleaded for age being given its due respect, he then advanced a more systematic case for considering Ayurveda to be scientific. He asserted that anyone with a truly scientific mind investigates everything before passing judgement. Thus Newton, he argued, had been able to connect the falling of the fruit with gravity because he was both observant and possessed an inquiring mind. Upon investigation, he further declared that medicine is universally focused upon six objects: 1) place (in the sense of soil); 2) time (in the sense of seasons); 3) patient (in the sense of constitutions); 4) materia medica; 5) air; and 6) water.

Ray's proposal of this six-fold classification bears some clarification. It seems to superficially resemble the robust Hippocratic tradition of *Airs, Waters, and Places*.[33] Here, it is also worth recalling that such an 'ecological theme' was also available in classical Ayurvedic texts.[34] What Ray was saying, however, was quite distinct from both of these. Summing up the Hippocratic tradition, at least in its medieval and early modern form in Europe, Andrew Wear points out that, a 'central assumption in *Airs, Waters, Places* is that there is a causal connection between a place, including its climate, season, water, and food, and the people born into it'.[35] Ray, by contrast, neither posits a fixed causal connection between place and the temperament, nor indeed does he insist that native-born people are the only ones whose health is shaped by their milieu. Ray's point was simply that medicine universally has six objects of enquiry.

Moreover, the link that connected all these six objects of medicine, according to Ray, was the Ayurvedic *doshas*. In subsequent sections we shall see why *doshas* are distinct from the Hippocratic notion of humours. This, in turn, will introduce another level of distinction between the superficially similar *Airs, Waters, Places* tradition and Ray's position. Though, here again, it is worth pointing out that Ray's version of the *doshas* was not identical to the classical *doshas* found in Sanskrit texts. Ray in fact, glossed his description of the three *doshas* as 'nervous influence' or 'electricity', 'body heat', and 'lymph'. This is again something I shall discuss more fully later, but for now it is worth noting the distinctive idea of *doshas*, transcreated by braiding together classical

Ayurvedic definitions with concepts such as electricity drawn from the nineteenth-century 'Western' scientific tradition.

Ray's argument, therefore, had two basic propositions. First, that medicine everywhere was defined by its attention to six objects of study, and Ayurveda did in fact focus on these six objects. Second, that in order to be scientific, any medical tradition had to explore these six objects systematically through an experimental framework. Again, he argued, Ayurveda had done this for longer than any other therapeutic tradition. Hence, he posited that Ayurveda was eminently scientific. In so doing, of course, he also subtly repositioned Ayurveda itself. He inserted into the Ayurvedic framework a new experimental orientation premised on observation and demonstration and linked it to late Victorian ideas of 'natural laws'. The new 'Ayurvedic nature' that emerged through Ray's braiding of Indic and Western ideas was a distinctive one. Just as it differed from classical Ayurvedic understandings of reality through its emphasis upon the experimental and the demonstrable, as well as its refractions through notions of electricity, lymph etc., it differed also from contemporary Western ideas by insisting on the three *doshas* as the basis of all reality. This latter insistence, in turn, as I will show later, pushed Western notions such as 'lymph' to acquire entirely new meanings as a heat-storing substance immersed in the blood.

The reticulated body

In 1908, Ray's versified text depicted the Ayurvedic body he had been describing in prose in his journal nearly twenty years earlier. This is what he wrote:

> Bayu Pitto Koph name dhatu tin jon,
> Jibdehe thaki' kore tahare dharon.
> Tripodi upore jotha thake drobyochoy,
> Todrup dehoti thake koriya ashroy.
> Morttyodhame shantiram telegraph jotha,
> Jei shoktite songbad bohe jotha totha.
> Temni tarit-shokti ache norodehe,
> Tahari bayu naam ayurbede kohe.
> Snayusutro ache dehe tarer soman,
> Tarit tahate – shanti, kore obosthan.

Mostishko janibe ta'r aphis prodhan,
Odhin aphis ache bohu-poriman.
Jalsomo dehe snayu royechhe beriya,
Tarit tahate ache dehoti dhoriya.
Tariter poriman kom beshi hole,
Songbader karjyo nahi somobhabe chole.
Dehete tarit jodi kom beshi hoye,
Karjyobighno ho'ye rog koribe ashroy.
Reler koler gari thanda jotokkhon,
Mritobot eksthane thake totokkhon.
Jol-ognijoge ushno hoibe jokhon,
Hoibe shojib dekho kolti tokhon.
Ognir obhabe thanda mritosomo ro'be,
Shojibota-bhab ta'r kotha cho'le ja'be.
Temni manob-deho ushno jotokkhon,
Shojib shey deho, shanti, thake totokkhon.
Roktomajhe ek drobyo diyachhi rakhiya,
Tahatei tap shoda rakhi'chhe dhoriya.
Bohiya shey tap rokto shorbottro chhoraye,
Tahate ushnota dehe shomobhabe boye.
Je drobyo roktete thaki' tap dhori' rakhe,
Ayurbbed-mote, shanti, pitto bole ta'ke.[36]

[Vayu, Pitta, Kapha are the names of three people,/ Residing in the bodies of the living they bear it./ Just as objects are placed on a three-legged table/ So the body remains upon them./ Just as on earth, Shantiram there is the Telegraph,/ The power that bears news here and there/ Similar electric-power is in the human body/ Ayurveda tells us its name is Vayu./ Nerve-threads are in the body akin to wires/ In them, Shanti, resides electricity./ The Brain is its main office, this you ought to know,/ There are many subordinate offices./ A web-like nerve encircles the body,/ Electricity in it bears the body./ Should the electricity increase or decrease,/ The work of news does not function smoothly./ So long as the railway engine remains cold,/ It remains stationary like a corpse./ When it heats up on adding water and fire,/ See the machine comes alive then./ Lacking fire it remains cold as a corpse,/ Its liveliness will disappear./ Likewise so long as the human body is warm,/ It is alive, Shanti, only so long./ I have kept a substance in the blood,/ That is what stores heat at all times./ Flowing in the blood, the heat spreads everywhere,/ Thus the body remains uniformly hot./ This, Shanti, is called Pitta in Ayurveda.]

Ray's metaphors were surprisingly stable over the period of nearly two decades between his journal and his versified text. In 1890 he had described the Ayurvedic body along almost identical lines. In the very first issue of his journal he had stated that, 'All our present glory is down to the single theory that the Aryans had discovered long ago in the distant past ... That theory is *vayu, pitta*, and *kapha* the three *doshas*'.[37]

Having established the centrality of *vayu, pitta*, and *kapha*, he then went on to describe what these three entities were. In living bodies, he explained there was a 'white-coloured bunch of threads'. They emanate from the brain and the spine before branching into numerous branches and sub-branches and covering the entire body. These were called *snayus*.[38] *Vayu* was the 'force' or *shakti* in these thread-like *snayus*. Explaining this mechanism Ray wrote that, 'we notice when a telegraph wire lies on the ground it lacks the power to transmit messages. But when it is connected to an electricity-producing machine, then news can be transmitted by it. That is why we call the telegraph wires things made by electricity-conducting materials and not simply electricity'.[39] Furthermore, 'Just as we have described the *snayus* as the pathway for electricity, so we will dub blood the conductor of heat'.[40] Explaining the importance of body heat, Ray wrote, 'The railway engine runs so long as it is hot, not when it goes cold. Our body is exactly like the railway engine'.[41] The description is almost identical to the one he versified eighteen year later in the 1908 text. In these descriptions heat is *pitta* and it is something akin to, but not identical to, electricity. It is the vital essence in the body.

Laura Otis has pointed out that railways and the telegraphs were frequently used as metaphors that allowed the worlds of physics and physiology to be connected.[42] Here we notice a third partner joining the duo in the form of Ayurveda. These metaphors in Ray's writings functioned to create a three-way connection between physics, physiology, and Ayurveda. Thus not only was electricity rendered as a force within the body, hence bridging the worlds of physics and physiology, but was also aligned with the Ayurvedic idea of *vayu*. Likewise, the heat of physics and the blood of physiology had to further induct the *pitta* of Ayurveda into their tightly knit families.

By thus redefining Ayurvedic ideas in terms of ideas from physics and physiology, a new Ayurvedic body was being crafted. This new body was essentially a reticulated body, crisscrossed throughout by *snayus* through which *vayu*-electricity and *pitta*-heat submerged in blood were constantly circulated. The newness of this body can only be fully appreciated once we compare it to earlier Ayurvedic bodies.

This is easier said than done. Two initial problems impede any efforts at clear comparison with earlier Ayurvedic bodies. First, Ayurveda is almost unique amongst the classical medical traditions of the world in not having developed a significant tradition of visually representing the body.[43] Second, from what we know about medical education in precolonial Bengal (which is the region Ray came from), for centuries – if not millennia – erudite Kabirajes seemed to have studied compilations based on the older canonical texts rather than the canons themselves. These compilations, of which Madhavakara's *Rogavinishchaya* was the best regarded, were organised according to diseases and gave no single crisp definition of the three *doshas*, namely, *vayu*, *pitta*, and *kapha*.[44]

If we look back to the core Ayurvedic canon with these caveats in mind, we find in the *Charaka-samhita*, the oldest and most canonical of Ayurvedic works, multiple, fairly distinctive meanings for each of the three *doshas*. The chapter on *vayu*, for instance, is framed as a conference of sages where different sages offer distinct definitions of *vayu* without contradicting each other. Thus one sage describes *vayu* as 'Rough, light, great, cold, sharp, and elaborate – these are the six normal qualities of Vayu'. A second sage, without in any way contradicting the former, has this to offer: 'The Lord Vayu is the primal cause of creation, the cause for the rise and demise of the mortal and immortal, he is the dispenser of joys and sorrows, he is death, he is Yama, he is the controller, he is the father of his subjects'.[45] The chapter makes no attempt to reconcile these two positions. Both definitions, along with others, are equally valid. This polysemy allows both substantive and deific meanings of *vayu* to co-exist. It is both a specific 'moribific entity', to use a term coined by Sanskritist G. Jan Meulenbeld, as well as a deity. It was this polysemy and the agentive/deified set of meanings that Maitreya was deploying when, to Ray's mild vexation, he insisted that *pitta*, another one of the *doshas*, was actually the god Brahma.[46]

Another aspect of premodern discussions of *doshas* was that, unlike the humours of classical Greek medicine, each of the three *doshas* had their own particular 'seats' or *doshasthanas*. Thus *vayu* is generally localised in the large intestine, *pitta* in the navel, and *kapha* in the chest.[47] Pathogenesis was not merely the result of increase or decrease of *doshas* but rather their displacement. The *Madhukosha*, a famous premodern commentary on the *Rogavinishchaya*, thus states that, 'when a [*dosha*] that maintains its proper measure is dragged away from its receptacle by the wind and moved to another seat, it generates even if maintaining its proper measure, a morbid alteration.'[48]

Finally, the *doshas* themselves are not monolithic, homogenous entities. Each of the three, *vayu*, *pitta*, and *kapha*, are internally differentiated by location and function into five subordinate types.[49] In some cases even the direction of their movement, that is, upward, downward, or lateral, is taken into consideration.[50]

Premodern ideas about *doshas* therefore had three significant aspects that I have highlighted here. First, they existed on a spectrum between being deified/agentive and substantive things in the body. Second, while they were capable of motion, they had very specific seats in the body. Finally, they were not homogenous entities. Their translation as either electricity or heat elided all these meanings and rendered them into fluid energies cognisable by Western physics and physiology. In so doing it also homogenised and rationalised the space inside the body. Instead of being an internally variegated and, one might say, 'suprarational' space where deities could reside, it was rendered into a mundane and uniform space organised around a reticulated network of *snayus*.

These *snayus* themselves are no less interesting. In Ray's writings they acquired a strong resemblance to nineteenth-century ideas about nerves. Sanskrit scholar Dominik Wujastyk points out, however, that 'Faced with the word *snayu*, one is virtually obliged to use its English cognate term "sinew". But the *snayus* seem sometimes to refer to what are today called nerves rather than to sinews or tendons.'[51] Ray's translation then, while not entirely wrong, is at best a partial reading. Structures that could simultaneously be sinews, tendons, or nerves are certainly different from what nineteenth-century physiology described as 'nerves'.

Elsewhere I have described the image of the body crafted by Ray and his contemporaries as a *Snayubik Man*.[52] I think of such images as 'physiograms', that is, 'materialized physiologies' or 'middle-level inchoate generalities (about the body) embedded in everyday forms of medical practice'.[53] In Ray's repeated descriptions of the workings of the body we catch a glimpse of this physiogram of the *Snayubik Man*. The reticulated and rationalised physiological space it occupied had been fashioned out of a three-way exchange between physics, physiology, and Ayurveda through the shared metaphors of the railway and the telegraph.

The *Snayubik Man*

Interestingly, the *Snayubik Man*'s fluid, undifferentiated energies did not last long in practice. Long-entrenched Ayurvedic belief in the internal subdivisions of the *doshas* re-emerged in Ray's writings, thereby complicating, if not undermining, his metaphors of electricity and heat. Yet these subdivisions did not re-emerge in their classical form. They, too, acquired new locations and functions.

Pitta, which Ray had equated with heat, is a good example of the new subdivisions within the *Snayubik Man*. According to the *Susruta Samhita*, the second oldest Ayurvedic treatise, *pitta* has five subtypes, namely, *pachaka-pitta* situated between the *pakkashaya* (stomach) and the *amashaya* (mucous receptacle in the belly), *ranjaka-pitta* located in the liver and spleen, *sadhaka-pitta* located in the heart, *alochaka-pitta* located in the eyes, and *bhrajaka-pitta* located in the skin.[54] Ray's description of the location of these five subtypes of *pitta* was different. He located *pachaka-pitta* in the gall bladder, *ranjaka-pitta* in the liver and spleen, *alochaka-pitta* in 'that part of the brain (*mastishka*) which is known as the optic thalamus', *aadhaka-pitta* in the brain (*mastishka*) more generally, and *bhrajaka-pitta* on the surface of the skin.

There is clearly a general tendency in Ray to map the location of the five types of *pittas* onto a biomedical anatomic space. While preserving a broad locational symmetry, he therefore tries to be more bio-anatomically specific. Instead of placing *pachaka-pitta* somewhere in between the *pakkashaya* and the *amashaya*, he located it precisely in the gall bladder. Similarly, in the case of *bhrajaka-pitta* he located it specifically on the surface of the skin. But in some cases Ray's attempts to find precise bio-anatomical correlates led him to radically alter the original location. Thus in the case of *alochaka-pitta*, he located it in the 'optical thalamus' – a bio-anatomic structure that made little sense in a classical Ayurvedic imagination of the body. What seems to have motivated him is his general reading of the Ayurvedic tradition to make this type of *pitta* responsible for visual cognition of form. Since the bio-anatomical body of Western medicine held that the actual act of visual cognition took place in the brain and not the eyes themselves, he had to relocate *alochaka-pitta* from the eyes to the optic thalamus. Even more dramatically, but motivated undoubtedly by a similar quest to reconcile the bio-anatomic body with the Ayurvedic body, he located *sadhaka-pitta* away from the heart and in the brain.

These relocations are significant in themselves. By depriving the eyes and the heart of cognitive functions and by consolidating these cognitive actions in the brain, Ray affected a significant shift in Ayurvedic anatomy. The 'mind' in Ayurveda had never been exclusively identified with the brain. As the *Charaka-samhita* stated, 'The mental faculty is indeed independently produced. It is what binds the life together with the experiencing body, and just before it departs, its behaviour alters, affection mutates, all the senses suffer, strength drains away, and diseases wax strong.'[55] It continues further that, it is this mind that is the apprehender of the senses. Clearly then, the act of cognition is not located in the brain, but rather in this independent mental faculty.

In fact, the close identification of the self with the mind, and the mind with the brain, is novel even within the Western tradition. Regarding this ascendancy of the brain as the prime location of selfhood under modernity, Fernando Vidal has dubbed it 'brainhood'. Vidal argues that the 'cerebral subject' was an anthropological figure inherent in modernity and one that ideologically motivated much of modern neuroscientific research, rather than emerging from such research.[56] Clearly, Ray was being driven by the same ideological propensities that were inspiring the emergence of Western 'brainhood' precisely at this time.

Yet, what is interesting is that this emergent brainhood in Ray is disrupted and left inchoate by his insistence of the circulatory nature of *pitta*. If *alochaka-* or *sadhaka-pitta* were the quintessential cognitive forces, their location in the brain must be balanced with their understanding as a form of 'heat' that can flow throughout the body. There was thus a fundamental contradiction in the *Snayubik Man* between its cerebral subjectivity that resonated with contemporary Western explorations in neurology and the more holistic subjectivity engendered in the hydraulic metaphors of electricity and heat.

The *Snayubik Man* was in effect pulled in two different directions. On the one hand, there was a bodily imagination that was clearly centred on the brain. On the other hand, there was an image of the body that was circulatory and did not privilege any one part over another.

Neither of these two possible imaginations had been available in this form in classical Ayurveda. They had both emerged through Ray's tryst with modernity. The fluid metaphors he drew from the physical sciences were as modern as the brainhood. But yoked together they did not always work in unison. As a result the *Snayubik Man* was an unstable, effervescent entity constituted in the cauldron of two opposing tendencies.

The contradictory pulls engendered in the *Snayubik Man* are clearly noticeable in the visual representations of the modern Ayurvedic body. While a familiar Western image of the circulatory system was progressively incorporated into modern Ayurvedic texts, these images conspicuously lacked a discrete brain, showing only a tangle of nerves in the skull, whereas the Western templates they were drawn from invariably possessed a distinct brain.

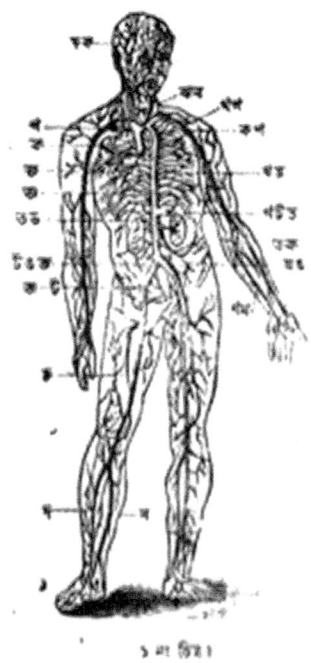

Figure 9.1 Nagendranath Sengupta, *Sachitra Susruta Samhita*.

From physiograms to cosmograms 235

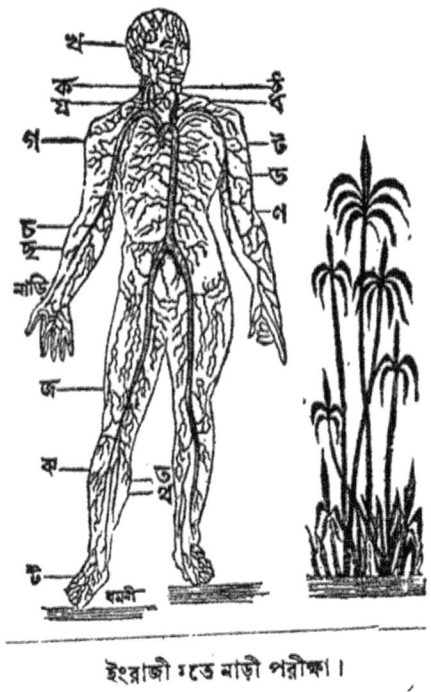

Figure 9.2 Gopalchandra Sengupta, *Ayurveda Samgraha* (Calcutta, 1871).

Experience and metaphors

By the time Ray began writing, the 'kinship of nineteenth-century physics and physiology' was well established through such eminent authors as Hermann von Helmholtz.[57] This kinship was engendered in a constant flow of metaphors, and a host of leading European scientists of the nineteenth century used the same metaphors of electricity, telegraphs, railways, and so on that Ray deployed. It was highly likely then that Ray himself had merely stumbled upon these metaphors in the course of his *daktari* education and redeployed them. Such a purely textual genealogy of Ray metaphors, however, would be misleading. Even if he had indeed picked up these metaphors from his readings in

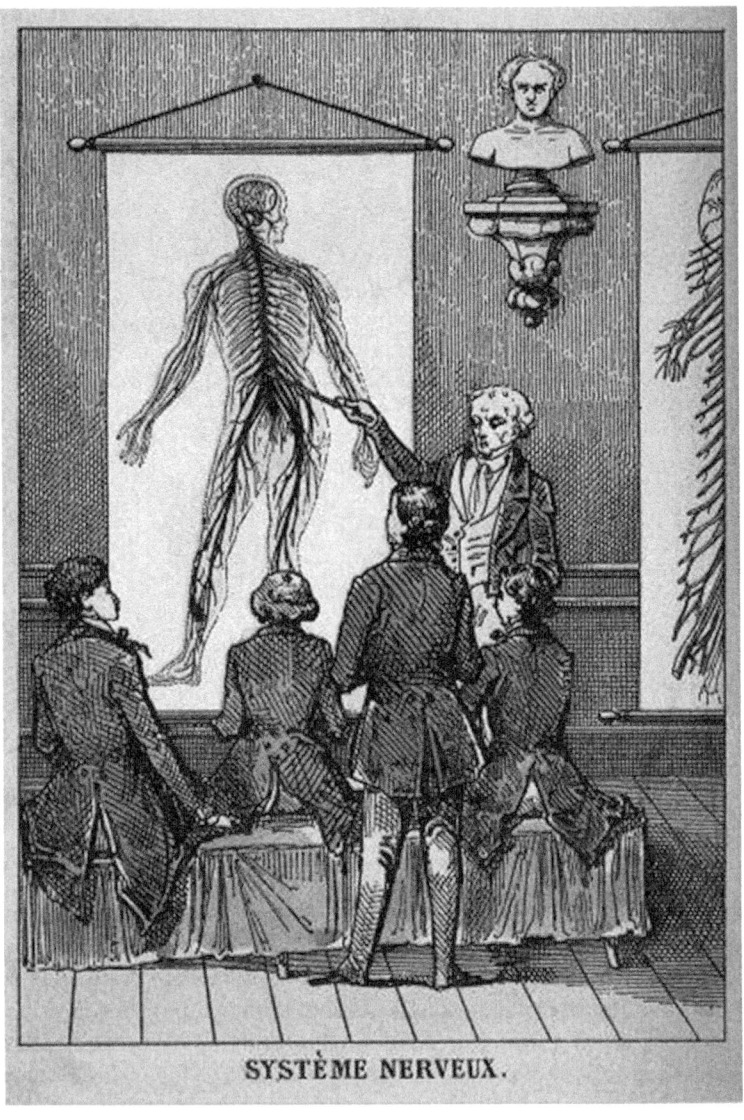

Figure 9.3 Lecture on the Nervous System from 1860. Wellcome Images.

Western scientific literature, how he used them was shaped by his own experiences of the material realties of colonial infrastructure.

Railways had been introduced in Bengal in the early 1850s and were quite well established by the 1890s.[58] After 1870, precisely the time when Ray was growing up, the railways began to grow at an exponential rate. Route mileage grew from a mere 4,771 in 1870 to 26,955 in 1905. Passenger traffic went up from 19,283,000 in 1871 to 231,283,000 in 1905.[59] The story of the telegraph system was broadly similar. After early experiments by the talented W. B. O'Shaughnessy in the 1830s, the first telegraph networks in India began to be built by 1851. By 1851, 4,000 miles of cables had been established in the major seats of British power. It was the great mutiny and rebellion of 1857 that spurred the British to speed up the building of telegraphic lines. Thus, within two years of the rebellion, and despite the damage done during that time, the mileage of telegraph lines had jumped to 11,000 by 1859. Like the railways, the telegraph had also been heartily embraced by the local people. In 1855 Kalidas Maitra, a Bengali intellectual, penned the first Bengali book on telegraphy which also gave detailed explanations about electricity.[60]

Ironically, even as the usage of the railways and the telegraphs grew, most Hindu Bengalis, such as Ray, were barred from technical proximity with these technologies. Particularly after the rebellion of 1857, anxious to keep the channels of communications in the hands of social groups whose loyalty the imperialists felt more confident about, the British followed a deliberate policy of employing Eurasians in both the railways and the telegraphs.[61] The scope for men such as Ray to get closely acquainted with these technologies was therefore limited by official policy. They were only allowed to consume the services provided by these technologies, not work with them closely.

Ray therefore knew of these communication networks as a consumer, not as an operator. Yet these communication networks remained the only ways he could interact with electricity. Domestic electricity was still a long way off in the 1890s for most people, even in the capital city of Calcutta, not to mention the village of Talanda in Rajshahi where Ray was based. Moreover, the consumer's relationship with this kind of large technological system could never be as intimate as the relationship of users with smaller, everyday technologies.[62] As a result, when Ray turned the railways and the telegraph into metaphors, his usage was marked by his own distant and mediated experience of these technologies.

Two major features of Ray's metaphoric usage mark him off from European men of science who also deployed such metaphors. For Helmholtz, and most of the other Europeans interested in such metaphors, the metaphoric interest in networks, circuits, and electricity led putatively to actual experimentation. This concrete experimental ethos, in turn, progressively produced a sense of electricity as something measurable. Measurements of time became particularly important.[63] They began to ask questions about how long it took for bodily impulses to travel through the body or produce a reflex action, etc. None of this happened in Ray's case, despite his overt enthusiasm for conducting experiments.

Over the years, Ray, as we have seen above, carried out numerous experiments. But not one of them involved electricity. All his experiments were essentially chemical experiments involving gases and liquids or anatomical dissections of goats and rats. The mismatch between his experimental vigour and his broad-stroke, impressionistic description of the railways and telegraphs is a testament to how his own mediated experience of these technologies from afar influenced his thinking. As Otis points out with reference to Charles Babbage, 'The better one got to know machines, the better one understood the body and mind. Technology suggested not just what questions to ask about the nervous system but how to perform the experiments and what sort of answers one might expect to find.'[64]

In the absence of hands-on experience with the technologies, Ray's metaphors remained overly generalised. Otis has demonstrated with great acuity how Helmholtz's researches led not only him, but also Friedrich Nietzsche, to eventually evolve a new theory of knowledge itself as being metaphorical.[65] In Ray's case, none of this happened. But what did happen was rather surprising.

From physiograms to cosmograms

In 1908, the same year that he published his versified Ayurvedic text, Ray also published his first cosmological text. Over the subsequent decades he went on to publish three more such texts with the last volume appearing as late as 1941, when Ray would have been touching eighty. These books were audaciously ambitious works wherein Ray attempted to recover the history of those 'times of which there are no records'.

He himself divided the themes covered in these books into four broad areas: first, the mysteries of creation and the end of the world; second, the question of the origin of man and his early history until records could be found; third, the history of the planetary system and the cosmos; and finally, the history of the origin of language and writing. When he published the first of these books in 1908, he claimed that he had already been working single-mindedly on these themes for fourteen years. If this were true – and there is no reason to doubt him – it would probably explain why so little of his thinking on the body had changed between 1890 and 1908. It would also mean that he spent nearly forty-seven years – from around 1894 to 1941 – completely ignoring his medical interests and dwelling instead on these large cosmological issues.

Why did he do so? How were these interests connected? And why did he make no effort to connect the cosmological writings to his earlier medical ones? I argue that it was precisely because of the mediated, distant, and hands-off way in which he began to use the technological metaphors that led him down this track. Unlike men such as Helmholtz, for whom the metaphors led to experimentation and experimentation led to a theory of knowledge itself as being metaphorical, Ray's metaphorics led him down a very different path. Since he never experimented with his metaphors upon the human body, there was little that the body could reveal to him. His metaphorical deployments thus became completely one-way. He used the world to understand the body and not the other way around. Thus, to him, the world at large increasingly seemed to be the source of all knowledge and secrets. There was nothing to be learnt within the body that could not be fathomed without it. This was in stark contrast to the centrality that Ayurveda affords to the body in thinking about the cosmos.[66]

Similarly, whereas Helmholtz, and following him Nietzsche, began to move away from a strictly referential and denotative idea of knowledge precisely because they began to interrogate the workings of the mechanisms of perception itself, Ray once again went in the opposite direction. Not only did he not interrogate how perception worked, he increasingly arrived at a strongly positivist idea that knowledge was to be gained, as he put it, by 'breaking through metaphors and allegories'.[67] Repeatedly, Ray reiterated the need to 'break through metaphors and allegories' to 'reveal the true history of nature'. Reading widely and eclectically from the texts of Pierre-Simon Laplace to Charles Darwin on the one hand, and a wide array of religious literature from across the world ranging from the Zoroastrian Zend Avesta to the Christian Bible as well as the Quran and the Indic Vedas on the other, Ray pursued his key strategy of 'breaking metaphors'. The fascinating cosmology he arrived at through his strategy and his elaborate mathematical calculations are too rich and complex to unpack here. But it included, amongst other things, an ancient race of man-lions, an extremely dark-skinned Aryan race inhabiting the Arctic regions at a time when the rest of the planet was simply too hot to sustain life, a global climate change attended by large-scale migrations, life on the moon, and much else. He even attempted to start a new calendar which, according to him, would be pegged to the actual geological age of the earth.

This elaborate cosmology that Ray worked out throughout his life was, of course, not simply an aimless, benign, and apolitical set of musings. It was as political as his physiograms of the *Snayubik Man* had been. It was in fact a 'performative assertion, [an] entr[y] into debates, points of reference for further elaboration'.[68] It was, in other words, what John Tresch has called a 'cosmogram', a materialised cosmology that bore the political and historical imprint of the milieu in which it was created.[69] Throughout these cosmological texts Ray sought to reveal the validity of what he called 'ancient Aryan knowledge'. To do so, he repeatedly spoke of 'Nature' as an objective entity out there whose 'history' had to be revealed by the application of 'science' to break open the 'metaphors and allegories'. Yet, all that this 'science' eventually proved was the glory of the 'ancient Aryans'. But along the way it also completely recast traditions about those 'ancient Aryans'. The movement from the modern to the ancient and back to the modern – in a way that created an alternative modernity orthogonal to the hegemonic colonial modernity which also managed to heap glory on the ancient Aryans – was almost identical to how the *Snayubik Man* had been figured. The only difference was that Man, *Snayubik* or otherwise, had now disappeared in the mists of the cosmos.

What led from the alternately modern man to the differently modern cosmos were metaphors. In the absence of experimental possibilities, and with the body being rendered a mere screen upon which metaphors played out their stories, Ray had come to seek knowledge not through, but beyond metaphors. Metaphors would be what would then connect the knowledge back to the body. But the truth itself stood beyond the reach of the metaphors, and without the confines of the body, in the depths of the cosmos. This position also broke with the earlier pattern of his embrace of a late nineteenth-century European notion of 'nature' and 'natural laws'. Whereas the former had consistently included the human body as a crucial constitutive element, Ray's cosmological writings entirely abandoned it.

Whilst Ray's early medical writings are fairly representative of late Victorian trends in Bengali Ayurvedic circles,[70] his abandoning the body altogether in the pursuit of a new cosmology is highly quixotic. In their idiosyncratic singularity, however, they illuminate how an enthusiastic engagement with Victorian technologies, without the possibility of hands-on access to them, could lead Ayurvedic modernity away from the concrete practicalities of the body and towards purely speculative contemplation of the cosmos.

Distinctive modernities were not simply imaginal formations engendered by the creativity of particular intellectual agents. Neither distinctive intellectual inheritances nor the mere fact of geographic distance were in themselves sufficient to produce alternative medical modernities. They were developed within particular social, political and material contexts. In colonial Bengal it was these practical exigencies that shaped Ray's singular version of an Ayurvedic modernity. On the one hand the colonial state's need for cheap medical manpower created the educational institutions that acquainted him and numerous others like him with new ideologies of scientific medicine. At these institutions Ray and his peers imbibed new ideals of curiosity and observation and embraced new images of 'science' and 'nature'. Likewise, it was the colonial state's economic and political interests that produced the large technological infrastructures, such as the railways and the telegraph, which informed Ray's thinking. On the other hand though, the possibilities for conducting original medical research or gaining practical operative experience with technological equipment were severely limited for lowly Bengali VLMS doctors like Ray. They were neither encouraged to undertake such experiments nor given access to material resources to pursue experimental programmes that Western scientists of the day could pursue.

The colonial state had hoped that these doctors would imbibe a modicum of 'Western science' and then be happy to apply their training in the service of state in either a military or civil posting in the vast subcontinent hinterland. For the state, these were not really men of science. They were just a cheap fix for a large administrative responsibility. But men like Ray had other ambitions. As upper-caste men who had enjoyed social status through their links to precolonial traditions of learning, they saw themselves as unique inheritors of two distinct traditions of knowledge. It was their self-appointed task to compare, contrast, translate, and evaluate these two traditions to which they alone seemed to have access. Both the eponymous 'grandfather' and the ghostly figure of the 'Western scientists' who flitted through Ray's writings were limited to only one tradition. But as legatees to both traditions, Ray, and quite a few like him, saw themselves as distinct from either. The colonial state's diminutive sense of Ray's role and his own grandiose sense of purpose were hence constantly forced to rub against each other. His singular medical modernity was cooked in the cauldron of these contradictory material realities established by the colonial regime.

Medical historiography, like the colonial state before it, imagines a singular medical modernity because it imagines the non-West as a *tabula rasa* upon which Western scripts could be authored. As we see in Ray's case, however, the non-West was not an intellectual *tabula rasa*. The script of Western medicine had to be written upon the palimpsests that bore the distinct marks of earlier therapeutic traditions. The way historical agents such as Ray read these two scripts, one slightly fading and another still emergent, depended upon the social, political, and material context within which they encountered the therapeutic palimpsest.

Notes

1 J. Fabian, *Time and the Other: How Anthropology Makes its Object* (New York: Columbia University Press, 2014).

2 WHO, *Traditional Medicine Strategy: 2014–2023* (Geneva: WHO Press, 2013).
3 L. S. Jacyna, *Medicine and Modernism: A Biography of Henry Head* (London: Routledge, 2015).
4 W. Bynum, *The History of Medicine: A Very Short Introduction* (Oxford: Oxford University Press, 2008).
5 R. Cooter, 'Medicine and Modernity', in Mark Jackson (ed.), *The Oxford Handbook of the History of Medicine* (Oxford: Oxford University Press, 2011), 100–16.
6 S. N. Eisenstadt (ed.), *Multiple Modernities, Daedalus*, 129:1 (Winter 2000).
7 P. Chatterjee, *Our Modernity* (Rotterdam/Dakar: Sephis/Codesria, 1997).
8 D. Chakrabarty, *Provincializing Europe: Postcolonial Thought and Historical Difference* (Princeton, NJ: Princeton University Press, 2009).
9 There have been a number of recent works on the history of modern Ayurveda. The majority of these works, however, tend to focus on institutional changes. See for instance, K. Sivaramakrishnan, *Old Potions, New Bottles: Recasting Indigenous Medicine in Colonial Punjab (1850–1945)* (New Delhi: Orient Longman, 2006); R. Berger, *Ayurveda Made Modern: Political Histories of Indigenous Medicine in North India, 1900–1955* (Basingstoke: Palgrave Macmillan, 2013). My own work places more of a focus on epistemic shifts: see P. B. Mukharji, *Doctoring Traditions: Ayurveda, Small Technologies, and Braided Sciences* (Chicago: University of Chicago Press, 2016).
10 On Western medicine in colonial India, see D. Arnold, *Colonizing the Body: State Medicine and Epidemic Disease in Nineteenth-Century India* (Berkeley: University of California Press, 1993). On vernacularised Western medicine, see P. B. Mukharji, *Nationalizing the Body: The Medical Market, Print and Daktari Medicine* (London: Anthem Press, 2009).
11 On modern Unani medicine, see N. Quaiser, 'Politics, Culture and Colonialism: Unani's Debate with Doctory', in B. Pati and M. Harrison (eds), *Health, Medicine and Empire: Perspectives on Colonial India* (Hyderabad: Orient Longman, 2001), 317–55; S. Alavi, *Islam and Healing: Loss and Recovery of an Indo-Muslim Medical Tradition, 1600–1900* (Basingstoke: Palgrave Macmillan, 2008); G. N. A. Attewell, *Refiguring Unani Tibb: Plural Healing in Late Colonial India* (New Delhi: Orient Longman, 2007). On modern Siddha medicine, see G. J. Hausman, 'Siddhars, Alchemy and the Abyss of Tradition: "Traditional" Tamil Medical Knowledge in "Modern" Practice' (PhD dissertation, University of Michigan, 1996); R. S. Weiss, *Recipes for Immortality: Healing, Religion, and Community in South India* (Oxford: Oxford University Press, 2009). On modern Tibetan

medicine, see L. Pordié (ed.), *Tibetan Medicine in the Contemporary World: Global Politics of Medical Knowledge and Practice* (New York: Routledge, 2008).
12 On the contemporary global career of Ayurveda, see F. M. Smith and D. Wujastyk (eds), *Modern and Global Ayurveda: Pluralism and Paradigms* (Buffalo: SUNY Press, 2008). See also, J. S. Alter (ed.), *Asian Medicine and Globalization (Encounters in Asia)* (Philadelphia: University of Pennsylvania Press, 2005).
13 P. Hehir, *The Medical Profession in India* (London: H. Frowde and Hodder & Stoughton, 1923), 9–10.
14 B. Ray, 'Abataranika' [Inaugural Preface], *Chikitshak*, 1:1 (1296 BE), 2.
15 *Ibid.*, 2–3.
16 *Ibid.*, 4.
17 B. Ray, 'Vayu Pitta Kapha', *Chikitshak*, 1:1 (1296 BE), 5.
18 T. R. Trautmann, *Aryans and British India* (New Delhi: Yoda Press, 2004).
19 *Ibid.*, 6.
20 B. Ray, 'Sharir Kriya Bigyan', *Chikitshak*, 1:1 (1296 BE), 9–12.
21 Ray, 'Vayu Pitta Kapha', *Chikitshak*, 1:3 (1296 BE), 54.
22 B. Ray, 'Rasayan Bigyan', *Chikitshak*, 1:3 (1296 BE), 49–52.
23 Ray, 'Rasayan Bigyan', *Chikitshak*, 1:2 (1296 BE), 25–9.
24 B. Ray, 'Sharir Kriya Bigyan', *Chikitshak*, 1:2 (1296 BE), 56–60.
25 Ray, 'Sharir Kriya Bigyan', *Chikitshak*, 1:4 (1296 BE), 80–5.
26 S. Shapin and S. Schaffer, *Leviathan and the Air Pump: Hobbes, Boyle and the Experimental Life* (Princeton, NJ: Princeton University Press, 2011), 79.
27 S. Kuriyama, 'Between Mind and Eye: Japanese Anatomy in the Eighteenth Century', in C. Leslie and A. Young (eds), *Paths to Asian Medical Knowledge* (Berkeley: University of California Press, 1992), 21–43.
28 Though popular writing on Ayurveda often emphasises its demonstrative basis, this is generally a bid to align Ayurveda with hegemonic contemporary notions of objectivity and scientificity. The actual demonstrations and 'practice' mentioned in the classical Ayurvedic texts were quite distinctive. For a fuller discussion of this point see Mukharji, *Doctoring Traditions*.
29 Ray, 'Rasayan Bigyan', *Chikitshak*, 1:2 (1296 BE), 26–7.
30 C. Merchant, *Autonomous Nature: Problems of Prediction and Control from Ancient Times to the Scientific Revolution* (Abingdon: Routledge, 2006), 9–10.
31 E. V. De Castro, 'Cosmological deixis and Amerindian perspectivism', *Journal of the Royal Anthropological Institute*, 4:3 (1998), 469–88.
32 B. Ray, 'Ayurbbed Baigyanik?', *Chikitshak*, 3:3 (1306 BE), 41–6.
33 C. E. Rosenberg, 'Epilogue: airs, waters, places. A status report', *Bulletin of the History of Medicine*, 86:4 (2012), 661–70.

34 F. Zimmermann, *The Jungle and the Aroma of Meats: An Ecological Theme in Hindu Medicine* (Delhi: Motilal Banarsidass, 1999).
35 A. Wear, 'Place, health, and disease: the *air, water, places* tradition in early modern England and North America', *Journal of Medieval and Early Modern Studies*, 38:3 (2008), 443–65 (p. 444).
36 B. Ray, *Podyo Ayurbbed-Shikkha* (Calcutta: Leela Printing Works, 1315 BE), 7–8.
37 Ray, 'Vayu Pitta Kapha', *Chikitshak*, 1:1 (1296 BE), 6.
38 *Ibid.*, 7.
39 *Ibid.*, 9.
40 Ray, 'Vayu Pitta Kapha', *Chikitshak*, 1:4 (1296 BE), 78.
41 Ray, 'Sharir Kriya Bigyan', *Chikitshak*, 1:1 (1296 BE), 10.
42 L. Otis, *Networking: Communicating with Bodies and Machines in the Nineteenth Century* (Ann Arbor: University of Michigan Press, 2001).
43 D. Wujastyk, 'Interpreting the image of the human body in premodern India', *International Journal of Hindu Studies*, 13:2 (2009), 189–228 (p. 189).
44 G. J. Meulenbeld, *The Madhavanidana and its Chief Commentary* (Leiden: Brill, 1974).
45 S. Sharma, *Caraka-Samhita: Mul o Bonganubad* (Calcutta: Bhaisajya Steam Machine Jantra, 1904 [1311 BE]), 104–7.
46 Mukharji, *Doctoring Traditions*, 149.
47 D. Wujastyk (ed.), *The Roots of Ayurveda: Selections from Sanskrit Medical Writings* (New Delhi: Penguin Books, 2003), 30–1.
48 Meulenbeld, *Madhavanidana*, 38.
49 Wujastyk, *The Roots of Ayurveda*, 162–3.
50 Meulenbeld, *Madhavanidana*, 39.
51 Wujastyk, *The Roots of Ayurveda*, 37.
52 Mukharji, *Doctoring Traditions*, 117–56.
53 *Ibid.*, 8–11.
54 G. J. Meulenbeld, *The History of Indian Medical Literature* (Groningen: Egbert Forsten, 1999), vol. IA, p. 214.
55 Wujastyk, *The Roots of Ayurveda*, 99.
56 F. Vidal, 'Brainhood, anthropological figure of modernity', *History of the Human Sciences*, 22:1 (2009), 5–36.
57 Otis, *Networking*, 25.
58 I. J. Kerr, *Engines of Change: The Railroads that made India* (Westport, CA: Greenwood Publishing Group, 2007), 17.
59 *Ibid.*, 67.
60 D. K. Lahiri Choudhury, *Telegraphic Imperialism: Crisis and Panic in the Indian Empire, c. 1830–1920* (Basingstoke: Palgrave Macmillan, 2010).

61 L. G. Bear, 'Miscegenations of modernity: constructing European respectability and race in the Indian railway colony, 1857–1931', *Women's History Review*, 3:4 (1994), 531–48; Lahiri Choudhury, *Telegraphic Imperialism*, 118.
62 On small and everyday technologies, see D. Arnold, *Everyday Technology: Machines and the Making of India's Modernity* (Chicago: University of Chicago Press, 2013) and Mukharji, *Doctoring Traditions*.
63 Otis, *Networking*, 25–9.
64 *Ibid.*, 29
65 *Ibid.*, 46–8.
66 Zimmermann, *Jungle*.
67 B. Ray, *Srishti-Sthiti-Pralay-Tattwa* (Calcutta: India Press, 1911), p. i.
68 J. Tresch, 'Cosmologies Materialized: History of Science and History of Ideas', in Darrin M. McMahon and Samuel Moyn (eds), *Rethinking Modern European Intellectual History* (New York: Oxford University Press, 2014), 153–72 (p. 163).
69 J. Tresch, *The Romantic Machine: Utopian Science and Technology after Napoleon* (Chicago: University of Chicago Press, 2012).
70 Mukharji, *Doctoring Traditions*.

10

From Schenectady to Shanghai: Dr Williams' Pink Pills for Pale People and the hybrid pathways of Chinese modernity[1]

Alice Tsay

I don't suppose there is a proprietary medicine manufacturer of importance in any part of the world who has not, at one time or another, encouraged his imagination to play with the idea of the prosperous business he might build up, and the wealth he might accumulate, if he could, by some means, convince a reasonable number of Chinese of the efficiency of his remedies.[2]

Pills on the move

The American folk-singer Pete Seeger tells a story about a girl who falls ill and is prescribed Dr Johnson's Pink Pills for Pale People by the doctor. Her father makes up a silly song for her while on the phone and is overheard by the inquisitive telephone wire, which replicates and disseminates the song to all its 'friends' until the communications infrastructure becomes so noisy that no one can hold a proper conversation. The government eventually cuts down the telephone poles and wires, throwing them overboard far from shore. In the watery depths, however, the wires continue to resonate with the sounds of the song:

Pink pills for pale people,
Pink pills for pale people.
Pink pills, pink pills,
Pink pills for pale people.
Ha, ha, ha, ha, ha![3]

The story takes its inspiration from a widely distributed patent medicine called Dr Williams' Pink Pills for Pale People. Though Seeger turns it into a fable about the white noise of commercialism in modern society, the tale also suggests the ubiquity and pervasiveness of the product to which it alludes.

In real life, Dr Williams' Pink Pills for Pale People never languished in the sea but made it across several oceans. This chapter examines advertisements for the product in Chinese-language publications in Shanghai during the early twentieth century, comparing them to English-language advertisements printed in Shanghai, England, and the United States. Much like the telephone poles that refuse to be silenced, the long advertising history of Dr Williams' Pink Pills in Shanghai represents survival against the odds. In marked contrast to the endlessly repetitive underwater song that Seeger describes in his story, however, Dr Williams' Pharmaceutical Company created a range of culturally adaptive approaches to selling their product. Other Western brands in Shanghai favoured one of two marketing strategies: dropping their product unchanged into the new environment or attempting to fashion a market for new tastes. In contrast, the advertisements for Dr Williams' Pink Pills insisted on the particularities of their specific product while evoking a familiar psychical world for their Chinese consumers. Taking the extensive history of the pills into account thus complicates the accepted narrative of advertising as the major driving force of urban modernity in Shanghai and offers a more nuanced account of the way hybridity – not only cultural, but also temporal – was strategically mobilised to articulate a distinctly Chinese vision of twentieth-century society.[4]

Studies of advertising content in this historical and geographical setting have tended to focus on the development during this period of a multivalent visual culture that promoted an aspirational or fictive reality. Tani Barlow claims that the 'sexy girl iconography' in 1920s and 1930s Shanghai presents 'the fantasy of modern social life in the colonial modern arena' even through products as mundane as insect repellent.[5] In *Selling Happiness*, Ellen Johnston Laing similarly argues for the role of calendar posters in transforming the visual culture of Shanghai and normalising Western-style art for the Chinese public.[6] Along the same lines, Weipin Tsai contends that advertising in the newspaper *Shenbao* helped to produce the idealised image of the housewife as at once 'consumer, domestic, and patriot' in the new vision of liberated femininity that emerged after the 1915 New Culture Movement.[7] Even in case studies in which the advertising medium consists primarily of text, emphasis is placed on the construction of an ideological position: Susan Glosser's study of the Shanghai Dairy Association's marketing campaign for milk, for example, tracks how a product originally 'so foreign as to be literally indigestible' for most Chinese was recast 'as the key to China's success in the evolutionary struggle to survive'.[8] Such scholarly accounts frequently align modernity in China with Westernisation and progressiveness in ways that diminish the role of internal forces in influencing the social, economic, and ideological shifts that took place in China in the decades following the fall of the Qing Dynasty in 1912. While historians such as Samuel Y. Liang and Marie-Claire Bergère have identified the need for more nuanced accounts of Shanghainese and Chinese modernity, their works do not focus on advertising culture as an important site of cultural confluence.[9]

The case study of Dr Williams' Pink Pills for Pale People advertisements in Shanghai suggests that modernity in China emerged through a more complex negotiation between old and new, local and global, rather than arriving as a fully fledged cultural export from the West. These widely popular pills were marketed in Chinese-language publications in Shanghai from at least 1913 to 1941, and from even earlier in the *North China Herald*, an English-language newspaper that was also based in the city. While these Shanghainese advertisements employed the cutting-edge strategies of representation of the time, this progressiveness belies other aspects of the Pink Pills story, most notably its sustained reputation as backwards and outdated in the West. The forgotten Chinese afterlife of this derided patent pills opens up an alternate version of global modernity that develops along hybrid cultural and temporal pathways. Beyond calling into question the sequential connotations implicit in the language of modernity, the deeply site-specific sense of the modern self that emerges in this case study of early twentieth-century China suggests the need to decentralise the role of the West in the historical narrative of modernity. One localised modernity implies the existence of others, each unique in its configuration.

A chequered history

A discussion of the history of Dr Williams' Pink Pills for Pale People helps to contextualise the inroads it made in Shanghai. Formulated in

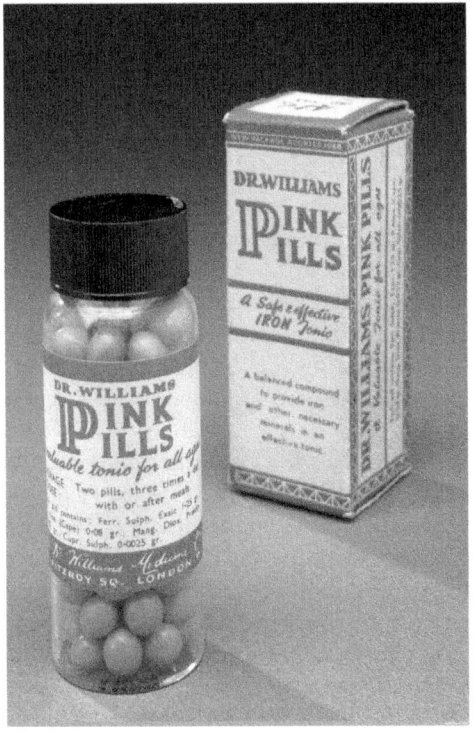

Figure 10.1 Dr Williams' Pink Pills for Pale People.

Canada by Dr William Frederick Jackson in 1886, the pills quickly spread to the United States.[10] Following the company's relocation from Ontario to Schenectady, New York, Dr Williams' Pink Pills were marketed extensively in England and around the world. By the early twentieth century, the product had been advertised in more than eighty countries.[11] A 1907 advertisement, for instance, listed branch offices in 'Rockville, Ont., London, Eng., Paris, France, Sidney [sic], N.S.W., Cape Town, South Africa, Bombay, India, Rio Janeiro, Brazil, Mexico City, Mex.'[12] George Fulford, who 'purchased Jackson's patent for the paltry sum of $53.01' in 1890,[13] reportedly amassed a fortune of over £1.6 million after just sixteen years of marketing the pills.[14] Though it had become an object of contempt and a symbol of quackery in England

and North America by the early twentieth century, the company existed until 1989.[15]

According to an 1899 *Illustrated London News* advertisement, Dr Williams' Pink Pills could cure a vast range of ills: anaemia, consumption, scrofula, rickets, fits, chronic erysipelas, bronchitis, lumbago, rheumatism, rheumatic gout, sciatica, eczema, paralysis, locomotor ataxy, neuralgia, St Vitus's Dance, and nervous headache.[16] This list of purported uses was not exhaustive, since other advertisements emphasised different sets of ailments. Another *Illustrated London News* advertisement from 1898, for example, claimed to have healed an ex-Royal Marines sergeant who had 'suffered more than most men in a lifetime' from myriad afflictions, among them 'disease of the lungs' and 'giddiness of the head'.[17] In short, Pink Pills were sold as a cure-all drug, adaptive to longtime medical concerns such as rickets as well as the proliferation of nineteenth-century anxieties about nervous systems gone awry.

Given these untempered claims to miraculous power, the actual efficacy of the pills should come as little surprise. Even as early as 1897, the brand had been dogged with accusations that its contents included harmful ingredients such as 'impure carbonate of iron, with a little arsenic, green copperas, and pearl ash'.[18] In March of 1902, the British publication *The Chemist and Druggist* published a virulent attack on Dr Williams' Pink Pills in the form of a coroner's inquest into the death of an unnamed cabdriver in an article appearing right before a piece entitled 'The Week's Poisonings'.[19] The results from pharmaceutical tests are less lurid, though not by much. Table 10.1 gives the results of a series of lab tests, reflecting the changes in the ingredients of the pills over the years.

In short, only the first formula seems wholly innocuous. Ferrous sulphate, listed as 'exsiccated iron sulphate' and 'iron sulphate' through the years, is an iron supplement.[20] According to the National Institutes of Health, however, the 80.99 milligrams present in the 1961 formula is nearly double what is now considered the tolerable upper intake level for adults, undermining the relative harmlessness of the caffeine and Vitamin B_1 (thiamine hydrochloride) it also contains.[21] The 1935 formula, which contains significantly smaller ferrous sulphate quantities, also contains manganese dioxide, used today in pyrotechnics and as a 'depolarizer in dry cell batteries', as well as copper sulphate, which

TABLE 10.1 Contents of Dr Williams' Pink Pills for Pale People

Formula, 1905		Formula, 1935		Formula, 1961	
Powdered liquorice	45.16%	Excipients	38.68%	Iron sulphate (exsiccated)	70.40%
		Iron sulphate	26.66%		
Iron sulphate (exsiccated)	24.19%	Sodium carbonate	26.66%	Caffeine citrate	28.17%
		Extract of gentian	3.33%	Manganese sulphate	0.01%
Anhydrous potassium carbonate	21.29%	Powdered aloes	2.66%		
		Manganese dioxide	1.77%	Copper sulphate	0.01%
Sugar	6.45%	Zinc phosphide	0.16%	Thiamine hydrochloride	0.01%
Magnesia	2.90%	Copper sulphate	0.08%		

Source: P. G. Homan, B. Hudson, and R. C. Rowe, *Popular Medicines: An Illustrated History* (London/Chicago: Pharmaceutical Press, 2008), 141–2.
Note: In the source, the formulas for the three years are each given in different units ('grains' in 1905, percentages in 1935, and milligrams in 1961) and have been standardised and listed in descending order in this table.

is toxic when ingested and used as a textile mordant and wood preservative.[22] In contrast, the earliest formula combined potassium carbonate and magnesia, both food additives, with a sugar- and liquorice-heavy mixture. While safe enough, this combination gives new force to the 1897 advertisement declaring, 'These are not like pills; they are like sweets'.[23]

In North America and Britain, the public tide had turned definitely against Dr Williams' Pink Pills by the first two decades of the twentieth century. Perhaps influenced by the many scathing pieces appearing in professional medical journals, the United States government seized large quantities of the pills in 1915 on grounds that the company had made 'false and fraudulent claims'.[24] While US advertisements subsequently worded their declarations more conservatively, the company was accused of continuing to make outrageous assertions in international advertisements over which the United States government held no jurisdiction.[25]

The divergence in advertising strategy across global markets was both more and less extreme than contemporary critics asserted, depending on the region being considered. In most foreign countries, Pink Pills advertisements aligned closely with their counterparts in England and the United States. However, the marketing of the pills in Shanghai – and in China more widely – presents an anomaly that suggests highly localised efforts to promote the products.

Foreign opportunities

While Dr Williams' Pharmaceutical Company sold its products in many global markets, its marketing history in Shanghai offers an unusual case in terms of timing, scale, and audience-specific strategy. Most foreign advertisements for the company appeared in the last decade of the nineteenth century and the first decade of the twentieth. This turn-of-the-century period roughly coincides with the company's heyday in North America and England but predates the widespread circulation of Pink Pills advertisements in Shanghai by several decades. For instance, in South Africa, the company trademarked the name by 1893 and was circulating advertisements in local publications such as the *Mafeking Mail and Protectorate Guardian* soon after.[26]

Additionally, the company generally focused on English-speaking audiences in these foreign territories, even in dual-language publications. While the South Africa-based *Mafeking Mail and Protectorate Guardian* was published in both English and Afrikaans, Dr Williams' advertisements only appeared in the English sections. The same was the case with the *Amrita Bazar Patrika*, a Bengali and English newspaper published in Calcutta. Many of these English advertisements were taken directly from Anglo-American publications and cited testimonies from England or the United States rather than drawing from a local customer base.

There were some foreign-language advertisements, but they were the exception rather than the rule. Between 1906 and 1907, three different Zulu advertisements for Dr Williams' Pink Pills ran in *Ilanga lase Natal*, a Cape Town-based newspaper that was the first Zulu newspaper. However, no more appeared in the publication thereafter. Spanish-language advertisements appeared on a greater scale around the turn of the century in a few South American publications, such as *El Comercio* in Peru and *Mercurio de Valparaiso* in Chile, but still in relatively limited numbers.[27] In comparison, as will be further discussed, the marketing of the pills in China established a scale of distribution and level of cultural tailoring that made it unique even within the global history of the company.

The belated but dramatic flourishing of Dr Williams' Pink Pills for Pale People in Shanghai suggests that the company's products can be read, in more ways than one, as holdovers from a bygone time. This interpretation even appeared in some contemporary accounts, including that of the North Carolinian agriculturalist and travel writer Clarence Hamilton Poe. After travelling through Asia from 1910 to 1911, Poe wrote angrily about a time in Shanghai when he discovered an advertisement for Dr Williams' Pink Pills for Pale People on the back of a religious newspaper. He interpreted this as a prime example of Western avarice preying on Chinese ignorance and vehemently criticised opportunists for 'coining the poor Chinaman's substantial shekels' using 'American patent medicines discredited at home by the growing intelligence of our people'.[28]

Poe's picture of the Chinese people trailing behind Americans in an ignorant past is undoubtedly problematic, part of a long Western tradition of mapping evolutionary progress onto cultural difference. More importantly within the context of this study, however, his comments situate the advertisements as temporally displaced. In Poe's reading, despite the contents of the patent medicine having been established as outmoded and inert, it continues to function as an active agent by 'coining' and conning Chinese citizens.

This case study seeks to examine the counterintuitive and continued pertinence of Dr Williams' Pink Pills in Shanghai long after the brand's obsolescence in other parts of the world. Advertisements for the pills in Shanghai combined hallmarks of their marketing in other parts of the world with a customised blend of references to longstanding healing traditions as well as modern Chinese culture. Questions of medical efficacy aside, these advertisements resist a linear and Western-centric account of modernity. Contemporary Chinese commentators anthropomorphically located the contributions of the West in the two figures of 'Mr Science' and 'Mr Democracy'. However, the study of modernity in early twentieth-century Shanghai must also account for 'Dr Williams' as a Western import that disrupts the narrative of unidirectional progress and influence. Instead, the extensive body of advertising for Dr

Williams' Pink Pills in Shanghai represents an archive of complex and occasionally contradictory negotiations of self and society during the first decades of the twentieth century in relation both to the outside world and to the past.

Pills for all people

In their initial encounters with Dr Williams' Pink Pills for Pale People, Chinese consumers would probably have been less mystified than by unfamiliar products like deodorant, powdered milk, or even porridge oats, which entered the market around the same time. A 1923 Quaker Oats advertisement had to assure consumers that it could be 'used in the same way as rice' (效用如米).[29] In contrast, the *wan* (丸) or pill form of medication dates back several centuries in China. Traditionally, a variety of medicinal powders were bound with water and honey, creating a round ball that was then covered with a protective wax coating.[30] Though there is no indication that Dr Williams' Medical Company revised the familiar 'ovoid' shape of its Pink Pills, they took other steps to ensure that their brand and product were appropriate for the intended audience.[31] In Chinese, 'Dr Williams' Pink Pills for Pale People' was translated as *Weilianshi Dayisheng Hongse Buwan* (韋廉士大醫生紅色補丸), or 'Doctor Weilianshi Red Supplement Pills'. Alliteration abandoned, the pink pills became red in name, a colour with greater cultural resonance and existing precedence in traditional medicine packaging.[32] During the Qing Dynasty, for instance, an apothecary company called He Ming Xing Tang (何明性堂) produced detoxifying *hong wan* (紅丸) or 'red pills' that appear to have been widely distributed.[33] Moreover, this Chinese name dropped the reference to being 'for Pale People' present in the English. Instead, the roundabout allusion to a sickly complexion was replaced in Chinese with an explicit declaration of the pills as *bu* (補), adopting the language of bodily nourishment and strengthening central to Chinese medicine.[34] In English advertisements for Dr Williams' Pink Pills, the frequent references to impure blood likely derived from the vestiges of belief in humoral theory.[35] Translated into the terms of Chinese corporal understanding, this was depicted as *xueqi chongying* (血氣充盈): sluggishness or thickness of the blood from problems with the circulation of *qi* (氣).[36] Incidentally, as a purported panacea, Dr Williams' Pink Pills were in a good position to fit the symptom-based rather than disease-based approach central to traditional Chinese medical treatment.[37] Sherman Cochran has argued, using the British-American Tobacco Company as his subject, that 'the transmission of culture was not simply a matter of an American business unilaterally exporting to China advertising that had been invented in America.'[38] In drawing on a long history of Chinese medicine, Dr Williams' Pharmaceutical Company fashioned implied lines of cultural transmission that ran not only between different places but also different times. On many levels, then, the Shanghai advertisements carefully situated the product as simultaneously new and known.

Available evidence suggests that Dr Williams' Pink Pills was a widely available and increasingly established product in Shanghai. While consumers always had the option of contacting the company directly with their orders, in the mid-1920s, the advertisements went from declaring that the pills could also be procured 'wherever Western medicines were sold' (凡經西藥者均有出售) to announcing that they were available 'at all pharmacies' (各藥局均有), a significantly wider claim.[39] By 1941, advertisements sent customers directly to the National Department of Health (國民政府衛生署) for their pills, suggesting integration into official distribution channels.[40] Given the beleaguered reputation of Pink Pills in North America and England, surely no one could have predicted the stamp of approval that Dr Williams' Pharmaceutical Company appears to have received in Shanghai from a governmental organisation whose focus on establishing public health and sanitation standards has been seen as a main component of developing modernity in China. The success of the product was particularly remarkable in the immediate wake of the New Culture and May Fourth Movements of the mid-1910s and 1920s, which reacted against both traditional Chinese culture and anything suggesting excessive imperialist influence, leading to a growing enthusiasm for *aiguo huo* (愛國貨), or patriotic products.[41] As a foreign product that had been familiarised through the form of traditional Chinese medicine, Dr Williams' Pink Pills should have been doubly pressured. It seems, however, that the pills' hybrid identity functioned as a strength rather than a liability.

Anatomy of an advertisement

For the most part, the complex cultural mixture underlying Chinese-language advertisements for Dr Williams' Pink Pills for Pale People were coded through a highly consistent set of content and formatting tropes. This happened despite the fact that they appeared in publications with a diverse range of orientations and intended audiences, including *Shenbao* (申報/*Shanghai News*), *Liang You Hua Bao* (良友畫報/*The Young Companion*), *Funü Zazhi* (婦女雜誌/*Ladies' Magazine*), and *Funü Shibao* (婦女時報/*Women's Eastern Times*). Excepting a few runs in *Liang You Hua Bao* in 1925, these advertisements tended not to be repeated within the same publication, suggesting that Dr Williams' Pharmaceutical Company had the financial means to hire a large staff to source and design new variations on their established patterns of layout and narration.

Chinese advertisements for the Pink Pills made use of personal testimonies as their main rhetorical technique, a practice that derived from overseas. In England and the United States, the earliest advertisements for the pills had sought to create an aura of objectivity around personal testimonies, framed in pseudo-investigative style. One *Ladies' Home Journal* advertisement, for example, had the following heading:

> An Illinois Miracle: A Case of Deep Interest to Women Everywhere: Saved Through a Casual Glance at a Newspaper – Weak, Pale, and in a Deplorable Condition when Relief Came – A Remarkable Narrative Carefully Investigated by a Dubuque Times Reporter.[42]

Other English-language advertisements for the Pink Pills in China replicate this textual encounter (i.e., 'a casual glance at a newspaper') that apparently brings about the 'Illinois miracle' mentioned above. For instance, the *North China Herald* of 18 January 1913 includes a two-column advertisement that narrates one Señora F. Palacio's recovery after 'a pamphlet telling of the many cures Dr Williams' Pink Pills have wrought' fortuitously arrives in her husband's post-box.[43] These advertisements emphasised authority derived from documentation (pamphlets, newspaper) or genre (investigative journalism) in order to legitimise their claims to the consumer.

In Chinese advertisements, this testimonial strategy was taken much further and given a slightly different focus. Antonia Finnane identifies a *Shenbao* advertisement from 1913 as featuring Madame Liu Pan, a Shanghainese sewing machine instructor.[44] Another *Shenbao* advertisement, which ran in April of 1915, includes two testimonies, one from Mr Cui Xiwu (崔錫鴻君), a clerk in the executive department of the

Ou-lu Company, and another by Mr Zhao Shaoqin (招少琴君) from the Guangdong Da Gong Bao news agency (Figure 10.2).[45] Advertisements for Pink Pills for Pale People in *Funü Shibao* included testimonies from 'the wife of Mr Ding Zhenzhi' (丁振之君之夫人) and 'the wife of Mr Liu Zhengxing' (劉振興君之夫人).[46] These lengthy personal testimonies were accompanied by woodcut portraits of the individuals. Explicitly labeled as *yüzhao* (玉照), or formal portraits, these images contributed to the cultural and personal specificity of the advertisements, particularly when compared to English-language advertisements that often used more generic imagery. Furthermore, with very few exceptions, the Chinese advertisements for Pink Pills always included a drawing of the packaging, most likely for promoting brand recognition, though this was often not included in advertisements in North America or England. In contrast to Chinese advertisements for companies like British American Tobacco, which initially featured 'illustrations to German fairy tales … American landscapes and American heroes like George Washington and Abraham Lincoln', Dr Williams' Pharmaceutical Company appears to have been early in adopting audience-specific advertising techniques in the Chinese market.[47]

Consequently, despite their heavy emphasis on text, Pink Pills advertisements in Shanghai tended to emphasise personal connection rather than written authority. A 1923 *Shenbao* advertisement, for example, alludes to a large populace who has 'confidence [in their product] from personal experience or the experiences of friends' (由其自己之經驗或由其友人之閱歷確知).[48] Similarly, multiple testimonials in *Liang You Hua Bao* refer to a friend (友人) who recommended the medicine to the sick man or woman.[49] Despite the obvious ironies of medium, the transference of knowledge was framed as happening not between text and person but between one person and another. This emphasis of word-of-mouth connection can be interpreted as a means of evoking the *guanxi* (關係), or interpersonal relationships, central to Chinese culture. This nuance marked a way in which the advertisements for Dr Williams' Pink Pills were more sophisticated than those for competing medicines, such as Sanatogen Tonic, which focused more directly on the product's properties.[50]

Framing the advertisement as a discourse among friends, family, and fellow Chinese nationals, moreover, may have allowed Dr Williams'

From Schenectady to Shanghai

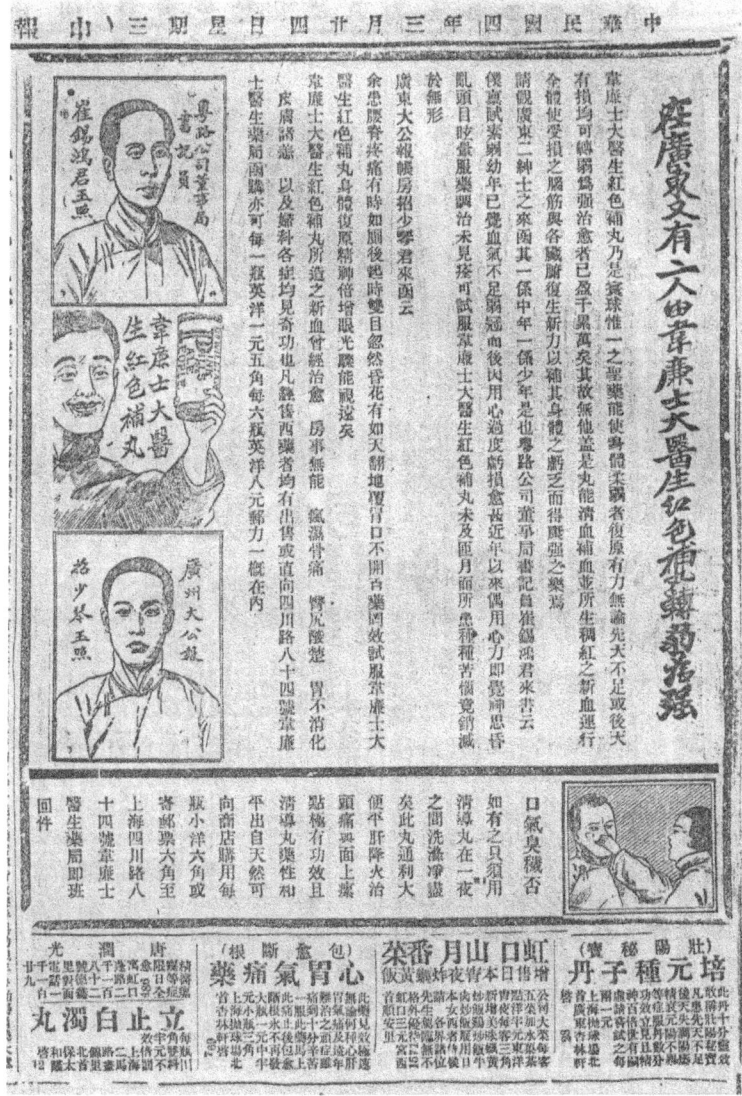

Figure 10.2 1915 *Shenbao* advertisement for Dr Williams' Pink Pills featuring testimonies from Mr Cui Xiwu (top) and Mr Zhao Shaoqin (bottom), 3 April 1915.

Pharmaceutical Company to circumvent anti-foreign sentiment by minimising the cross-cultural origins of their product. While the May Fourth movement of 1919 catalysed resistance to traditional Confucian values and rejected the veneration of the elderly, the emphasis in the media of the late 1920s that a modern housewife must also be a 'mother of good citizens' meant that a good deal of attention remained on the nuclear family, though now shifted to the younger generations.[51] The trend of pairing Pink Pills with other Dr Williams Pharmaceutical Company products in advertisements after the 1930s likely reflects this trend, particularly as Baby's Own Tablets were often the secondary product of choice. A *Liang You Hua Bao* issue in 1933, for instance, included an advertisement for both the Pink Pills and Baby's Own Tablets entitled 'The whole family of Mr. Wu Jinqing' (吳俊卿先生闔府), featuring a couple with their four children.[52] While the English-language advertisements for Dr Williams' Pharmaceutical Company hewed closely to the portraits of solitary suffering that seemed particularly symptomatic of the Western experience of modernity, these Chinese advertisements drew a wider orbit around the company's various products and the people who used them.

At the same time, these gestures towards new values were countered in the advertisements by features more closely associated with the traditional. Linguistically, the Chinese used in these advertisements appears not to be in *baihua* (白話), or the vernacular register that was gaining traction in writing during this time. Instead, Classical Chinese phrasing and textual markers give a formal inflection to the language. The previously mentioned 1923 *Shenbao* advertisement described its wisdom as 'coming from personal experience or those of friends' (由其自己之經驗或由其友人之閱歷), employing *zhi* (之) as a possessive marker. Similarly, *ye* (也) appears with some regularity at the end of sentences for emphasis, as do compressed four-word phrases. These features, along with highly formal diction throughout the body of these advertisements, suggest Classical language registers.

Similarly, while women were sometimes portrayed progressively as nation-building mothers, at other times they were shuffled out of the limelight, as in the case of a 1929 *Liang You Hua Bao* advertisement that includes a testimony about the wife of a certain Mr Fung.[53] In the text, he speaks on her behalf and refers to her using the phrase *neizhi*

(內子), a traditional term for 'wife' that men used when addressing outsiders, literally translating to 'the one inside'. Moreover, the Chinese advertisements appear not to target women, as the various English-language advertisements for Dr Williams' Pink Pills seemed to do. Barbara Mittler notes that advertisements directed toward women in *Shenbao* frequently used punctuation marks within the text – a newer writing style influenced by Western practices.[54] However the Chinese Pink Pills advertisements that have been found are written in continuous text blocks without punctuation, following the assumption in most traditional forms of Chinese writing – much akin to the practice of *scriptio continua* in Classical Latin and Greek – that the educated and predominantly male reader will automatically recognise clausal and sentence breaks without the need for spaces and punctuation. The media and advertising culture of early twentieth-century Shanghai certainly offered women a new prominence in the public sphere. Such visual prominence did not necessarily equal progressiveness, however, but could just as easily be employed to re-affirm rather than reform the old.

Tailored and culturally adept, the advertisements for Dr Williams' Pink Pills for Pale People in Shanghai represented extended and groundbreaking efforts by a Western company to inhabit the social and cultural world of its new audience. As the advertisements themselves show, however, this world was itself one of conflicting forces. The company's linguistic and cultural touchpoints often drew heavily on traditional visions of language, gender, medicine, and authority, even as the product's prominent commercialisation and implied association with the National Department of Health suggested that the company sought to push against many of these same traditional structures in order to take advantage of new systems for mass marketing and distribution.

Where she stands

One of the most striking illustrations of the complex position given to the Chinese subjects featured in advertising for Dr Williams' Pharmaceutical Company products appears not in newspaper advertising, which has been the main focus of this chapter, but in a 1922 *yuefenpai* (月份牌), a type of calendar poster that served as a major medium

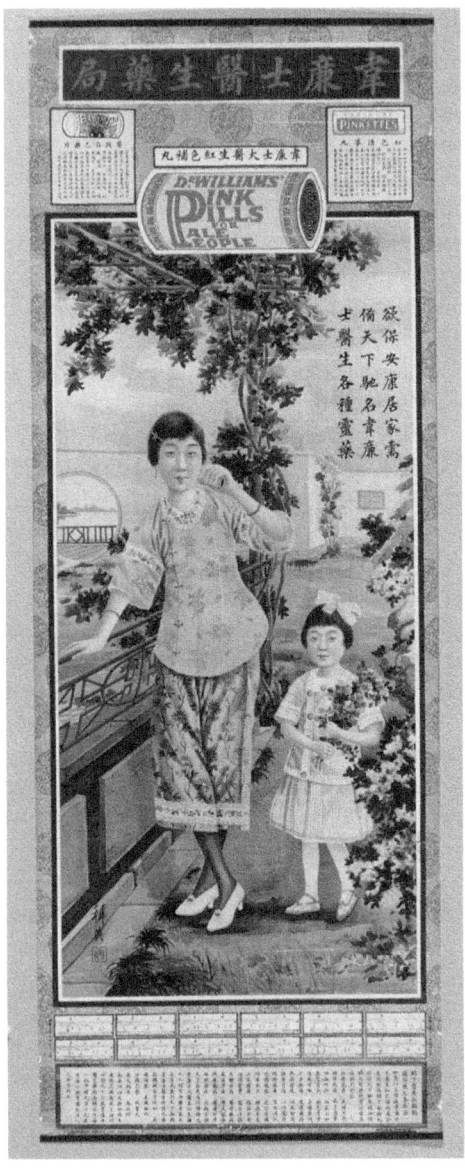

Figure 10.3 Dr Williams' yuefenpai poster designed by Hang Zhiying, 1922.

for advertisement in China during the early twentieth century (Figure 10.3). Designed by Chinese artist Hang Zhiying, this poster includes a prominent image of the Pink Pills for Pale People packaging, along with smaller inset images of two other products from Dr Williams' Pharmaceutical Company: Baby's Own Tablets, the infant supplement mentioned above, and Pinkette's, a laxative. In the image itself, a woman dressed in blue patterned silk stands next to a little girl in a Western-style pink outfit with a matching bow in her hair and Mary-Jane shoes. The woman appears to be wearing black silk stockings, which became popular among Chinese women during the 'sudden flurry of interest in Western fashions' following the 1911 Revolution.[55] She leans on an iron fence wrought with a Chinese-style design, but this fence is linked to an arbour of wisteria growing on a Western-style trellis. Thus, the picture ties together imagery from a wide range of origins, reflecting the cultural fluidity that was central to the lifestyles of Shanghai's privileged classes.

At the same time, this poster contains many hallmarks of the text-heavy print advertisements discussed earlier. The colophon text to the upper right of the image declares, 'To keep your family safe and healthy, you must be prepared with the world-renowned medicines of Dr Williams' (卻保安康居家需備天下馳名韋廉士醫生各種靈藥). The word used for 'medicines', interestingly, is *lingyao* (靈藥). While *ling* can mean 'highly effective', it also has connotations of the spiritual or magical. Another translation of *lingyao* could be 'miraculous cure', which would seem closer in emphasis to the *xiandan* (仙丹) or mystical elixirs of Chinese folklore than to Western medicine and scientific progress. Moreover, the image is not left to speak for itself, which may be wise considering that the woman portrayed looks fairly frail. Instead, it contains far more text than appears on the usual calendar girl poster, which sometimes includes only the brand name and company details. Located at the bottom of the calendar and in the two inset boxes at the top, these blocks of text anchor the calendar and prevent it from being a solely visual advertisement. The font is far too small to be taken in from a distance, and thus it forces the close reading encounter that was central to the early English advertisements of Dr Williams' Pink Pills for Pale People discussed earlier. Just as the clothing and surrounding of the figures in the advertisement reflect a complicated mixture of influences, the woman's stance seems to reflect the same ambiguous poise. Does she stand on her own two Western-shod feet, bolstered by the strength given to her by the packet of Pink Pills in her left hand? Or does her weight actually fall on a symbol of tradition, the elaborately wrought red fence? The semiotic space of this *yuefenpai* resists easy decoding, its sense of modernity signalled more through its fluid integration of varied cultural points of reference than in the fact that it is a Western product she clasps in her hand.

While the colourful, rich imagery of the *yuefenpai* stands out against the stark, black-and-white newspaper advertisements that were the main medium for Pink Pills advertisements, the indeterminacy of the calendar poster is highly characteristic of the brand's resistance to clean geographical and teleological narratives about cultural influence and historical progress. Spanning several decades, the advertisements for Dr Williams' Pink Pills in Shanghai clearly demonstrate how the transmission of a Western product resulted in the creation of culturally hybrid modes of expression and self-identification, producing a deftly accommodating visual and linguistic vocabulary. While excoriated and dismissed in Northern America and England, the product's counterintuitive survival in Shanghai seemed to lend truth – psychologically, if not medically – to its dubious claims of being everything to everyone. Moreover, the dexterous blend of cultural references found in these advertisements illuminate varied, oftentimes frictional forces that produced change and moulded selves in early twentieth-century Shanghai. In particular, for a port city that had been home to a significant foreign presence since the Opium Wars of the previous century, it is critical to emphasise that this hybridity represented not only inter-cultural but also intra-cultural confluences. The inhabitants of Shanghai could choose between an array of possibilities for self-definition, between being oriented toward the future and influenced by the past, between being conclusively 'Western' and adaptively 'Shanghainese'. In revealing the interwoven pathways of cultural influence defining early twentieth-century Shanghai, the unlikely revitalisation of Dr Williams' Pink Pills for Pale People in the international marketplace also demonstrates the need to recognise how socio-cultural changes taking place around the globe in this period produced heterogenous and localised versions of modernity that differed markedly from its emergence in the West. The marketers examined in this chapter figured this out and generated a rich body of work in response; it is now time for scholars to follow their lead.

Notes

1 I am grateful to Pär Cassel and David Porter for their comments on earlier versions of this chapter.
2 C. Crow, 'Pills for the Ills of China', in *Four Hundred Million Customers* (New York/London: 1937), 202.
3 P. Seeger and P. Dubois Jacobs, 'Pink Pills for Pale People', in *Pete Seeger's Storytelling Book* (San Diego/New York/London: Harcourt, 2000), 48.
4 Shanghai functioned as the centre for publishing and cultural production in Republican-era China (1912–49), a period coinciding with the timeframe covered here. This was true for publishing in both Chinese and English. As a result, a discussion of cultural production in China during this period, including the history of advertising, inevitably focuses on Shanghai. While the city is often seen as the locus of shifts and trends taking place in the nation more widely during this time, Shanghai's cultural influence permeated the nation's other provinces and cities to differing degrees. Thus, I have attempted to restrict my argument to Shanghai.
5 T. Barlow, 'Buying in: Advertising and the Sexy Modern Girl Icon in Shanghai in the 1920s and 1930s', in A. E. Weinbaum et al. (eds), *The Modern Girl around the World: Consumption, Modernity, and Globalization* (Durham, NC/London: Duke University Press, 2008), 288–319 (p. 289).
6 E. J. Laing, *Selling Happiness: Calendar Posters and Visual Culture in Early Twentieth-Century Shanghai* (Honolulu: University of Hawai'i Press, 2004), 1, 3.
7 W. Tsai, *Reading* Shenbao: *Nationalism, Consumerism and Individuality in China, 1919–37* (London: Palgrave Macmillan, 2010), 73.
8 S. Glosser, 'Milk for Health, Milk for Profit: Shanghai's Chinese Dairy Industry under Japanese Occupation', in S. Cochran (ed.), *Inventing Nanjing Road: Commercial Culture in Shanghai, 1900–1945* (Ithaca, NY: Cornell University Press, 1999), 207–33 (pp. 207, 209).
9 See Liang, *Mapping Modernity in Shanghai: Space, Gender, and Visual Culture in the Sojourner's City, 1853–98* (London: Routledge, 2010) and M.-C. Bergère, *Shanghai: China's Gateway to Modernity* (Stanford, CA: Stanford University Press, 2009).
10 Though the history of the pills makes it clear that they were named after the inventor's given name, even in late nineteenth-century advertisements, the product name is given as 'Dr Williams' Pink Pills for Pale People', punctuated as if based on a surname.

11 'Cool Things – Pink Pills for Pale People', Kansas Historical Society, n.d., www.kshs.org/kansapedia/pink-pills-for-pale-people/10240. Accessed 28 November 2016.
12 'W.T. Hanson Co. v. Collier et. Al', *The New York Supplement: Containing the Decisions of the Supreme and Lower Courts of Record of New York State. June 3–July 15, 1907*, vol. 104 (St Paul, MN: West Publishing Co., 1907), 792.
13 P. G. Homan, B. Hudson, and R. C. Rowe, *Popular Medicines: An Illustrated History* (London/Chicago: Pharmaceutical Press, 2008), 138.
14 L. Loeb, 'Doctors and patent medicines in modern Britain: professionalism and consumerism', *Albion: A Quarterly Journal Concerned with British Studies*, 33:3 (Autumn, 2001), 404–25 (p. 418 n.).
15 Homan et al., *Popular Medicines*, 142.
16 *Illustrated London News* 3118 (21 January 1899), 107.
17 *Illustrated London News* 3107 (5 November 1898), 685.
18 Australasian Medical Association, 'Public Health', *The Australasian Medical Gazette* (20 August 1897), 416.
19 'Mr. Braxton Hicks on Nostrums', *The Chemist and Druggist*, 60 (March 1902), 330.
20 United States Pharmacopeial Convention, *Food Chemicals Codex*, 7th edn (Rockville, MD: United States Pharmacopeial Convention, 2010), 402.
21 'Iron', *National Institutes of Health*, 7 December 2018, https://ods.od.nih.gov/factsheets/Iron-HealthProfessional/. Accessed 25 January 2019.
22 R. J. Lewis, Sr, *Hawley's Condensed Chemical Dictionary*, 15th edn (Chichester: Wiley, 2007), 336.
23 *Illustrated London News* 3107 (5 November 1898), 685.
24 American Medical Association, 'The propaganda for reform', *JAMA: Journal of the American Medical Association* (10 November 1917), 1638.
25 Ibid., 1637–8. Many British and American writers complained that the lack of direct legislation in England meant that patent medicine companies could continue making exaggerated claims.
26 A. F. Russell and P. S. Twentyman-Jones, 'Dr Williams Medicine Co. vs. Alexander', *Cases Decided in the Supreme Court of the Cape of Good Hope During the Year 1905*, vol. 22 (Cape Town: J. C. Juta & Co., 1907), 589.
27 These foreign-language advertisements did employ testimonies from local residents, but no artwork. As I will later discuss, visual images formed a central component of Chinese-language advertisements for Dr Williams' Pink Pills for Pale People.
28 C. H. Poe, *Where Half the World is Waking Up* (Garden City, NY: Doubleday, 1912), 135–6.
29 *Shenbao* 188 (26 February 1923), 1006.

30 S. Go, *Hong Kong Apothecary: A Visual History of Chinese Medicine Packaging* (New York: Princeton Architectural Press, 2003), 33.
31 The descriptive word comes from Homan et al., *Popular Medicines*, 140.
32 Go, *Hong Kong Apothecary*, 38. The other two colours are yellow and black.
33 Ibid., 35.
34 Dropping the phrase 'for Pale People' from the product name feels like a curious choice within a contemporary Chinese – and indeed broadly Asian – marketing context, in which beauty products often promise to *mei bai*, or beautify and whiten the skin. These associations of paleness with beauty and virtue run deep in East Asian history. 'In ancient China, Japan, and Korea', writes Lori L. Tharps, 'pale skin – besides being a prerequisite for beauty – was an indicator of elevated economic status for both men and women. In other words, dark skin was the marker of the peasant class, whose work kept them outdoors toiling under a hot sun.' However, within the original Anglo-American cultural context of Dr Williams' Pink Pills for Pale People, paleness was meant as shorthand for signifying illness. The largely iron-based pills were supposed to restore the flush of good health to the consumer. This misalignment of values was likely the reason why the Chinese translation of the product name made no mention of skin tone. See L. L. Tharps, *Same Family, Different Colors: Confronting Colorism in America's Diverse Families* (Boston: Beacon Press, 2016), 98.
35 See, as an example of this, *Illustrated London News* 3118 (January 1899), 107.
36 This language appears, for instance, in an advertisement in *Liang You Hua Bao* 5 (15 June 1926), 18.
37 Go, *Hong Kong Apothecary*, 8.
38 S. Cochran, 'Transnational Origins of Advertising in Early Twentieth-Century China', in S. Cochran (ed.), *Inventing Nanjing Road* (Ithaca, NY: Cornell University Press, 1999), 60.
39 See, for instance, *Shenbao* 133 (3 April 1915), 423 for an example of the former and *Liang You Hua Bao* 34 (January 1929), 36 for an example of the latter.
40 See *Liang You Hua Bao* 167 (June 1941), 27.
41 Bergère, *Shanghai: China's Gateway to Modernity*, 163.
42 *Ladies' Home Journal* 10:4 (March 1893), 35.
43 *North China Herald* (18 January 1913), 208.
44 A. Finnane, 'The Fashion Industry in Shanghai', in A. Finnane (ed.), *Changing Clothes in China: Fashion, History, Nation* (New York: Columbia University Press, 2008), 101–38 (p. 118).
45 *Shenbao* 380 (April 1915), 133.
46 See *Funü Shibao* 4 (1911), 6 and *Funü Shibao* 6 (1912), 6.

47 Laing, *Selling Happiness*, 30.
48 *Shenbao* 659 (February 1923), 188.
49 *Liang You Hua Bao* 5 (15 June 1926), 18; *Liang You Hua Bao* 34 (January 1929), 36.
50 Advertisements for these, for instance, appear in *Shenbao* 210 (1 March 1925), 8.
51 Tsai, *Reading* Shenbao, 101.
52 *Liang You Hua Bao* 74 (29 February 1933), n.p.
53 *Liang You Hua Bao* 34 (January 1929), 36.
54 B. Mittler, *A Newspaper for China?* (Cambridge, MA: Harvard University Asia Center, 2004), 262–3.
55 Finnane, *Changing Clothes in China*, 97.

11

Poisonous arrows and unsound minds: hysterical tetanus in the Victorian South Pacific

Daniel Simpson

When the Royal Navy sloop and flagship of the Australia Station HMS *Pearl* returned to Sydney harbour on 23 August 1875, it brought with it sad and disturbing news. On the journey home, three sailors, including the Station's popular and well-respected commodore, James Graham Goodenough, had died from wounds sustained a fortnight earlier at Nendö Island, part of the Santa Cruz group in the South Pacific Ocean. On 12 August, Goodenough and five members of his crew were shot with reputedly poisonous arrows following an unsuccessful attempt to interview Nendö people as part of their investigation into the Pacific Islands labour trade, which Goodenough considered a modern form of slavery. In an echo of the death of Captain James Cook almost one hundred years before, the men came under attack while fleeing the beach for the relative safety of the *Pearl*'s whaleboats, pursued by islanders who had long since grown wary of British intrusion. Diligently recorded by the *Pearl*'s surgeon, Adam Brunton Messer, the symptoms suffered by at least three of the wounded sailors were undoubtedly those of tetanus. Though the disease had long since been associated with open wounds and tropical climates, the tetanus bacterium *Clostridium tetani* had not yet been discovered; the poisonous arrows' power to tetanise their victims was therefore unexplained. This chapter explores how Messer subsequently utilised the ambiguous aetiology of tetanus in order to dispute claims that the arrows were poisonous and to argue instead that the sailors of the *Pearl* in reality suffered from a 'hysterical' form of the disease. In doing so, Messer imbricated mid-Victorian concern about stress and nervous breakdown with imperial efforts to 'civilise' the South Pacific. Sympathetic to missionary proselytisation in the region, and desirous to bolster the standing of the Medical Department of the Navy, Messer suggested that tetanus was most likely to occur in victims possessing a 'superstitious dread' of poisonous arrows. The social, physical, and mental health of the inhabitants of the Santa Cruz group, and of those who visited, were therefore said to be contingent upon the spread of Christian belief and modern medical understanding.

Only one year previously, Goodenough had sought to associate himself with Cook rather less literally by unveiling a memorial to the famous navigator at Randwick, in Sydney.[1] It was owing to the contemporary predominance of such conventions of 'naval hagiography' that the specific nature of the Santa Cruz poisons met with an initially uncritical reception.[2] The throng which greeted the *Pearl*'s unhappy return to Sydney in 1875 was more enthused by the opportunity to mourn its fallen commodore. Reporting a week later, the *Sydney Morning Herald* declined even to mention that poison had been involved.[3] Of greater significance to the crowd was the fact that Goodenough's party had been 'massacred', in further proof of the 'savage' and 'cruel' nature of a people who, four years before, had murdered the first bishop of Melanesia, John Coleridge Patteson, on nearby Nukapu.[4] The intensity of popular ill-feeling, helped along by reports of the failing missionary endeavour, occurred within a period otherwise distinguished, according to Jane Samson, by an emerging sense of 'imperial benevolence' in which 'Christian piety, public duty and particular constructions of race and culture' informed 'a powerful alliance between humanitarian activism and naval power'.[5] The clamour which surrounded the perceived martyrdom of the Royal Navy's 'strikingly modern' and Christian luminary thus underlined the dialectical and introspective nature of the much-championed humanitarian ethos; as with rumours of cannibalism, reports of poison were fleeting, vague, and requiring of little evidentiary support.[6]

Much of Messer's argument was therefore controversial at the time. Lauded not only in Sydney society but throughout the British Empire as a paragon of the rational, moral, and Christianly virtues then thought to exemplify the 'modern' condition, Goodenough was an inauspicious target for the surgeon's claim that a 'civilised' state could be lost as well as gained. Safely beyond the range of Santa Cruz arrows, colonists living in Australia were far from curious about their true nature, and did not necessarily sympathise with claims that Nendö people could be 'improved'. Nevertheless, Messer undoubtedly sought to appeal to public and learned audiences alike. A pamphlet outlining his theories was distributed in 1877, seemingly with government assistance, to 'all museums' in Australia, where it sought to draw the venom from popular displays of poisonous arrows, and the lurid claims of their efficacy often made in accompanying texts.[7] The pamphlet was a much abbreviated version of two striking reports published by Messer, 'An enquiry into the reputed poisonous nature of the arrows of the South Sea Islanders', and a 'Continuation' of his enquiries, which appeared in the Admiralty's *Statistical Report of the Health of the Navy* for 1875 and 1876.[8] Owing to the considerable interest with which it was received, the surgeon also published a summary of his work in an 1878 edition of the journal of the Anthropological Institute of Great Britain and Ireland, of which Messer had become a fellow in 1877.[9]

Messer's reports, and in particular his argument for 'hysterical tetanus', offer valuable evidence of the application of psychophysiological theory to constructions of modern and civilised behaviour, civilisational progress, and mental illness in the late nineteenth century. However, the fate of Messer's work also highlights the challenge which the emergence of germ theory posed to understandings of the relationship between good mental and physical health. Arthur Nicolaier's 1884 experiments with bacteria, and the first isolation of the tetanus bacterium by Robert Koch and others in 1889, challenged theories of tetanus, including Messer's, which blamed eccentric systems of thought for the muscular stiffness and spasms associated with a disordered nervous system.[10] Soon disputed, the evasions and contradictions of Messer's work, which I explore below, had also the unintended effect of dramatically increasing concern about the manufacture of poisonous weaponry by the indigenous populations of the South Pacific Ocean. Largely alone in thinking that fear of poison was superstitious, and unable convincingly to rule out Nendö people's use of plant-based poisons such as strychnine, Messer appears, by giving substance to the issue, to have single-handedly transformed what was formerly a vague suspicion of indigenous toxins into something approaching a colonial and imperial crisis. This is apparent, for example, in a series of fearful editorials thereafter published in British and Australian newspapers.[11]

Never comprehensively resolved, the legacy of the debate endured into the late nineteenth and twentieth centuries, especially within comparable, albeit literary, 'murder mysteries', which perpetuated the notion that contact with isolated and 'primitive' peoples threatened at best to prejudice a modern and civilised visitor's moral condition, and at worst to inflict sudden death. Many readers are likely to recall the character Tonga, a man from the Andaman Islands, who accompanied the antagonist Jonathan Small in Arthur Conan Doyle's Sherlock Holmes story *The Sign of Four*, first published in 1890.[12] Weakened first by the lure of an oriental treasure and thereafter imprisoned for stealing it, the narrative tells of Small's encounter with Tonga in an Andaman penal colony, and of his subsequent use of the 'little Andaman Islander' to wreak revenge. Significantly, Tonga's deadly poisoned 'darts', shot from a blowpipe, were found by Holmes and John Watson to contain 'some strychnine-like substance which would produce tetanus'.[13] This conflation of an unknown poison with tetanic spasms suggests strongly that Conan Doyle was inspired by the well-publicised research into Santa Cruz arrows which occurred in the aftermath of Goodenough's death. In so doing, Conan Doyle influenced further stories about strychnine poisoning (a poison derived from certain plants), and its association with a sudden, mysterious, and violent fate. Examples include Agatha Christie's 1920 novel, *The Mysterious Affair at Styles*.[14]

Naval medicine and imperial modernity, c. 1875

The peculiar combination of inductive logic, careful rationalism, and fascination with strange and exotic phenomena which suffused Conan Doyle's life and writings, and indeed the late Victorian period more generally, was present too in Messer's enquiries into the attack on the *Pearl*.[15] Eager from the start to exploit the incident as an opportunity to investigate the poisonous character of Santa Cruz arrows, the surgeon recorded in his journal a detailed 'epitome' of the condition of the wounded sailors in the eight days from 13 to 20 August.[16] At sea, Messer's treatments were limited; in the manner of responding to snakebites, the puncture wounds left by the arrows in their victims were at first sucked by whichever volunteers were immediately to hand. Thereafter, the care given by Messer comprised of linseed poultices, cupping, morphine, carbolic acid (for cleaning wounds), and silver nitrate (for cauterising them). The men's wounds were varied; fired from a mere five yards, two arrows had pierced Goodenough's thin frock coat and straw hat, leaving a scratch to his head and a deeper injury to his left side. Further arrows hit two ordinary seamen named Edward Rayner and Frederick Small, causing injuries to their legs and scalps that were also eventually to prove fatal. The coxswains Thomas Jones and Allen Jervis, and the ship's cook, Thomas Satchwell, suffered similar arrow wounds but recovered after the second day. A sub-lieutenant, Henry Hawker, 'accidentally came in contact with an arrow in the hand of a native and received a slight scratch of the skin' before the attack occurred. Hawker and Jervis complained of twitching, and the latter suffered two 'epileptiform fits', but both recovered by the eighth day. A final sailor, the engineer Alfred Belts, also demanded treatment after handling some of the arrows which had been brought on to the ship, but was not included in the epitome.

Tetanus did not become apparent in Goodenough, Rayner, and Small's wounds until the sixth day, at which stage Messer attributed the disease to their insomnia and worsening spasms. By 21 August, these symptoms had proven fatal in all three patients. Messer's actions following the *Pearl*'s arrival in Sydney two days later are not recorded, but the surgeon's records show that it took until March 1876 to complete his first official report of the incident.[17] Making the most of Sydney's ready access to imperial networks, Messer's research was eclectic; his report drew upon a reading of sixteenth-century naval journals, correspondence with the Melanesian Mission, recent psycho-physiological theories of the nervous system, and an emerging expertise in toxicology sourced from the Melbourne and Sydney universities in order to dismiss the reality of Santa Cruz poisons and to argue that a form of mental illness was instead responsible for the sailors' and commodore's deaths. Rejecting strychnine-based explanations, which nonetheless later gained prominence, Messer argued that several of his patients had in reality suffered from 'hysterical tetanus'; a prevailing terror of the reputed poisons among medically uneducated British sailors predisposed them to a nervous irritability which mimicked or encouraged the onset of the disease.[18] By the same mechanism, Messer claimed that an 'ignorant' belief in poison both illustrated and perpetuated the enduring state of backwardness and mental abnormality then said to characterise Nendö people, and so compounded the difficulties of the Melanesian Mission.[19] Messer's 'chief object', he later wrote, was therefore to 'dispel this belief in the poisons, and thereby minimise the risks of tetanus; for it is asserted by many missionaries and others that this and other allied diseases of the nervous system, have become much less frequent among those islanders who have renounced superstition and have embraced Christianity'.[20]

The tone and message of Messer's reports are best understood in relation to the Royal Navy's contemporary efforts to distinguish itself as an engine of modernity and an affiliate of imperial expansion. Implicit in much of the surgeon's writing is an argument concerning the relevance of then emerging understandings of stress and nervous breakdown to constructions of civilisational progress and the modern, rational self. These themes reflected the Medical Department of the Navy's then ongoing struggle to police the mental health of its sailors, as much as they did naval surgeons' broader desire to associate themselves with the extension and consolidation of imperial control.[21] The particular elegance of Messer's study was that one of its main subjects, the late commodore Goodenough, had formerly embodied a growing trend of humanitarian activism within the navy distinguished by determinedly 'benevolent' efforts to improve and to Christianise South Pacific peoples. Posthumously immortalised in 1876 as 'The Christian hero of Santa Cruz', Goodenough was, according to Samson, a 'staunch modernizer', who sought to associate muscular Christianity and Victorian notions of patriotic duty with the navy's efforts to colonise and to civilise the South Pacific.[22] Following the attack at Santa Cruz, the subjection of the wounded Goodenough to Messer's ministrations neatly underlined the need for medical interventionism to operate in parallel. By 1875, Messer had become a firm advocate of the argument that civilisational progress mapped the subjugation to rational thought of ignorance, stress, and superstition. Proper regimes of thought expressed a sound psycho-physiological state, the main guarantors of which were Christian belief and a modern medical understanding of the mind.

Though it is difficult to be certain, there is an intriguing possibility that the surgeon's arguments were therefore to some degree opportunistic. Messer's analysis of Goodenough's mind, which is explored in more detail below, sought through the language of volitional and non-volitional mental reflexes to lessen the aspersions which the surgeon's diagnosis of hysterical tetanus cast upon the commodore's Christianly character and masculine virtues. It did not, however, do so completely. Since Goodenough had come, by 1875, to represent imperial British exploration to a degree almost comparable with that earlier achieved by Cook, Messer perhaps hoped to increase perceptions of the significance of his report by revealing the commodore to be vulnerable to malign and superstitious influences. What is certain is that the *Pearl* had recently become a site of peculiar significance to debates concerning the best means of 'modernising' South Pacific cultures; as experts in unrelated fields, it is tempting to imagine Goodenough and Messer arguing for the relative merits of paternalistic protection and medical intervention over dinner on the ship's quarterdeck. The commodore and surgeon had, for instance, each developed their own close links with imperial officials in the British metropole during the *Pearl*'s earlier visits to Fiji in 1874. As Samson observes, the British government was persuaded to carry out its subsequent annexation of Fiji partly in consequence of Goodenough's investigation of the local labour trade.[23] At a time in which the Royal Navy was increasingly evangelical and pious, Goodenough's Christian, humanitarian, and anthropological insights formed a potent mix.[24] Contemporaries also recognised, however, the distinct contribution made by Messer himself. A report by the surgeon on the climate and inhabitants of Fiji, which he sent to the Colonial Office in 1874, was even said by some to have been the dominant factor in its subsequent annexation.[25] There, Messer spoke of Fiji's healthy climate as a means to encourage colonisation. 'Dysentery', he argued, 'is the only disease which Europeans have to fear in Fiji and to guard against, as can generally be done by observing a few simple precautions'.[26] In a manner which foreshadowed the interventionist style of his later work, the surgeon suggested that the local popularity of native kava root was a symptom of poor education, and a cause of delirium.[27]

Messer was one of many nineteenth-century surgeons trained to show scientific initiative, and to develop independent investigations of this kind, while on naval voyages. Born in Edinburgh in 1838, Messer had studied medicine at the University of Edinburgh, and in 1859 joined the navy as a surgeon.[28] In so doing, he formed part of a large diaspora of Scottish medical graduates in the naval service. The Royal Naval Hospital Haslar in Gosport lay at the centre of this network, and it was to here that Messer's draft report on Santa Cruz arrows was first sent. Since 1827, the hospital had maintained a museum and library under the direction of the Edinburgh graduate and naval Inspector of Hospitals, William Burnett. With the encouragement of two further Edinburgh graduates, the phrenologist James Scott and, after 1855, the navy's Director-General John Liddell, Haslar supported and trained the navy's surgeons in a manner reminiscent of the broad curricula which flourished within Scottish universities in the aftermath of the Scottish Enlightenment.[29] The museum and library reflected not only pathological and anatomical interests but also promoted anthropological treatises and collections, thus supporting and extending colonial interest in the joint study of exotic climates, cultures, and peoples. After the mid-1850s, surgeons at Haslar seeking cures for a growth in toxic injuries inflicted against the navy's sailors became increasingly interested in the use of plants to manufacture poisonous weapons; relevant botanical specimens were displayed in the hospital museum alongside examples of the objects themselves.[30] The study of poison, about which almost nothing was known, thus increased in tandem with the British Empire's incursion into tropical climates.

Messer was influenced too by the study of so-called 'naval lunatics'. Haslar, where a 'Naval Lunatic Asylum' opened in 1815, had been central to the medical investigation of the minds of the navy's sailors since 1807, when the Edinburgh graduate Thomas Trotter, a former Haslar physician, published his essay on the 'increasing prevalence' of nervous diseases in Britain.[31] The seamen of the navy, who were supposedly more 'manly' and thus less susceptible to mental illness than the general public, had alarmed Trotter by exhibiting signs of a weakened 'nervous temperament' then thought to be widespread.[32] Though Trotter argued that 'savage races' tended to possess a healthier mental state than 'civilized' Europeans, he followed a convention later used by Messer in remarking that the 'inhabitants of some of the South Sea Islands are examples to the contrary'.[33] Citing the 'mania' associated with the collapse of the South Sea Company in 1720, Trotter also preceded Messer in commenting upon the dangers the region posed for those of an unsound mind.[34]

In November 1836, naval surgeons first began to study mental illness in an imperial and systematic manner following Burnett's publication of a 'nosological synopsis' designed to be filled out in conjunction with their standard medical journals. In the synopsis, surgeons were asked to record 'neuroses' such as apoplexy, dyspepsia, and mania.[35] Although the synopsis was designed only to record mental ailments suffered by sailors of the Royal Navy, surgeons were encouraged to extend their commentary in the space provided for 'General Remarks' at the back of naval medical journals. Here, surgeons could make observations on a range of imperial affairs. Every two years, gold medals were awarded to the surgeons whose journals were 'most approved of by the principal Medical Officers of the Navy, and the Presidents of the Colleges of Physicians and Surgeons'.[36] The medals, funded since 1830 by a bequest from the Scottish physician Gilbert Blane, bore the inscription *mente manuque*, meaning 'with mind and hand', and thus encouraged scientific research.[37] In 1874, Messer used this space to make his report on the colonial potential of Fiji. In 1875, he won the Blane medal for his work on poisonous arrows.[38]

Sailors, 'savages', and poison

Messer's 1875 report used historical, ethnographic, and medical allusions similar to those employed by Trotter as a means to encourage support for the Melanesian Mission and the Royal Navy's humanitarian endeavour. Whereas sailors had previously been compared with 'savages' as a means to point them toward more 'civilised' behaviour, Messer was arguably attempting the opposite. By linking sailors' belief in poisonous arrows with that of Nendö people, Messer sought to equate missionaries' efforts to bring Christianity to the South Pacific with a better-established consensus about the need to educate the Royal Navy's 'ignorant' and 'superstitious' workforce. Following the attack on Goodenough, the Melanesian Mission was much in need of such a defence. Missionaries had hardly dared to visit Nendö Island since 1864, when Patteson narrowly escaped an arrow attack himself, and it was reportedly with Nendö people's encouragement that he was later killed at Nukapu.[39] Reporting the commodore's death on 28 August 1875, the *Sydney Mail and New South Wales Advertiser* observed that 'the Santa Cruz group has acquired for itself a savage pre-eminence' as a place of 'inhuman massacre', and cast doubt upon missionaries' ability to redress the 'peculiar hostility to white men among the savages'.[40] As an antidote to such feeling, Messer's reports on poisonous arrows emphasised the importance of a well-functioning nervous system for rational behaviour, and argued that this was wanting in sailors and Nendö people alike. Notions of racial difference were thereby undercut in favour of an argument for the latent capacity for civilisation that resided in the mind; behaviour befitting of the modern age could only be brought about by Christian belief and medical understanding, and could easily become threatened if they were neglected.

The Victorian period was one of pronounced concern with the 'enigma' of nervous breakdown, as Janet Oppenheim has shown.[41] The relationship between civilisation, stress, and depression being much contested, Messer's effort to conflate religious instruction with a functional nervous system, and a functional nervous system with sane and civilised behaviour, offered a powerful physiological apparatus and vindication for missionary work. Premised, too, upon an attempt to promote the abilities and influence of naval surgeons, Messer's argument was helped by the fact that allusions to mentally unstable or superstitious sailors were used frequently in the nineteenth century to promote Christian belief and theological education. The Christian magazine *Leisure Hour*, published by the Religious Tract Society, for instance, interpreted the problem of 'naval lunatics' from a moral and educational angle in its long-running series on the 'Superstitions of Seamen'. In 1852, the magazine observed that 'seamen are perhaps the most superstitious of mortals', and that 'ignorance is undoubtedly the mother of superstition'.[42] The Society offered libraries to sailors as a possible solution. 'Much has been done of late years to improve the condition of seamen', it wrote, and 'to communicate to them that religious knowledge which is the best counter-agent of superstitions'.[43]

The salubrious qualities of 'moral and religious instruction' were similarly promoted within the navy's asylums, which experienced an epidemic in cases of mental illness between 1874 and 1875. In this period alone, the Royal Naval Lunatic Asylum at Great Yarmouth was forced to hire extra attendants in order to cope with an influx of 268 patients exhibiting 'mania' and 'insanity', twenty-two of whom died from 'Diseases of the Nervous System'.[44] Messer would therefore have had reason to assume the sympathy of Admiralty officials when he began his 1875 report on the Santa Cruz arrows with a deliberate reference to the unhealthy superstitions of sailors. 'It has been the popular belief from the earliest times', he wrote:

> that many of the more savage races which Europeans have met in different parts of the world are in the habit of using poisonous arrows and darts, both in warfare and in the chase. This belief has, in many cases, been accompanied by an amount of dread of these weapons, which has led to the subject of poisonous arrows being obscured by numerous mysterious and improbable stories. Nowhere perhaps at the present day does so much of this sensational and unscientific rumour exist as among the Islands of the South Pacific, owing partly to the fact that most of it has been derived from uneducated sailors.[45]

In 1873, another of the Australia Station's surgeons, Godfrey Goodman, similarly remarked in his medical journal that it was 'generally believed by the traders to Santa Cruz, that all the arrows there are poisoned.'[46] Following an arrow attack, Goodman noted how one ship's mate had recovered after pouring 'strong hydrochloric acid, which he kept for cleaning shells, into his wound.'[47] Goodman was nevertheless at a loss to describe the nature of the poisons involved, or to explain the efficacy of this drastic solution. In his own reports, Messer resorted to eighteenth-century observations made at Santa Cruz by the British naval explorer Phillip Carteret for medical insights. 'In the writings of the early voyagers numerous instances are given of their men being wounded among the South Sea Islands "by deadly flights of poisonous arrows"', he wrote, 'but they are not so well known to modern voyagers.'[48] This had allowed superstition to replace scientific analysis, and in consequence members of the Australia Station's fleet had developed a tendency toward nervousness and hysteria comparable with the 'peculiar mental constitution of ignorant and savage races.'[49] At Santa Cruz, this was demonstrated by Nendö people's supposed indulgence in 'superstition, witchcraft, and sorcery in their most debasing forms.'[50]

Key to Messer's argument was his observation that the painful spasms suffered by sailors wounded by Santa Cruz arrows did not resemble the known effects of blood poisoning, or of contact with the region's plants. The methods by which Nendö people reportedly poisoned the arrows also seemed to point more to superstitious belief than to any developed knowledge concerning the production of poisons. According to Messer, the sailors of the *Pearl* were most particularly afraid of a method said to involve immersing the arrows 'in a dead decomposing human body'.[51] Rumours focused on the story of a sailor who had reported seeing:

> one or two dead bodies lying in a state of decomposition, with several arrows sticking in them 'like porcupines, sir', while sitting by them was a native, with a fire of wood, and a pot of vegetable poison, who drew the arrows from the bodies dripping with viscid animal matter, held them over the fire till they were partially dry, then smeared them with the contents of the pot.[52]

Messer argued that the method of poisoning there described suggested certain misunderstandings of botanical and pathological science; the story was also so fanciful that sailors who were willing to believe it demonstrated a poor education, comparable with that of those who attempted to manufacture poison in this way. In 1866, the French morbid anatomist Victor Feltz had demonstrated that injections of 'putrid matter' could cause symptoms of blood poisoning in animals, but Messer noted that septicaemia had not likewise emerged in the arrow wounds.[53] Though strychnine poisoning from certain plants was known to cause tetanus-like symptoms, Messer ruled this out on the basis that it usually did so immediately, and that in any case none of the necessary plants grew in the Santa Cruz region. George Britton Halford, a professor of medicine and expert on snake-poisoning at the University of Melbourne, had reassured Messer that his own experiments with poisonous arrows from the neighbouring Solomon Islands had suggested no indigenous knowledge of, or access to, any dangerous plants.[54]

It is revealing that Messer was prepared to rule out the presence of poison on this basis. The tips of the arrows were, he noted, coated in a strange substance, and often dyed red; various interviews with missionaries confirmed that Nendö people possessed a strong belief in the arrows' power to poison wounds[55] Messer's own knowledge of blood poisoning was seemingly poor, for he referred to Feltz only briefly, and called him 'Felty'.[56] Such was the surgeon's wish to claim that superstitious belief was the only potent poison associated with the arrows, his dismissal of the presence of toxins was therefore spurious. Although Messer's second report investigated Santa Cruz plants more systematically, it too contained flaws. Messer wrote to the Melanesian Mission

Poisonous arrows and unsound minds 281

to enquire into indigenous uses of plants, and in return received several specimens, which he sent to the Royal Botanic Gardens at Kew. Upon their arrival, however, the plants were in no condition for adequate testing.[57] Messer instead based his results on experiments which involved poking dogs and rabbits with collected arrows, and feeding them indigenous plants, which in some cases produced symptoms of tetanus comparable with those suffered onboard the *Pearl*.[58] The animals made for inconclusive subjects, however. 'Three quarters of an hour after swallowing the dose [a] dog vomited', Messer wrote, 'but at once ate all the vomited matter.'[59] On this dubious evidence, Messer concluded that 'we may be justified in looking upon these reputed poisons with the gravest doubts as to their potency.'[60]

Disciplining fear: understandings of tetanus and the nervous system

Having cast into doubt the existence of Santa Cruz poisons on these grounds, Messer set out his theory that the wounded men onboard the *Pearl* in reality suffered from certain varieties of tetanus. The surgeon's attempt to associate the suffering caused by poisonous arrows with poor education, stress, and superstition depended upon a nineteenth-century understanding of the relation of the disease to the nervous system about which very little has since been written. Indeed, the history of tetanus in this period is almost completely unexplored.[61] In the years which preceded the first isolation of tetanus bacterium, the aetiology of the disease was highly uncertain. The symptoms of tetanus, in particular muscular stiffness and spasms, were assumed to be the manifestation of one or more disorders in the nervous system, which might themselves have any number of causes. As Messer himself noted, warm climates were strongly associated with the disease; John Hunter, the well-known eighteenth-century surgeon and collector, had suggested that climate alone might be sufficient to produce tetanus.[62] What would now be recognised as the bacterial form of the disease was often also associated with, or mistaken for, conditions such as strychnine poisoning and a raft of neurological disorders such as non-epileptic or dissociative seizures. For this reason, Messer considered the sporadic but short-lived fits suffered by Jervis, Hawker, and Belts to be just as significant as the considerably more serious symptoms exhibited by Goodenough, Rayner, and Small.

Messer's conflation of tetanus with poor education and an ignorance of Christian teaching drew upon an earlier tradition of partisan diagnoses of hysteria made by religious authorities in Britain. Such diagnoses targeted, in particular, outbreaks of religious revivalism, spiritualism, and other ostensibly eccentric superstitious or supernatural practices.[63] In 1846, Hector Landouzy first coined the term 'hystero-epilepsy' to bring together medical investigations of the physical ailments which manifested in patients suffering extreme mental excitement, but it was only in 1881 that the neurologist William Gowers developed a method for distinguishing between epileptic seizures and 'pseudoseizures'.[64] This ambiguity allowed Messer to wield diagnoses of tetanus as part of a wider struggle for the control of the indigenous inhabitants of Santa Cruz, in a manner comparable with that identified by Christopher Lawrence in relation to the political history of scurvy.[65] Despite the shared context of naval medicine, however, the moral conventions of discipline and hygiene associated with scurvy's treatment did not feature significantly in Messer's discussion of tetanus; ideas of cleanliness were mentioned in his reports only in the most superficial terms.[66] Tetanus's capacity to affect sailors of all ranks and temperaments, from Goodenough to the ship's cook, seemingly made a mockery of the cohesive and longstanding vision of moral behaviour which Lawrence describes. 'Habits of life, such as temperance, and the reverse', Messer noted, 'have no apparent connection with its production'.[67]

The potency of Messer's argument accordingly lay in his access to a new psycho-physiological language of the nervous system, which permitted him to claim that certain forms of tetanus were easily avoided. As suggested above, the important thing about Messer's theory was that it could be applied universally; his was a treatment of the mind and spirit. The surgeon's various references to 'voluntary, reflex, sensory, and motor functions', and more generally to 'the well-known power of the mind over the body in inducing insanity and other allied diseases of the nervous system', betrayed an association with the influential theories of the Unitarian physician William Carpenter.[68] In 1874, Carpenter had first published *The Principles of Mental Physiology*, in which he stressed the interrelation of psychological and physiological behaviour, and thus the importance of the 'training and discipline of the mind'.[69] Here, Carpenter explained that tetanus was a symptom of the breakdown of the nervous system, which itself occurred in consequence of 'an undue excitability of the *Emotions* [and] their known influence on the "vaso-motor Nerves".[70]

In a line of thought earlier developed in his *Principles of Human Physiology* and an essay on the 'Voluntary and Instinctive Actions of Living Beings', Carpenter argued that the progress of civilisation could be read in terms of the development of man's powers of 'internal volition' over those of 'external stimuli'.[71] In a sign of divine providence, the human nervous system had been imbued with sufficient complexity to allow the expression of willpower.[72] Involuntary and therefore irrational behaviour, which often manifested in spasms, was the consequence of a subversion of the reasoning process, and an affiliated disease of the nervous system. The rationale for strange behaviour, wrote Carpenter, 'is simply as follows. The continued concentration of Attention upon a certain idea gives it a dominant power, not only over the mind, but over the body; and the muscles become the involuntary instruments whereby it is carried in to operation'.[73] Contrary to those, such as the philosopher George Henry Lewes, who assumed 'that a Physiological Psychology strikes at the root of Morals and Religion', Carpenter argued that models of the mind based in materialist science were no obstacle to religious faith or the idea of a conscious self.[74]

For Messer, the problematic dominant 'idea' among sailors and Nendö people was that of fatal and incurably poisoned arrow wounds, which considerably heightened the stressful nature of the navy's increasingly violent Pacific encounters. Fear of poison weakened the nervous system, and was a symptom of the superstitious belief which resulted from an ignorance of Christian education. Should a man with a fear of poisons proceed to encounter a suspected poison, his already fragile nervous system would be placed in a perilous state. In a departure from Carpenter, this was the condition Messer called 'hysterical tetanus', which he distinguished from the disease's 'idiopathic' and 'traumatic' forms.[75] The surgeon borrowed the latter two subdivisions from the early work of the military physicians Robert Willan and John Hennen, who had, in 1801 and 1820 respectively, identified the role of anxiety and terror in 'inducing the traumatic, as well as the idiopathic form of the disease, as seen in its frequent occurrence after battles, earthquakes, etc'.[76] In such cases, fear and allied conditions encouraged a form of tetanus which ultimately derived from wounds or exposure to dangerous environments. Hysterical tetanus could occur without such provocation, but remained just as dangerous. It was a sign, perhaps, of the contemporary growth of professional interest in what Carpenter called 'Physiological Psychology' that Messer cited no particular authority in his discussion of this latter form of the disease. References to 'hysterical tetanus' in texts published in English appear to date back at least as far as an 1844 translation of the German homeopathist Andreas Joseph Friedrich Ruoff's 1837 *Repertorium für die homöopathische Praxis*, but were becoming increasingly frequent at the time of the attack on the *Pearl*.[77] Short summaries of the condition appear, for example, in Timothy Holmes's 1870 text, *A System of Surgery: Theoretical and Practical*, and in Frederick James Gant's 1871 treatise, *The Science and Practice of Surgery*.[78]

Making only a very subtle allusion to the fact that hysteria was then commonly considered a feminine trait, Messer's 1875 report sought to demonstrate the truth of his theory that hysterical tetanus was responsible for the suffering of the *Pearl*'s crew by sorting Goodenough and the six other men wounded by Santa Cruz arrows according to their relative nervous temperaments. This gave the semblance of a controlled scientific experiment:

> five men were wounded by arrows fired at them by the natives of that place, in a treacherous and unprovoked attack, while another officer on the same occasion accidentally received a scratch by coming in contact with the point of an arrow in the hand of one of the natives. Here, then, was suddenly afforded an opportunity of observing the effects of these arrow wounds, and testing the truth of their poisonous reputation in seven cases, two officers and five men. It is worthy of record, that Commodore Goodenough was an officer of the very highest intelligence, possessed of a most powerful and deeply cultured mind, free, one would suppose, from any weakness or dread of uncertain danger, and in whom the *mens sana in corpore sano* was most fully illustrated. In the other officer, a different and very highly nervous disposition, was combined with a weakly and rather delicate body. As for the five men, every difference in age, disposition, and habit of life was represented. The wounds themselves were in every case slight.[79]

The 'slightness' of the wounds made the hysterical form of tetanus the most likely culprit for the men's suffering, once the poisons themselves were proven fantastical. The disease, Messer argued, had been abetted by certain environmental factors; 'favourable' conditions for the production of tetanus, whether traumatic, idiopathic, or hysterical, had appeared at Santa Cruz in the form of 'punctured wounds… an unusual amount of excitement after an attack, together with much anxiety of mind, fear of poison, and consequent despondency. To these must be added an exceedingly hot, damp, relaxing climate'.[80] References to 'inward' and 'outward' behaviour, likely inspired by Carpenter's success in reconciling divine willpower with mechanistic models of the mind, allowed Messer to overcome the contradiction between his diagnosis of a hysterical mental state and Goodenough's reputation as a rational, masculine, and Christianly explorer. The commodore's mind had exerted a sinister and seemingly autonomous agency in its fixation on the existence and deadly nature of indigenous poisons:

> In the commodore's case, as before mentioned, we would not have expected to find that the influence of the mind over the body was of a hurtful nature, but rather the reverse. Unfortunately, however, from the very first, although apparently disbelieving in the danger of the poison, his mind never left the subject, but at once began to look forward to and prepare for a fatal result. This, however, he did in all outward calmness, and with a courage and resignation which others have well described.[81]

Messer may have acknowledged that too overt a challenge to Goodenough's character was likely to have a negative impact on the dissemination and publication of his report. The last sentence of the extract above likely refers to the work of Henry Goldfinch, one of the *Pearl*'s lieutenants, who had written a moving account of Goodenough's illness and death.[82] There, Goldfinch emphasised the manner in which the commodore accepted and made a virtue of his fate:

> 19th August. This afternoon I witnessed the saddest scene possible we had been greatly alarmed all day about the state of the Com at 5pm he sent for all the officers into his sleeping cabin he spoke to us all generally at first telling us the great comfort he had in dying was the love of God and exhorting us to love *him* more then he said goodbye & spoke a few kind words to each of us kissing us all round every one in tears.

If Goodenough had not resigned himself to his death from poisonous wounds, Messer implied, he may have survived the attack; lack of medical education and a consequent superstition had encouraged the commodore's fate. Whereas Rayner and Small similarly suffered from a hysterical mental state with few outward symptoms, the 'delicate' officer, Hawker, and the engineer, Belts, had by contrast exhibited it in full. Though Hawker received only a slight scratch to his shoulder, Messer reported that 'unusual and irregular symptoms of tetanus set in very early, his mind becoming extremely excited'.[83] Convinced the presumed poisoning meant 'he must surely die', Hawker refused to leave his cabin and 'adopted strange and eccentric methods to prevent his jaw becoming locked … He nearly succeeded in producing real tetanus, and probably would have done so had his wound been anything beyond the merest scratch.[84] Belts, who was 'extremely nervous and timorous', suffered similarly after he 'allowed himself to imagine' that a wound on his thumb 'was caused by one of the arrows he had accidentally touched'.[85] Messer's published report states that Belts's fear of poison was so extreme that he was ultimately invalided from the navy, being 'actually considered insane'.[86] In his original notes, however, the surgeon noted more candidly his suspicion that Belts in fact 'exaggerated his symptoms for his own purposes'.[87] The surgeon's desire to establish cases of hysterical tetanus may therefore have been acknowledged, and exploited, by devious elements of the *Pearl*'s crew.

Conclusion

It has not been my intention here to offer a final diagnosis of the sufferings of the *Pearl*'s wounded sailors, but it is as well to observe that Goodenough, Rayner, and Small almost certainly died from an infection caused by tetanus bacteria. Strychnine poisoning appears an unlikely explanation, as Messer observed, because it took more than a week for the men to die. Nevertheless, it should be noted that since Nendö people were undoubtedly aware of the association between arrow wounds and tetanus, the arrows could indeed be considered poisonous. As no attempt has lately been made to settle this question, Santa Cruz arrows now held at the British Museum are pragmatically considered toxic, and have their points carefully wrapped.[88] With respect to the 'outward symptoms' of what Messer called hysterical tetanus, in the case of Hawker, Jervis, and perhaps Belts, the condition might now be referred to as a form of non-epileptic seizure; these can be stimulated by anxiety and depression, and may well have been less prevalent in sailors who, in consequence of Christian faith or otherwise, did not believe in the indigenous manufacture of poison.[89]

The caution afforded to the arrows now in the British Museum speaks to Messer's contradictory legacy. The surgeon was the first explorer of the British Empire to undertake a detailed study of exotic poisons, and incidents of poisoning, but he failed to make a significant impact upon medical research. Furthermore, though Messer sought to establish that no viable poisons were manufactured in the Santa Cruz Islands, his references to decomposing bodies, witchcraft, and painful death lingered long in the imagination of his contemporaries. The problem was that Messer's case for hysterical tetanus, about which he himself called for more research, was not strong enough to convince physicians, sailors, and the public that poisonous arrows could safely be ignored. 'Is it certain', came one typical response in the contemporary press, 'that the Polynesians never soak their arrows in a solution of strychnia or some analogous vegetable poison?'[90] The Gilbert Blane medal, it may fairly be concluded, in truth rewarded Messer's deft weaponisation of the Victorian concern with nervous breakdown, and his novel use of emerging psycho-physiological explanations for tetanic spasms. By proposing that the most dangerous and enduring barriers to the development of the South Pacific region were the stress and hysteria of superstition, the surgeon consolidated the Medical Department of the Navy's influence within a triumvirate of imperial encounter, humanitarian activism, and Christian proselytisation. Though never explicit, the doubts Messer cast upon Goodenough's mental state challenged the stability of contemporary formulations of 'modern' civilisation and its forms of behaviour; poisonous arrows, like Conan Doyle's Tonga and his darts, had the power to disrupt and to terrorise civil societies. In 1877, an editorial in the *Australian Town and Country Journal* revealed that the political significance and religious symbolism of Messer's reports had not been missed. 'At present the prayer to be delivered from "the arrow that flyeth by day" has a peculiar significance', it observed. Should Messer's discoveries offer an antidote to terror, 'they will rank high among the services conferred by explorers upon mankind.'[91]

Notes

1 'Statue to Captain Cook, at Randwick', *The Sydney Morning Herald* (28 October 1874), 5.

2 C. I. Hamilton, 'Naval hagiography and the Victorian hero', *Historical Journal*, 23:2 (1980), 381–98.
3 'Death of Commodore Goodenough and two seamen of H. M. S. Pearl at Santa Cruz', *Sydney Morning Herald* (3 September 1875), 5.
4 *Ibid.* T. Kolshus and E. Hovdhaugen, 'Reassessing the death of Bishop John Coleridge Patteson', *Journal of Pacific History*, 45:3 (2010), 331–55.
5 J. Samson, *Imperial Benevolence: Making British Authority in the Pacific Islands* (Hawaii: University of Hawai'i Press, 1998). J. Samson, 'Hero, fool or martyr? The many deaths of Commodore Goodenough', *Journal for Maritime Research*, 10:1 (2008), 1–22 (p. 1).
6 *Ibid.*, 7.
7 'Poisoned Arrows and Their Antidotes', *Australian Town and Country Journal* (21 April 1877), 18.
8 A. B. Messer, 'An Enquiry into the Reputed Poisonous Nature of the Arrows of the South Sea Islanders', in A. Egerton (ed.), *Statistical Report of the Health of the Navy for the Year 1875* (House of Commons, 1876), 149–63. A. B. Messer, 'Continuation of an Enquiry into the Reputed Poisonous Nature of the Arrows of the South Sea Islanders', in A. Egerton (ed.), *Statistical Report of the Health of the Navy for the Year 1876* (House of Commons, 1877), 184–98.
9 A. B. Messer, 'On "An inquiry into the reputed poisonous nature of the arrows of the South Sea Islanders."', *Journal of the Anthropological Institute of Great Britain and Ireland*, 7 (1878), 209–11.
10 S. M. Blevins and M. S. Bronze, 'Robert Koch and the "golden age" of bacteriology', *International Journal of Infectious Diseases*, 14 (2010), 744–51.
11 See, for example, 'Poisoned Arrows', *Tribune* (28 April 1877), 3.
12 A. Conan Doyle, *The Sign of Four* (London: Spencer Blackett, 1890).
13 *Ibid.*, 99.
14 A. Christie, *The Mysterious Affair at Styles* (New York: John Lane, 1920).
15 M. Saler, '"Clap if you believe in Sherlock Holmes": mass culture and the re-enchantment of modernity, c. 1890–c. 1940', *The Historical Journal*, 46:3 (2003), 599–622.
16 Messer, 'An enquiry', 160–1.
17 The National Archives, London (hereafter TNA), ADM 101/246, A. B. Messer, 'Medical and Surgical Journal of HMS Pearl for 1 January to 31 December 1875', 38.
18 Messer, 'An enquiry', 158–9.
19 *Ibid.*
20 Messer, 'On "An Inquiry"', 210.
21 R. Pietsch, 'Hearts of oak and jolly tars? Heroism and insanity in the Georgian navy', *Journal for Maritime Research*, 15:1 (2013), 69–82.

22 Samson, 'Hero, fool or martyr?', 3; R. I. S. (ed.), *The Christian Hero of Santa Cruz* (London: S. W. Partridge & Co., 1876).
23 Samson, *Imperial Benevolence*, 167.
24 R. Blake, *Religion in the British Navy 1815–1879* (Woodbridge: The Boydell Press, 2014).
25 'Obituary', *British Medical Journal*, 2:3073 (1919), 692.
26 TNA, ADM 101/243, A. B. Messer, 'Medical and Surgical Journal of HMS Pearl for 1 January to 31 December 1874'.
27 L. Forbes, 'Notes on Fiji', *The Lancet*, 107:2732 (1876), 75–8.
28 'Obituary', 692.
29 D. Simpson, 'For Science, Friendship or Personal Gain? Alexander Collie and the Origins of Naval Ethnography at Haslar Hospital Museum', in G. Sculthorpe and M. Nugent (eds), *Yurlmun: Mokare Mia Boodja* (Albany: Western Australian Museum, 2016); D. Simpson, 'Medical collecting on the frontiers of natural history: the rise and fall of Haslar Hospital Museum (1827–1855)', *Journal of the History of Collections*, 30:2 (2018), 253–67; L. Kontler, 'Mankind and its histories: William Robertson, Georg Forster and a late eighteenth-century German debate', *Intellectual History Review*, 23:3 (2013), 411–29.
30 Simpson, 'For Science, Friendship or Personal Gain?', 31.
31 T. Trotter, *A View of the Nervous Temperament* (Newcastle: Edward Walker, 1807).
32 *Ibid.*, 153.
33 *Ibid.*, 20.
34 *Ibid.*, 156.
35 TNA, ADM 101/38/5/1, 'Copy of an instruction dated 1 November 1836 from W. Burnett, Physician General'.
36 *London Medical Gazette*, vol. 17 (London: Longman, Rees, Orme, Brown, Green, & Longman, 1836), 542.
37 *Ibid.*
38 'Obituary', 692.
39 Kolshus and Hovdhaugen, 'Reassessing the death', 345.
40 'The Massacre at Santa Cruz', *Sydney Mail and New South Wales Advertiser* (28 August 1875), 265.
41 J. Oppenheim, *'Shattered Nerves': Doctors, Patients, and Depression in Victorian England* (New York: Oxford University Press, 1991).
42 'Superstitions of Seamen', *Leisure Hour*, 44 (28 October 1852), 692–4.
43 *Ibid.*, 694.
44 W. Macleod, 'Annual Report of the Royal Naval Lunatic Asylum at Great Yarmouth', in A. Egerton (ed.), *Statistical Report of the Health of the Navy for the year 1875*, 122–30.

45 Messer, 'An enquiry', 149.
46 TNA, ADM 101/242/1A, G. Goodman, 'Medical and Surgical Journal of HMS Basilisk for 1 January to 31 December 1872'.
47 *Ibid.*
48 Messer, 'An enquiry', 153.
49 *Ibid.* 150.
50 *Ibid.*
51 Messer, 'On "An Inquiry"', 209.
52 Messer, 'Continuation of an enquiry', 180.
53 L. Coze and V. Feltz, 'Physiologie pathologique', *Gazette Médicale de Strasbourg*, 26:61 (1866), 115–208; Messer, 'An enquiry', 154.
54 *Ibid.*, 164.
55 *Ibid.*, 153.
56 *Ibid.*, 154.
57 *Report on the Progress and Condition of the Royal Gardens at Kew* (London: George E. Eyre and William Spottiswoode, 1879), 27.
58 Messer, 'Continuation of an enquiry', 196–8.
59 *Ibid.*, 196.
60 *Ibid.*, 195.
61 For an exception, see I. Read, 'A triumphant decline? Tetanus among slaves and freeborn in Brazil', *História, ciências, saúde—Manguinhos*, 19:1 (2012), 107–32.
62 J. F. Palmer (ed.), *The Works of John Hunter, F.R.S.* (London: Longman, Rees, Orme, Brown, Green, & Longman, 1835), 585; Messer, 'An enquiry', 157.
63 R. Noakes, 'Natural Causes? Spiritualism, Science, and the Supernatural in Mid-Victorian Britain', in N. Brown, C. Burdett, and P. Thurschwell (eds), *The Victorian Supernatural* (Cambridge: Cambridge University Press, 2004), 23–43.
64 H H. Landouzy, *Trait de l'hysterie* (Paris: J. B. & G. Balliere, 1846); W. R. Gowers, *Epilepsy and Other Chronic Convulsive Diseases* (London: J. & A. Churchill, 1881).
65 C. Lawrence, 'Disciplining disease: scurvy, the navy, and imperial expansion, 1750–1825', in D. P. Miller and P. H. Reill (eds), *Visions of Empire* (Cambridge: Cambridge University Press, 1996), 80–106.
66 Messer, 'An enquiry', 152. See, for example, M. Harrison, 'Scurvy on sea and land: political economy and natural history, c. 1780–c. 1850', *Journal for Maritime Research*, 15 (2013), 7–25.
67 Messer, 'An enquiry', 157.
68 *Ibid.*, 154.
69 W. B. Carpenter, *Principles of Mental Physiology* (London: Henry S. King & Co., 1874).

70 *Ibid.*, 70. Emphasis in original.
71 W. B. Carpenter, *Principles of Human Physiology* (London: John Churchill, 1842); W. B. Carpenter, 'On the voluntary and instinctive actions of living beings', *Edinburgh Medical and Surgical Journal*, 48 (1837), 22–44.
72 For a related discussion, see A. Crabtree, '"Automatism" and the emergence of dynamic psychiatry', *Journal of the History of the Behavioural Sciences*, 39:1 (2003), 51–70.
73 Carpenter, *Principles of Mental Physiology*, 293.
74 *Ibid.*, p. xii.
75 Messer, 'An enquiry', 152.
76 *Ibid.*, 157; R. Willan, *Reports on the Diseases in London* (London: H. L. Galabin, 1801); J. Hennen, *Principles of Military Surgery* (Edinburgh: Archibald Constable and Co., 1820).
77 A. J. F. Ruoff, *Repertorium für die homöopathische Praxis* (Stuttgart: Hallberger'sche Verlagshandlung, 1837); A. Howard Okie, *Ruoff's Repertory of Homoeopathic Medicine, Nosologically Arranged* (Philadelphia: J. Dobson, Kay & Brothers, & H. Hooker, 1844).
78 T. Holmes, *A System of Surgery: Theoretical and Practical* (London: Longmans, Green, and Co., 1870); F. J. Gant, *The Science and Practice of Surgery* (London: J. & A. Churchill, 1871).
79 Messer, 'An enquiry', 151.
80 *Ibid.*, 157.
81 *Ibid.*, 151–2.
82 The British Library, RP 5181, H. Goldfinch, 'Account by Lieut H E Goldfinch of the fatal wounding of Goodenough by the Natives of Santa Cruz', 12 August 1875.
83 Messer, 'An enquiry', 152.
84 *Ibid.*
85 ADM 101/246, 65.
86 Messer, 'An enquiry', 152.
87 ADM 101/246, 66.
88 See, for example, British Museum object Oc1981, Q.2442.
89 For a survey of recent debate, see A. M. Kanner and S. C. Schachter, *Psychiatric Controversies in Epilepsy* (Amsterdam: Elsevier/Academic Press, 2008).
90 'Poisoned Arrows', *Tribune* (28 April 1877), 3.
91 'Poisoned Arrows and Their Antidotes', *Australian Town and Country Journal* (21 April 1877), 18.

IV
Reflections and provocation

12

What is your *complaint?* Health as moral economy in the long nineteenth century

Christopher Hamlin

Unlike most other forms of historical writing, histories of public health are moral narratives. For more than a century, historians of the infectious diseases that were long its chief focus have been able to unfold the drama of heroic social and scientific achievement over complacency and ignorance. That narrative is possible because author and reader share metrics of progress – through microbiology and epidemiology. One knows what needs to happen. Suffering from faecal-oral diseases? Stop ingesting … But what and who will facilitate, or retard?

By this standard the pathologies of progress are at a disadvantage. George Beard's neurasthenia, flagship of the conditions considered here (can we even call them diseases?), is no longer a medical entity, only a curious conceptual relic. Given that we have decided that the persons thus diagnosed had no such disease, must we throw out their whining? Without a way to validate what brings suffering persons to clinical encounters, we risk doing that. One sort of validation comes from subjectivity: we have suffered from analogous conditions – perhaps depression, stress, or anxiety. But all these too are controversial terms in negotiations between subjects, practitioners, and societies. For as Charles Rosenberg has pointed out, translation is not always validation.[1]

I have no solution to validating general, amorphous, or sub-clinical suffering beyond reorienting the writing of medical history to make such pathologies of progress less anomalous. That means exploring dynamisms. What, in these cases, evokes response? Not – as elsewhere in public health, fear of catching plague or disgust at rot or ugliness.

This chapter explores the powers of medical expression – i.e., whatever a supplicant must say to elicit an adequate response – in nineteenth-century Britain. Plainly, the responder must know the codes too; coadaptation between supplicants and responders will presumably vary by place and time and perhaps, too, by race, age, gender, or class. Here I focus mainly on class, defined not in terms of objective socio-economic status nor modes of discursive engagement, but in terms of expectations of suffering. And I am concerned not with particular injury but with general affliction – with forms of expression which equate to: 'I can't stand it', 'I can't live like this'. The statements have no definite relation to the afflictions/conditions themselves, which may be life-threatening in the near term or debilitating in the longer. They may be intensely irritating or involve incursion of risks.

Historians of medicine will find context for such concern in classic works by Michel Foucault and by Nick Jewson: both explore how social and professional structures affect the expression of affliction and perhaps the experience of it too.[2] Some voicings of pain bring sympathy and soup. Others bring indifference, impatience, or contempt (especially if there are significant costs in responding to my whining). In that case I may learn to deny or suppress those pains.

Of the seven parts of this chapter, the first four are foundation, the next two application, and the last an assessment. My first task is to expand/adapt E. P. Thompson's concept of a 'moral economy', developed to explain features of social relations at the beginning of the long nineteenth century, to the domain of social medicine. Next, à la Raymond Williams, I begin to consider 'keywords', here verbs of existential unacceptability. These are probes for social practices, and good ways to chart change.[3] The first is the 'complaint' of my title. Sections three and four explore the nineteenth-century antecedents of general patho-physiological processes that served, and in some cases still serve, as currency in the moral economy of health: we use versions of them to validate suffering. Sections five and six are literary-historical case studies. With the help of Charles Dickens, I seek to show the limits of a medical moral economy in the 1830s and 1840s; with the help of D. H. Lawrence, I explore dynamic aspects of that moral economy in late-century public health/social medicine: its use not merely to enforce standards but also its potential to raise them. In the conclusion I assess this sort of analysis as a narrative foundation for the social history of health.

Health as moral economy

The protests I have alluded to are equally moral and economic expressions (they involve assertions of obligation and appeals for resources to relieve). For my period and for Britain, E. P. Thompson's concept of 'moral economy' is a good starting point. Thompson was seeking to explain so-called 'bread riots' of the late eighteenth and early nineteenth centuries – episodes in which crowds, largely led by women, acted against purveyors who had raised the prices of staple foodstuffs. These crowds did not loot; they took what they needed and paid what they saw as the just price.[4] Thompson was challenging narrative and analytic practices prevalent in one wing of Marxist historiography – that class conflict was incessant and unlimited, a zero-sum game, and that such explosions simply reflected a critical mass of tension and a circumstance. This Thompson challenged with two points. First that riots occurred not at the height of desperation but in anticipation of the price changes that would lead to it, and second that they were restorative not revolutionary. While, in Chapter 1 of this volume, we saw the shock of revolution interpreted and treated within emergent psychiatric practice as a form of therapy, here the crowds were not maximisers but moral enforcers, acting conservatively to maintain familiar social relations and stations of life.

Thompson did not extend the concept to health, yet such extension is implicit. Bread prices are proxies for survival; rioters were acting rationally, recognising that the debility of hunger would ultimately make it impossible to act.[5] And the concept is particularly apt for health. Unlike markets generally, where the marginal utilities are morally neutral and the participants value them as they please, health assessments involve perceptions of obligation and entitlement as well as allocation of scare communal resources. In the broader terms of welfare, such assessments are familiar – treatment and experience of children in the child reform movement discussed in Chapter 3; in the endless debates in charity organisation societies or about poor laws; in tergiversations about sturdy beggars or the deserving poor; and about moralising or demoralising forms of relief.

Thompson, however, was focusing not on obligation but entitlement. Concerned to humanise the writing of social history by directing it toward subjects and cultures rather than material conditions and determinisms, he did not consider what particular moral code rioters were seeking to enforce; 'moral' was important chiefly as a category. Prices, however, are quantitative; not so states of health. Here real questions arise about what the operant moral principles were on which people made medical claims. For rioters were taking risks. Their actions might be grudgingly tolerated by the magistracy or might not: a 'moral economy' might as readily be invoked to sanction price rises, not only by political economists defending the market, but by merchants passing on wholesale price increases. Why did rioters think they would be successful?

First, probably, because their demands were specific, modest, transitory, and local. To be deliverable, entitlements (or, more directly, 'rights'), must be well defined. The 'state of complete physical, mental and social well-being and not merely the absence of disease or infirmity', which the World Health Organization (WHO) obliges states to guarantee their citizens is indefinite.[6] The mandate offers no way to move from an expressed deficit of well-being to mediatory medicalisation, nor of prioritising harms to health. Nor does it acknowledge trade-offs in which delivering the right to some might require taking it from others. Instead, health is treated as an inalienable entity, akin to the right of conscience. The point is important: for 'moral' does not come as the antithesis of 'economic'; we should recognise that bargains are being struck, and allocations of costs and benefits will be occurring.

To make sense of the nineteenth-century medical moral economy – and the bread riots – would require a sharper definition of cultural conditions. Two sorts of explorations would be critical – one conceptual, and the other rhetorical, but also sociological. There must be an authoritative conceptual metric into which suffering may be translated, and hence claims of entitlement assessed and adjudicated – that is, a moral economy must have a currency. Since obligation, not price, is at issue, we cannot expect a market to make incommensurables commensurable, but something must do so. In fact, there were integrative biomedical concepts that did, though they changed radically over the course of the century. (By contrast, the WHO's 'well-being' lacks a clear currency.) But we also need to understand the situations and speech acts through which people could successfully invoke those conceptual frameworks. In the absence of objective tests of suffering – and there were more of these than we may realise – by what magic words does one establish one's claim? And how does this vary by speaker, place, and conditions? We might hope to discover too the determinants of the quality of response a claim elicited – minimal, grudging, and brief, or sympathetic, long-term support? For my goal here is to explore not only the kinetics of the medical moral economy but also its dynamics for progressive change. How was that moral economy made to grow in terms of the modestly rising entitlements and obligations for the public's health that occurred during the period (though never to the asymptotic levels imagined by WHO visionaries in 1948)?

This approach differs from a common view in which public health provision is a gift of policy made in the aftermath of social investigations to those too dull to demand it themselves. The questions it involves are formidable. Many historians have avoided them, or have looked at them from one side only – that of the providers of relief, with their concerns about epidemic diseases and their institution-building practices. Mathias in Chapter 5 demonstrated various means by which fictions of the period provoked and explored imaginative extensions of public health concerns. But 'moral economy' points us toward mandated exchanges, exchanges that are not merely permissible but obligatory.[7]

An essential beginning is the status of 'complaint'. Any claim on the moral economy will come as a complaint – bread rioters were complaining unambiguously about unacceptable prices. To complain, however, requires many things: recognition of suffering, the energy and capacity to express it, and perhaps the presumption of social sanction for the complaint's legitimacy. For we must not mistake complaint for power. Along with the question of who can complain is the question of what they can complain about and to whom.

Here I shall use 'complaint' and 'annoyance' as the terms traders use in the moral economy of medicine – they express conditions crowds (including crowds of one) find morally objectionable. In turn, I shall use 'stress' and 'overwork', and their nineteenth-century predecessors as the integrative conceptual metrics that serve as currency. Effacing the border between subjectivity and biomedical objectivity, these validate and delimit the complaint.

Irritations and agonies

Much of the history of moral economies is encapsulated in the changing valences of 'complain' over the course of the long nineteenth century. Earlier uses enforce seriousness and subjectivity: to 'complain' was 'to give expression to sorrow or suffering' (*OED* #1). It was linked to lamentation and wailing. This heritage lives on in the 'plaintive' 'pleading' of our 'plaint', registering pain and powerlessness.[8] There is nothing accusatory here, no grounds to second guess the suffering of the term's user. In medicine, too, a complaint is taken at face value as an existential expression: the recording medic writes, 'patient complains of' (#4a) and in further references translates these into the patient's 'complaint'. Usually the term is a hybrid between the conditions the patient objects to and the healer's understanding of the (quasi-diagnostic) entity to be remedied.[9] Here, medicalisation helps to legitimise: the complaint is recognised as a departure from well-being, a situation that may be fixable and perhaps could have been prevented.[10]

The most familiar modern usage is quite different: 'To give expression to feelings of illusage, dissatisfaction, or discontent; to murmur, grumble' (#6). These all point to blameworthy external causes: the complainer is simultaneously alluding to an injury, identifying responsibility for it, and appealing to a presumed entitlement. The valences differ from other ways of expressing injury and reparability: 'I have a suggestion', 'I have a problem that needs fixing', or even 'this case falls under the moral precept' may all be respected, even welcomed.

Yet with its overtones of sulkiness, 'grumble' suggests that by designating one's expression as a 'complaint' one has pushed a presumed 'moral economy' too far. We lose even more legitimacy if expressing a 'complaint' puts us on the slippery slope from 'subject who has complained' to the identity of 'complainer', a term for a habitual maker of such statements. Hence to have one's dissatisfaction registered as 'complaint' may be so counterproductive as to be the basis for dismissing one's imperative, as the *OED*'s illustrations suggest. Thus Robert Burns writes of one 'always compleenin frae mornin to e'enin' (4b). Evelyn Waugh writes: 'Everyone I met complained bitterly about the injustice of having to earn a living and the peculiar beastliness of his own profession' (6c). Here 'complaint' is self-indulgent kvetching.[11] However *discontented* we may be, no one wants to labelled a '*malcontent*'.

And those who say 'X is complaining again' are themselves complaining – expressing exhaustion and exasperation at being expected to fix what is too hard to fix, or to deliver special treatments that the complainers have no right to ask for. Though they may have the greater complaints, theirs may go unvoiced if, in the economy of exchanged rather than essential deference, they are paid to hear ours, as persons in customer service certainly are.

What shall we make of this evolution of heartfelt distress into barely tolerated moaning? I think the change reflects the coming of equality. 'Complaint' has become less moral and more economic. The tone of powerlessness (at least of some) in the face of misfortune – human or divine – is gone, replaced by a jealousy about status in societies that purport to deride class and deny station. The situation is that depicted by Norbert Elias in his famous analysis of the history of manners. According to Elias, in complaining we are expressing aspirations appropriate to the imperial (and imperious) identity we would like to be granted.[12] A lump under a mattress will no longer register if someone can respond: 'you're not a princess; you're lucky to have a bed at all'.

Complaining then may represent not a rebalancing of the moral economy, but its collapse, through an amplifying infection of irritability as people complain about complaining – a 'mood contagion', as Kowalski puts it.[13] The 'moral' in 'moral economy' was fragile. The equilibration Thompson's actors seek depended on some shared notion of the legitimacy of some complaints. These were in part functions of the supposedly objective biomedical currencies that circulated in this 'moral economy'. If current enlistments of 'complaint' often bring loss of social capital, it behooves us to look more closely at the conditions of its creation. Perhaps those very ripples of dissatisfaction we label as complaint can, in other circumstances, generate rising expectations that translate into healthful aspiration.

The afflictive world

Probably the most common contemporary expression for medicalised complaining is 'stress'. And, as Waugh suggests, its chief cause is the grind of (over) 'work', not merely from paid employment but as manifestion of the composite exhaustion of modern living (the titular 'pathologies of progress'). Used together, the terms are especially helpful in uniting physical conditions with emotional responses.[14] And both refer, sometimes simultaneously, to conditions and causes, and to perceptions, interpretations, and expressions. Both are critical terms. As with 'complaint' itself, an utterance of 'stress' signifies not only as diagnosis, but as accusation and explanation. Some nineteenth-century medical writers who spoke of stress were borrowing the notion of the forces that reshaped an object, while others drew from the vernacular 'distress'.[15] 'Work' too was an activity, a human identity, and a physical quantity.

Given these foundations, it is easy to see how the terms might translate subjectivity into objectivity. In doing so they functioned on three levels: to the individual they provided a way to articulate a state of being and adopt an appropriate identity on the basis of a self-assessment; to society they represented a demand for renegotiation of the terms of participation; and to the physician they offered a generic explanation that may guide both that sense of identity and that negotiation.

For contemporary scholars, that generic explanation is based in mid-twentieth-century physiological research chiefly by Walter Cannon of Harvard and Hans Seyle of McGill. They translated the heritage of 'neurasthenia', the quintessential pathology of progress, into hormone biochemistry. That translation broadened symptoms. In addition to providing a biomedical underwriting of subjective elements – mood changes, fatigue, trouble sleeping – it objectified and quantified injury in terms of elevated blood pressure, arthritis, ulcers, cancer, autoimmune conditions, coronary disease, or even suicide, though none was exclusive to 'stress'.[16]

There were other changes. First, some of these harmful changes were imperceptible. Thus stress validated complaint but was not limited to the ability to express. Second, physiological research provided a better conceptual basis for distinguishing recovery – the 'homeostasis' that allowed mammalian bodies to maintain stability in changing and in extreme situations – from irreversible damage: for overstressed bodies lost their ability to re-equilibrate. Remarkably, Cannon–Seyle managed to be explanatory and validating without being reductive. Just as there were stressors and manifestations of stress measurable but not felt, so there were some that might be felt but not measured: stress was emotional as well as physiological. Remarkable too is the cultural credit the concept acquired. In terms of declarations of illness accepted without biomedical confirmation, stress and anxiety come close to carrying the power of nausea or diarrhoea.

Discovery of 'stress' was not accidental. Concerned with understanding the dynamics of human performance, Seyle and Cannon drew from medical history and saw themselves as elaborating an equilibration agenda that had dominated classical (or 'humoural') clinical medicine since Hippocrates.[17] In turn their concept may serve as a currency. The explorations below suggest how it might be possible to apply that concept despite lack of confirmation from the usual epidemiological sources. For usually these concentrate either on immediate causes of death or on incidence of particular diseases. They obscure integrative conditions manifest in dissatisfaction or dysfunction. And leaving aside categories, the high incidence of infections will have masked stress-related conditions that would become visible only after an epidemiologic transition made so-called 'lifestyle-related' causes of death more prominent.[18]

'And all must have prizes'[19]

A medicalised 'stress' may seem the solution to the complainer's problem of how to register one's distress without being branded a malcontent. Yet it is equally possible that, linked to 'complaint', 'stress' will be swept into the same abyss. If it is to liberate or legitimise, medicalisation must first overcome a filtering based in class (and perhaps in gender, life stage, or race).

The irony is especially sharp for class. If those who complain the most about stress *also* possess the greatest means to avoid it, what of those without such means? Presumably they must be suffering more acutely. One may filter claims in two ways, both de-legitimising. One is to view 'stress' (or 'complaint') as peevishness. The other is the exoticisation of some persons as too dull to experience the refined anguish that plagues the more sensitive and vocal.

Prior to 1700 I find little class-specificity in discussions of constitutional illnesses in European medicine. The predominant notion is that any person will need periodically to rebalance the so-called non-naturals

– air, diet, activity, sleep, excretions and secretions, and passions of mind. The circumstances of stress vary by class and occupation as do the remedies – Mme Sévinge's accounts of mid-seventeenth-century Versailles life allude to the strain of courtly deference. Those of her rank can retire to their chateaux. That others cannot is simple fact, but the lack of any sharp demarcation between normal and pathological existence brings with it a presumption of universalism: we each in our way suffer from more or less the same strains.[20]

Diseases of affectation, or to James Adair, of 'fashion', begin to be evident shortly after 1700, with the emergence of the 'valetudinarian', one (usually a man) of such delicacy that health requires avoiding any 'annoyance' (a term I explore later). Other terms, 'spleen', 'vapours', 'hypochondriasis', 'hysteria', or merely 'febricula' did much the same work, though many had distinct class, life course, or gender implications. These would evolve by late in the century into a 'nervousness' endemic among wealthy young women and attributed in part to what are recognizably social stresses.[21]

Yet remarkably, these concepts took root first in a Newtonian cultural context, in which cause must have effect.[22] That view is even more prominent in another heritage of stress, also recognised in early modern medicine: the environmental, economic, and psychic stresses of poverty. Indeed, these, and not emotional stresses, were Seyle's primary concerns, and they were explored further by postwar physiologists studying starvation.[23] Bodies must respond lawfully to a variety of acute and chronic nutritional stresses, to dehydration, extremes of temperature (both hypothermia and heat stroke are kinds of stress), and sleep deprivation, but also to the anxieties which all of these incur. The manifestations of hunger, for example, are equally somatic, psychic, and social.

Such stress is axiomatic for Karl Marx, for whom health, bodily and mental, is a liquefiable asset, which capital will convert into surplus value. In discussing the working day in the first volume of *Capital*, Marx quotes contemporary investigators of the mid-Victorian workplace. He need not be a diagnostician of overwork, merely a compiler: these authorities recognise the slow destruction – of 'frames dwindling ... faces whitening ... humanity absolutely sinking into a stone-like torpor'. Some note stress-related conditions: 'dyspepsia ... disorders of the liver and kidneys ... rheumatism'.[24]

All are products of a lengthening work day. Capital burns individuals as fast as it can. It will extract time from eating, resting, or simply living, stopping only when the labouring population is no longer able to reproduce a future workforce. Marx quotes Benjamin Ward Richardson, writing, long before Seyle, on the 'stress of work'. Richardson imagines a blacksmith, capable of some number of hammer blows during a fifty-year working life, being 'made to strike so many more blows, to walk so many more steps, to breathe so many more breaths per day and … producing for a limited time a fourth more work', and dying earlier by exactly that proportion.[25]

Yet the protests do not come from the victims who 'silently pine and die', but from humanitarian investigators.[26] In his extended treatment, *Diseases of Modern Life* (1882), Richardson embraced the stresses of intellectual and artistic work. In the case of manual labourers, 'who wear out by such action itself, or by the addition of certain surrounding influences which add to the exhaustion', it was plain that work (and thus life) was stress. Of these 'sons of slavish toil', Richardson declared that 'the misery of their lives is only ameliorated by the shortness of the trial' – the hammer blows should be struck as rapidly as possible. As Rabinbach has shown, commodifying human lives had become a fetish by the end of the century.[27]

In converting stress into a currency of historical assessment – and not merely a crotchet of self-indulgent modernity, we face three central challenges.

I have considered the first, the palaeo-epidemiological. That the term 'stress' is grounded both in experiment and expression; that something like it was diagnosed in severe cases does not necessarily allow us to link the expression of stress to physiological stress in sub-clinical cases. Stressors manifest in many ways and over a long period; and surely we can't fit eighteenth-century persons with blood-pressure cuffs.

The second concerns expressibility. Can we assume that there will there be languages for stressed persons to say they are stressed? We have no basis for thinking that what is felt can and will be stated, much less recorded, nor any right to expect a transparent or uniform language of pain. Perhaps, if verbalising distress is forbidden, there will be other forms of protest, biomedical analogues to James Scott's 'weapons of the weak'.[28]

Last, and most important here, are the conditions outlined earlier with regard to successful enlistment of the moral economy: issues of universality, targeting, and responsiveness. If language is available, who gets to use it, on which targets, and with what expectations of response?

These questions may be asked of any illness, but are harder to answer for stress. Yet we can find bodies of evidence that bear on them in periods before the modern era of stress-expressibility. For various reasons, late medieval and early modern historians have been more comfortable exploring such issues.[29] Indeed, by integrating religious anxieties, their studies have sometimes approached the asymptote of a comprehensive accounting of stresses – psychic, physical, and spiritual. By contrast, nineteenth-century historians have often reduced the biomedical to epidemic infections – notably to cholera and tuberculosis. In British history in particular, the public health movement dominates. It is (correctly) seen as preoccupied with faecal-oral diseases.

But public health, as the WHO reminds us, involves more. One of the two cases I explore below concerns the desperation of unsettledness; the other the stultifying stuckness of settledness in a dehumanising environment. In each I use contemporary fiction to interrogate an ambiguous historical record. Literary artists claim access to characters' senses of self and world, including individuals' understandings of and responses to the stresses of their lives. Historians rarely aspire to such intimacy; rarely do our sources encourage it.

Cold women

To illustrate the importance and potential of 'complaint', it may help to consider its absence in conjunction with a minimalist concept of a moral economy. Thus: in the aftermath of the infamous New Poor Law of 1834, a nameless gravid woman is found 'lying in the street' by a local overseer. She has evidently 'walked some distance' and has been admitted to a workhouse where she gives birth, asks to see her baby, states that she will then die, and does so. She is overworked ('labouring' may apply equally to birthing, labouring under fever, and to walking and carrying – all heavy caloric demands). That she has undertaken a long journey on foot during her third trimester suggests desperation – mental as well as physical stress. Knowing what we know of contemporary mores and bastardy laws we may assume ostracism too: she is in need among persons who may despise her. Tea and sympathy might help but no one offers. How does she die? Not apparently from any single disease entity: the sequence of events rules out puerperal fever, but it is plausible to understand her death in some broadly accumulative sense. She suffers from exhaustion and exposure compounded with abjection and hopelessness. She has neither strength nor will to live.

You may know this woman as Agnes Fleming, mother of Oliver Twist, and the events as those of the first two pages of Dickens's novel. The modern reader only learns her name and background hundreds of pages later, while the first readers of this serialised novel were presented with her effective anonymity: they had to wait *two years* for a scanty backstory.

It is hardly possible to acknowledge, and yet dismiss, deadly stress more effectively than Dickens does here. In contrast with the 'wellbeing' guaranteed by the WHO, here obligation is asymptotic as it approaches nullity. Dickens comes close to denying her the personhood of speech. Agnes gets seven words. 'Let me see the child, and die'. Her postpartum condition and behaviour get fewer than 200 words, her background (discovery by the overseer, shoe wear indicating long journey, lack of identity), only forty-six. Her social status – 'No weddingring, I see' – takes just five. Here Dickens, perhaps sharing contemporary views, permits Agnes no complaint, except perhaps about herself, evident in her intent to die.[30] Not so David Lean, who concentrated on her complaint in filming the book. He opens with a tiny figure cresting a hill, with rising wind followed by rain and thunder. We see a thornbush, an exhausted face, a distant light toward which she staggers, and later a waking Agnes who smiles with delight at her baby.[31]

Here, none of the three conditions are met: the group to which Agnes is assigned – fallen women – is one in which complaint is forbidden; she is too stressed even to muster the strength to complain, and the targets of her complaint would be diffuse. Finally, this is a legal, not a moral economy: the parish officials do only what the poor law requires.[32] To the degree that a moral economy underwrites this, it is that of Thomas Malthus, whose analysis of human population dynamics indicated a need to minimise the population-inflating stimulus of obligation.[33]

Given Dickens's outrage at the physical and nutritional stress the New Poor Law imposes on Oliver, his neglect of his mother is striking.

But the very absence of a moral economy here invites consideration of the enormous range of obligations that might be recognised. Given a slug of brandy, and then asked, as a parish surgeon might, 'what is your complaint', where would Agnes begin? She might say, 'Isn't it obvious?' But what would she be targeting? Would she be admitting that she is, as Dickens later labels her, a 'weak and erring' fallen woman? Or might she fulminate at the sources of stress – God, men, or a society that so signally despises isolated pregnant women? Or perhaps she would be protesting a more general frailty of nature – the cold and exhaustion that bring on hopelessness, or even the nature of the body of a fertile female.

Accrediting Agnes's experience requires giving her a vocabulary. What might be the keywords for converting experience into protest? Two would be 'misery' and 'miserable'. Yet, as with 'complain' and 'complaint', the *OED* chronicles confusion: both conflation and inversion of moral valences. Originally 'misery' was objective: 'A condition of external unhappiness, discomfort, or distress; wretchedness of outward circumstances; distress caused by privation or poverty.' (*OED* 'misery', #1a). The subjective version, 'Great sorrow or mental distress; a miserable or wretched state of mind; a condition characterized by a feeling of extreme unhappiness', only begins to be (ambiguously) evident in the seventeenth century and takes hold only in the mid-nineteenth (#3a).[34] If this evolution may seem to humanise the physical condition of misery, it also allows its trivialisation: the well-off can now claim 'misery'.

'Miserable' evolves on a similar schedule (*OED*, 'miserable', #1a, #1c), but acquires even more nuances.[35] It can refer to external stressors as in 'miserable weather' or 'miserable working conditions' (#2b) but also to opposing representations of a person: either as 'contemptible, despicable' (#3b) or as 'poor, unhappy, or wretched' (#5b). The opportunity for confusion/inversion is evident. Both Agnes and a poor law official might call her 'miserable', but the first would mean 'unhappy' and the second, 'contemptible'. Even more sharply than with 'complaint' the very word with which one makes a claim on a moral economy subverts the claim.

For two reasons we should not regard Agnes an 'everywoman', even for early nineteenth-century Britain. Her pregnancy and marital status are factors in the operation of a moral economy; so too is the New

Poor Law itself, which in England, but not Scotland (or yet in Ireland) transferred much of the domain of entitlement/obligation into public policy. Agnes (and later Oliver) get care from the infamous workhouse of the New Poor Law, where an 'experimental philosophy' is in operation to determine the minima of human survival. But one may ask how other overworked and stressed persons – friendless, travelling on foot, perhaps in bad weather – negotiate their complaints with themselves and with medical or charitable institutions? How did this moral economy work for them? For here too there were gatekeepers and magic words.

This is a matter both of ideas and of institutions. With regard to ideas, a holistic Hippocratic-Galenic heritage, still ascendant in British medicine in the first half of the nineteenth century, emphasised individualistic causation of illness and gave exhaustion primacy as a cause. The key theorist was the popular Edinburgh medical teacher William Cullen. He and his successors trained many of the practitioners active in the north of England and in Scotland and Ireland.[36] Though his integrating entity is 'debility', a condition jointly physical and mental, Cullen's model anticipates Seyle's 'stress'. For Cullen 'cold' (a term implying too the lack of nutriment needed to withstand it) effectively stands for physical, and 'fear' for psychic stressors, with the latter including anxiety about meeting physical needs as well as 'watching' or sleeplessness, whose significance has been highlighted by modern stress theorists.[37] When these factors, operating collectively, reached a threshold, fever would result. That misery-induced fever might then spread to non-miserable persons. Via the emergent-contagion doctrine the poor became a threat to the rich.[38]

In the first half of the nineteenth century the most important medical institutions of a moral economy of health were dispensaries, infirmaries, and fever hospitals, particularly in Scotland and Ireland, where no legal obligation to support the destitute existed for most of the period. It may seem that this Cullenian paradigm will underwrite any complaint Agnes might make: to be exhausted, hungry, cold, or scared is to be dangerously ill. Therapy too was commonsensical – provision of the 'necessaries' (food, warmth, and shelter).

But there are ambiguities. With respect to expressibility, exhaustion exhausts reflection; fever (or hypothermia) undermines reason and behaviour – the very dignity we need if we expect accreditation of our protests. While acute irrationality would be noticed as delirium – itself interpreted as exhaustion – less serious cases might be unrecognised and unarticulated.[39]

Nor, even when it became serious enough to trigger a clinical response, did that composite debility imply culpability. Indeed, 'soup kitchen' medicine – the common practice during epidemics of distributing soup, blankets, and coals – has been denigrated as temporising: a patching-up that neglects underlying causes of social problems.[40] And yet there are hints that even where no legal provision existed, soup kitchens and other 'medical charities', providing relief – rest and food – did come to be seen as entitlements, as one would expect in a conservative and restorative 'moral economy'. Without acknowledging the agenda of culpability, they compensated reliably for oscillations in the conditions of survival. I have examined patient records from Dublin, Glasgow, Edinburgh, and Carlisle. In them are bits of Agnes-like stories, with Cullenian detail of exposure/exhaustion. Thus some examples from 127 cases described in Dominic Corrigan's service at the Hardwicke Hospital, Dublin, in 1840–41, and in 1844.[41]

A servant, 28, unable to shake a cold, with debility and loss of appetite, reports much 'mental anxiety and bodily exertion'.

A servant, 19, attributes lightness and giddiness, loss of appetite to a cold from sleeping in a damp room. A laundry maid, 37, attributes pains, cough, and cold feet to going out in the cold while hot. Two others refer illnesses to neglecting to change from wet clothes (had they a change available?). So too does a groom, ill from cold and wet on a February crossing from England.

A tailor, 24, having caught cold from wet, reports 'cold trembling all over, and general weakness. He wishes for something to eat'. The medic writes: 'he has merely to complain of weakness and thinks appropriate nutriment would quickly restore his health'.

A shoemaker, 27, has headaches and abdominal pains from 'falling asleep outside'.

An 'intemperate' cabinet maker, 29, of 'wretched appearance and feeble emaciated frame', has chest pain, but was 'observed not to suffer so much from cough as from want of food for which he had a good appetite'.

A woman, 39, having recovered from bronchitis, is discharged, but returns four days later with a relapse. On readmission she is found to have 'slight symptoms of common inflammatory fever – [but] to suffer more from the effects of want of care and of food'. Following a treatment of 'warmth. Food and some diaphoretic medicines, ... she was discharged well' two-and-a-half weeks later.

A shoemaker, 26, with pain in small of back and 'extreme mischief all over' cannot sleep. 'His Countenance ... expressive of distress rather than of illness'.

And, finally, an Agnes, 22, eight months pregnant, delivers and dies on the day of admission. She is described as 'cross and irritable', the only occasion in these notebooks where mood is mentioned.

How should we hear such summaries? Are patients accusing or simply explaining? Are doctors hinting that such problems are social and political, not medical, or simply acquiescing in the realities of their practices? Or even, does the privilege of hearing 'complaint' inhere only in critics, distant in time, situation, or both?

Usually we don't know. In July 1840 a woman, 21, attributes her fever, by then pretty well over, 'to having over-worked herself, and when very much heated ... having exposed herself to cold'. The language (if we can trust the recorder) seems to assert choice, to admit error. Yet how free is she? Depending on the expectations of an employer or the demands of a market in which she engages, not overworking may not be an option.

The Hardwicke was a state fever hospital. Because it might be, or become, contagious, incipient fever was taken especially seriously. And yet few of these patients have the most serious fever, typhus, and several have no fever at all. Some stay for weeks. A woman, 28, described as 'almost convalescent on admission ... [and] without any particular complications' stays two weeks.

Dublin's fever hospitalisation practices are unique, reflecting an oversupply of beds subsidised by a state fearful of masses of hunger-generated fever moving across the Irish Sea. Institutional responses differed in Glasgow, Edinburgh, and Carlisle. With fewer beds, they relied more on organised home care (as with Edinburgh's Society for the Relief of the Destitute Sick), or on intermediate institutions (like Glasgow's Town's Hospital).

Nosy neighbours

My second case explores the vocalising of chronic complaint rather than the negotiation of desperation. Do people come to recognise and protest the invisible stresses of debilitating conditions? To challenge the responsible moral economy when sudden changes threaten survival is not especially remarkable; to challenge it on a broad front in times of normality is more so.

Yet imagine a truly complaint-encouraging world. 'I am annoyed', I say, 'and stressed too, by rubble in the street, or the smell of sausage-making, or simply by filth'. A minor official, possessed of some obscure quasi-medical authority by virtue of the title of 'inspector of nuisances' appears, confronts the irritating parties, and makes their nuisance stop – by summons, fines, and mandamus action if necessary.

The Victorian nuisances inspector was the foot soldier of sanitary reform. What ultimately became the profession of Sanitary, or later Environmental Health inspector, was not wholly the brainchild of Edwin Chadwick, but he had much to do with ensuring the universal appointment of such officers by English local authorities in the two decades after the pioneering Public Health Act of 1848. Their odd work was not only to respond to complaints, but also to declare conditions to be nuisances.[42]

That their pronouncements were seldom contested is less a matter of expertise than of the cultural capital with which they operated. 'Nuisance' was both a vague and a powerful term. Its derivation is from 'annoyance', which, in turn, went well beyond private pique or insufferable affectation to refer to real condition. Thus, well into the eighteenth century, we see references to roads 'annoyed' by trash.[43] They are not being personified with capacity for taking offence; rather, 'annoy', like 'injury' or 'harm' united human with non-human. To the degree that nuisances were real, their discovery was a matter of perception, not of heightened sensibility.

Nuisances were legally real too. Under the broad heading of trespass, common law underwrote annoyance. A nuisance might be private or public, remediation of the latter being the responsibility of the magistracy or other appropriate local authority. One need not show harm to health, merely transgression of public standards. In many towns, moreover, there was a centuries-long tradition of citizen-based environmental enforcement through courts leet or assizes of nuisance. These relied on juries to inspect and adjudicate. To physical, customary, and legal authority, Chadwick added biomedical authority. The stench from next door was not just a violation of community standards or an impairment of one's enjoyment of property, but potentially deadly under the 'all smell is disease' maxim.

By ingeniously grafting a central government functionary onto the heritage of local self-government and common law, Chadwick and his successors were creating a role rife with a tension common to many forms of policing. As its appointed 'nose', the inspector was to represent the community; however, as representative of state- and science-based biomedical expertise, the inspector must be outside it, able to dictate the standards necessary for collective (and individual) well-being.

Inspectors were not miracle-workers transforming industrial towns into garden suburbs. The grand question is not so much *what* they did but *how* – both how they mitigated distressing conditions in nineteenth-century towns and transformed expectations and attitudes, instilling a culture of complaint. As with food riots, enlistment of communal standards was essential – as Elias and Mary Douglas remind us, 'dirt' is a communal declaration and a powerful social motor, just as a proper sense of annoyance was a key mark of class identity. By marshalling these forces the inspectors, prodding and praising on behalf of health, beauty, decency, and community, might hope gradually to produce change.[44]

Survival of inspectors' records is spotty, but among the best series is that for the east Midlands brewing and coal town, Worksop, for which there are weekly summaries in fine hand from 1871 to 1886. There the first inspector we meet is Henry Mellars, who shares a surname peculiar to the region with D. H. Lawrence's fictional gamekeeper, Oliver Mellors, aka Lady Chatterley's lover.[45] Lawrence's Mellors hails from the fictional Tevershall, a Nottinghamshire coal town based on Lawrence's boyhood home of Eastwood, about thirty miles from Worksop. However facile, juxtaposing the fictional Mellors with the real Mellars is a fruitful way to explore responses to the stresses of life in industrial towns.

Lady Chatterley's Lover is a novel of oppositions: living and dead, nature and artifice, beauty and ugliness, masters and servants, capital and labour, cleanliness and squalor, hope and despair, and, of course sensual engagement and dull acceptance. 'Tevershall' applies equally and interchangeably to town, coal pit, and people. There what Marx anticipated has come to pass: work drives out all else, including ability to challenge the conditions of existence.[46]

To outsider Connie Chatterley, Tevershallian conditions preclude the 'spontaneity' and 'intuition' of full 'humanness' (205). Not only is a stroll in the woods impossible, to feel annoyance and to complain, preconditions of any moral economy, are too. Describing 'blackened brick dwellings ... black slate roofs ... mud black with coal-dust ... pavements wet and black', she reflects: it seemed 'as if dismalness had soaked through and through everything. The utter negation of natural beauty, the utter negation of the gladness of life, the utter absence of the instinct for shapely beauty which every bird and beast has, the utter death of the human intuitive faculty was appalling' (204).

For Connie, horror gets the better of any sympathy, for it is she, not the Tevershallians, who experiences stress. Of 'the industrial masses', she is 'absolutely afraid'. They seem 'so *weird*' – 'incarnate ugliness'. All this brings 'a queer feeling ... all over her, like influenza' (213). But 'if you were poor and wretched you *had* to care', insists insider Mellors. In fact, there was too much life, 'a terrible, seething welter of ugly life' (146) behind the 'flat drabness'; lives of 'misery, bitterness, and ugliness', and of 'futility, futility to the nth power'. His pathology was not, like flu, a dangerous corruption of passing innocents, but internal – a malignancy, a 'great cancer' (193).

Capitalists Connie and Clifford Chatterley may choose how to engage with Tevershall – Connie with revulsion; Clifford, as a progressive industrialist, creatively. The responses of Mellors and of the other main character, the nurse Ivy Bolton, are necessarily more complicated. Being of Tevershall and dependent on it, they have fewer degrees of freedom. Yet each, crossing boundaries of class, encounters the same ambiguities that inspectors experienced. Like the inspectors, gamekeeper Mellors is expert yet servile. His education and experience would allow a middle-class career of local civic leadership, yet as much as possible he has abandoned Tevershall for a life in the woods raising pheasant chicks.

Not so Ivy Bolton, miner's widow, parish nurse, and finally nurse-companion to Clifford, a role in which she is both above and of Tevershall. Her story is complicated. Were Sophocles in charge, it might be one of vengeful karma. Ted, the husband she loved, had died in an explosion in Tevershall pit (before Clifford inherited). On the grounds of his independence – he stood while others crouched – compensation had been minimal (122–3). Ted had hated that life; he could not escape it even in sex with a caring partner seeking to relieve his anguish (217). After his death, Ivy finds the means to train as a nurse and reintegrates into Tevershall as 'one of the governing class of the village' (122) until her appointment to care for the paraplegic Clifford.

Here questions do arise about moral economies. 'What justice will she enforce?' Lawrence wonders. Her relationship with Clifford is deep, intimate, and multidimensional, yet ultimately she is a labourer, though one who, like Thompson's riot leaders, controls in quiet ways the terms of the relationship. And, like the inspectors, she mediates as a double agent, interpreting Tevershall for Clifford. If she is his spy, she is also its advocate, defending the workers against the masters. As to what stresses *she* feels from being a sounding board of Clifford's complaints and being chiefly responsible for Clifford's well-being (no less than Mellors is for his baby pheasants), Lawrence is silent.

In Worksop, Henry Mellars too must be both outsider and insider, dictator of propriety for the public's good and sensitive to the practicalities of life in a coal town. Worksop had about 11,000 people by the mid-1880s. Even before discovery of coal in the 1860s, it had been viewed as a sanitary disaster, a place of high death rate and squalor.[47]

It is in the first instance as a physical entity that Mellars confronts Worksop: persons appear in regard to structures. His moral economy must bypass any *grand mal* issues of class conflict. Wages and strikes, rents and prices, those factors that concentrate humans into small and dirty spaces and their most important means of protests, are off-limits for him. Instead, he will disturb this universe by modest architectural alterations, public and private. Want to stop the contemptuous gesture of male public urination? Remove corners to piss in, thus dulling the edge of class conflict by, literally, removing edges. Yet prostates and distended bladders still rule and urban settings must accommodate.[48]

The surviving notebooks begin in 1871. They show Mellars already busy seeking a standard of acceptable living – how many persons per privy? One, for twenty-one people on Church Walk, is too few. So are two for more than thirty, and 'the tenants are strongly of this opinion', he notes.[49] Indeed.

Water quality is a common complaint:

- 'unfit to drink ... has been ... for some months. The tenants declare that the drainage gets into the well'. This affects seven cottages, fourteen adults, and twenty-three children.
- Again, 'The tenants declare' – 'unfit to drink, being muddy and of nasty taste', with 'soap suds'. 'Tenants are much distressed to procure that required for drinking and cooking'.
- Or the 'inhabitants of the row ... complain much'.
- Or tenants 'complain greatly of the water ... It makes "*awful*" tea. ... I examined a large pot which had been filled over night; (the owner assured me that it was previously perfectly clean), a greasy, filthy smelling sediment was collected. Forty Two persons ... are supposed to drink the water'.
- Or water 'green in colour and nasty smell ... inhabitants are at ... wits end ... Several children have had slight fever'.[50]

This last is not epidemiology: that residents – who have not, we may presume, read John Snow – find the water that bad is authority enough for Mellars, though his successor Sampson White will routinely seek the authority of analysis. If, sometimes, Mellars associates bad water with disease, it is more as reminder: behind the work of defending decencies that should need no defense are health dangers too.

Accident prevention is a concern. Parents and Mellars worry about children falling into open wells. Or loose bricks or a sign may fall. Sometimes Mellars endorses tenants' direct action, as when, during a dry summer, they have 'wisely filled up the gullies with soil' as 'the stench was unbearable'. Yet they may need tutelage: women throw 'soap suds and dirty water into a field opposite houses, ... causing a Nuisance. ... Asked ... to *discontinue the same*'. Or he may mediate: whose turn to clean a common privy? The inspector must intervene.[51]

We should not assume that rules of sanitary propriety are obvious – to anyone. Why, after the stable has burned, can the horse not be buried in the garden? Are doors on privies the public's concern? Yes, his Board declares.[52] That raises the question: 'whose decency does Mellars enforce?' He respects local power, giving much time to the bishop's complaint of an obscure smell, while insinuating its frivolousness. But he also pushes, suggesting policy initiatives (the banning of pigsties), challenges developers of unsound housing – 'a discredit to the Town and its Sanitary Authorities', demands major repairs ('entire reconstruction' of a row of privies and wash-houses), and regulates nuisance industries (gas lime must be instantly barged out of town).[53] Ironically, among the malefactors is a non-complying landlord, Mr. Edward (not Edwin) Chadwick. (And Connie Chatterley visits Chadwick Hall.)[54]

Mellars defies classification. He is more than policeman, yet not quite activist. It may help to think of him as a live-in architect, always alert to what might be changed. Consider the following assessment of structure, circumstance, and use. A set of wash-houses and privies in the afternoon sun: 'in one corner of the Wash-house (that next to the privy pit) is a small ... set-pot for heating water for washing ... . [But] when used, the fire warms ... the contents of the pit, making the whole place unbearable. The ventilation also is inefficient. When the collier ... retires into the wash-house to strip and wash, for decency's sake the door is closed. The effect on an empty stomach may be imagined.'[55]

'Imagined', perhaps, but evidently not complained of. Much like Connie, Mellars has imported sensibility into a setting where it has been blunted by familiarity and lack of possibility. But here that sensibility generates not revulsion, but sympathy and possibility. Will (and should) anyone care if he gets these privy-wash-houses rebuilt? No grand sanitary problem will have been solved. Lawrence, who ignores sanitation in Tevershall, will still sneer: more fiddling with nth degree futility.

Here, however, the half-century separating Mellars from Lawrence's novel may matter. Whether or not class stratification was sharper in Lawrence's day, it was different: unions, a Labour Party, and concepts of inevitable struggle had transformed class consciousness. By contrast Mellars's notebooks remind us of an earlier paternalism in which seemingly incidental elements of the physical environment were both mark and means of moral progress. The idea of nuisance inspectors as counter-revolutionary cadres may seem far-fetched, but Chadwick's 1842 *Sanitary Report* was presented to a government terrified of Chartism, and for good reason: later in the summer the 'plug plot' rioters would make parts of the north ungovernable. Such a 'moralising' thrust continued: it would be central in late-century reformism – evident in the Charity Organisation Society and in Beatrice Webb's career as a lady rent collector.[56]

Given the emphasis in modern public health on the quality of communities, best known in the Healthy Cities movement, we should not dismiss such work.[57] However, I am less concerned with the impossible task of measuring Mellars's social-capital production, than simply with the recognition implicit in the public work that nuisance inspectors did – that the built environment (like the natural one that soaked and chilled Dubliners) strains health and may become a domain of moral economy.

Conclusion: recovering bodies

Each of the bodies of documents I have explored reaches randomly into matters both quotidian and intimate. Each of the many persons who come into our gaze arrives bearing some complex burden of exigency, which has precipitated a crisis. Each asks to be taken seriously. Often the tragedies they describe move us in their familiarity – travellers overcome by cold, wet, and worry; parents worrying about accident-prone play-spaces. These records remind us of irritants that always assail existence – hunger and thirst; weariness and the need for darkness, quiet, and rest; the many impediments and distractions to our movement, efforts, or attention; the discomforts of convenient elimination; the gasping for breath; the shivering and sweating from sun, cold, humidity, rain, or wind; and the incessant demands of impatient others. All these come with varying doses of fear. Rarely are the backstories detailed but we do the in-filling. We can overcome, too, the literary practices of probing junior doctors or officious inspectors. They bypass the most immediate and powerful expressions of pain, despair, or frustration – sobbing or yelling – though, inadvertently, the effect of their omission may dignify their subjects.

But what to *do* with these records? Learning what the Dublin doctors or Mellars did is all very well, but I am more concerned with those with whom they were interacting, persons often overlooked as too ordinary to be interesting, as if, in such lives, nothing happens that might be registered in complaint and/or stress. How they have come to be lost may be understood by considering two axes of interpretive practice: the axis separating social history from the social history of medicine, and that separating 'soft' from 'hard' Marxist interpretive practices. I will touch briefly on each, then on their intersection.

At the risk of over-generalisation, it is probably right to say that a commonplace of contemporary historical narrative is the awarding, and even the fetishising, of full 'agency' to historical subjects, as if all are wholly healthy mid-life adults living in constitutional polities and accountable accordingly. By contrast, the subjects of medical history (even after two generations of social historians seeking access to the experience of illness), remain largely doctor-defined. Usually being recognised as a medical subject has required diagnostic confirmation, whether by modern or by past professional standards, no matter how poorly that diagnostic status registers the existential complaints these persons may have had. Those poles suggest a missing middle – of people who complain and who have much to complain of, like those we meet in these records, and who live lives that are strained, but who cannot be written off as 'diseased'. Susan Lynn Smith's wonderful title, *Sick and Tired of Being Sick and Tired*, captures that existence. If the latter 'sick and tired' represents a draining of agency, the former reminds us of the further stress that comes from reflecting on that despair.[58]

We have invited ourselves into these lives via the bridging concepts of stress and overwork. But these terms, especially the former, a product of mid-twentieth-century physiology, are not fully adequate to liberate the experience of sufferer/complainer from the categories imposed by states or doctors. There is first the epistemic problem. Even were stress (or overwork) well defined, we have no obvious way to measure them in past populations, particularly for acute episodes.[59]

Marx's analytic, the presumptive monetisation of lives through conversion into surplus value, was too crude for that purpose – biologically, because life histories cannot be reduced simply to energy, and historically because struggles to control lives could not be reduced to that conversion either. Rather, as so-called 'soft' Marxists pointed out, class relations were contingently historical. Each formation of class relations would constitute a unique 'political culture' that would mediate historical processes. As a part of this more fluid approach, Thompson's 'moral economy' concept fostered rich empirical studies of how identities and interests emerged and evolved, but it went further. The 'cultural turn' of the 1980s, evident in the history of medicine as well as in social history, replaced bodies and conditions with linguistic practices, for articulation and restoration of the just balance of misery was a linguistic achievement.[60] To some radical medical historians, however, notably Roger Cooter, the cultural turn gave up far too much.[61]

For many of its latter day explicators, the subject and substance of justice of the moral economy was unimportant: what mattered was that there was a moral economy. Not so for Thompson. The moral economy concerned food. He saw himself as supplementing economists and old-style social historians – 'ineducable positivists' for whom behavior was a function of grain prices – but not as denying the biological foundation of their concern. '*Of course* food rioters were hungry', Thompson thundered, 'but this does not tell us how their behavior is modified by custom, culture, and reason' – factors which mediated the psychic and physical aspects of stress.[62] Yet practitioners of the cultural turn would go further. Consider James Vernon's view: 'that even hunger, that most material of conditions, was also the work of culture'; 'that how hunger was understood shaped who actually experienced it, and how'.[63]

For Thompson, culture 'modified'; for Vernon, it comes close to supplanting. What then to do with nine-year-old Oliver Twist, taken from the baby farm where he was 'atrociously presuming to be hungry' and transported to the workhouse, where the boys, 'voracious and wild with hunger' and contemplating cannibalism, pick him to lead a food riot by asking for more gruel? Both Thompson and Vernon can show us that Oliver has violated the moral economy of 'hunger' as Bumble and his Board understand it, but to stop there leaves us without access to Oliver's experience. Simply to say he has misunderstood that experience would be the height of callousness. Or one could respond that there is no issue: we are hearing only Dickens; Oliver is only words on paper. Yet the same applies to the representations of Thompson or of Vernon. In part these omissions reflect choices of gaze, for one may examine 'hunger' without denying hunger. Yet they reflect also the broader problem I have alluded to of the dependence of imagination on expressibility.

For Thompson, more than historical precision was at stake in correcting the economists. He was seeking an approach both sympathetic and analytic. Yet in the rarefied atmosphere of 'political culture', the morality of 'moral economy' simply evaporated: people acted and they talked about why they acted; that talk, coupled with the mysterious magic stimulant of 'agency', became a sufficient accounting.

What Thompson had overlooked was the need for a moral economics, a circulating currency.[64] Here it is worth keeping in mind the limits of relying on *Capital* for an understanding of the stakes in converting humans into surplus value. Marx (and Engels) were appallingly ignorant of the medicine of their day, particularly the post-Cullenean medicine relating poverty to disease, and being practised in Scotland and Ireland. Rarely too have later Marxist theorists appealed to biomedical metrics, though social (or social medical) theorists certainly have done.[65]

This chapter has explored whether stress might play a role akin to that of 'marginal utility' in economics. The complaints which express our stress are, after all, expressions of desire that presumably reflect determinations of marginal utility. Expressing and responding to them has both costs and benefits. Might we then theorise the pursuit of low-stress 'health and happiness hours' as the primary motor of moral economies? In recognising positive and negative forms of stress, Seyle and others were exploring such a possibility. Yet however tempting, this will not quite work (other than by definition). While marginal utility is an axiom in economics, stress is an empirical entity, loosely defined though supported by plausible theorizing. Conceiving it as a currency is complicated by its ambiguous relation to complaint. It might be nice if complaining were a proxy of harm, but it is not. Expressibility is problematic, equally between soma and psyche and between self and culture. Moral economies of complaint do matter, but as noise rather than signal.

How to respond? The current polarisation between biomedical objectivity and cultural interpretation omits an enormous missing middle of embodied subjectivity. Historians have been baffled to know what to make of someone who says 'I'm hungry', 'I'm cold' (hypothermia and heatstroke are invisible in histories of medicine and public health), 'I'm tired', 'I'm sad', or 'I'm afraid.' A phenomenologist's perspective may help, but the issue ultimately is an acceptance of embodiment: 'experience' should open a door to explaining, not merely to explaining away.

Notes

1 C. E. Rosenberg, 'The tyranny of diagnosis: specific entities and individual experience', *The Millbank Quarterly*, 80 (2002), 237–60; C. E. Rosenberg,

'Contested boundaries: psychiatry, disease, and diagnosis', *Perspectives in Biology and Medicine*, 49:3 (2006), 407–24, https://doi.org/10.1353/pbm.2006.0046.

2 M. Foucault, *The Birth of the Clinic: An Archaeology of Medical Perception* (New York: Pantheon, 1973); N. D. Jewson, 'The disappearance of the sick-man from medical cosmology, 1770–1870', *Sociology*, 10 (1976), 225–44.

3 R. Williams, *Keywords: A Vocabulary of Culture and Society* (Oxford: Oxford University Press, 1976).

4 E. P. Thompson, 'The moral economy of the English crowd in the eighteenth century', *Past & Present*, 50 (February 1971), 76–136.

5 E. P. Thompson, 'Moral Economy Reviewed', in *Customs in Common* (New York: New Press, 1991), 259–305, esp. 262–3.

6 'Appendix 1. World Health Organization, "Mission Statement"', http://healthydocuments.org/appendices/doc49.html. Accessed 14 March 2017.

7 An exception are the finely grained analyses of S. King, '"Stop this overwhelming torment of destiny": negotiating financial aid at times of sickness under the English Old Poor Law, 1800–1840. Author Abstract', *Bulletin of the History of Medicine*, 79:2 (22 June 2005), 228–60, https://doi.org/10.1353/bhm.2005.0072; S. King, 'Regional patterns in the experiences and treatment of the sick poor, 1800–40: rights, obligations and duties in the rhetoric of paupers', *Family & Community History*, 10:1 (1 May 2007), 61–75, https://doi.org/10.1179/175138107x185256; S. King, 'Negotiating the law of poor relief in England, 1800–1840', *History*, 96:324 (2011), 410–35, https://doi.org/10.1111/j.1468–229X.2011.00527.x

8 Notably, the French *se plaindre* is reflexive and there were once reflexive uses in English too (see *OED* 'complain' ##2, 4a), including in a medical context, but they have disappeared: I may 'feel myself discontented', but to say 'I complain myself' will bewilder – certainly it does not mean 'I complain about myself.'

9 Rosenberg, 'Tyranny of diagnosis'; Rosenberg, 'Contested boundaries'; A. Kleinman, *The Illness Narratives: Suffering, Healing, and the Human Condition* (New York: Basic Books, 1988).

10 In law, too, a 'complaint' is a technical term for dissatisfaction dire enough to undertake the expense of civil litigation (*OED* #8a).

11 This is the primary context in which Kowalski understands 'authentic' complaining. R. M. Kowalski, *Complaining, Teasing, and Other Annoying Behaviors* (New Haven, CT: Yale University Press, 2003), 25–52.

12 N. Elias, *The History of Manners* (New York: Pantheon Books, 1982).

13 Kowalski, *Complaining*, 47–8.

14 J. W. Scott, 'The evidence of experience', *Critical Inquiry*, 17 (1991), 773–97.

15 M. Jackson, *The Age of Stress: Science and the Search for Stability* (Oxford: Oxford University Press, 2013), 38.
16 Jackson, *The Age of Stress*, 3, 11.
17 Jackson (*The Age of Stress*, 2, 14, 63, 81–5, 97) notes the interest of the early twentieth-century pioneers of stress physiology, including Cannon, Henderson, and Seyle in 'Hippocratic ideas of balance and self-regulation'. For broader continuities, see K. Faber, *Nosography in Modern Internal Medicine* (New York: Paul Hoeber, 1922); W. Riese, *The Conception of Disease: Its History, Its Versions, and Its Nature* (New York: Philosophical Library, 1953).
18 D. Fox, *Power and Illness: The Failure and Future of American Health Policy* (Berkeley: University of California Press, 1993).
19 Lewis Carroll, *Alice's Adventures in Wonderland*, Chapter 3.
20 C. Hamlin, *More than Hot: A Short History of Fever*, Johns Hopkins Biographies of Disease (Baltimore, MD: Johns Hopkins University Press, 2014).
21 J. Adair, *Essays on Fashionable Diseases* [...] (London: Bateman, n.d.); R. Porter, 'Nervousness, Eighteenth and Nineteenth Century Style: From Luxury to Labour', in M. Gijswijt-Hofstra and R. Porter (eds), *Cultures of Neurasthenia from Beard to the First World War* (Amsterdam: Rodopi, 2001), 31–49; H. Beatty, *Nervous Disease in Late Eighteenth-Century Britain: The Reality of a Fashionable Disorder* (London: Pickering and Chatto, 2012).
22 A. Guerrini, *Obesity and Depression in the Enlightenment: The Life and Times of George Cheyne* (Norman: University of Oklahoma Press, 2000).
23 Jackson, *The Age of Stress*, 81–2; University of Minnesota: Laboratory of Physiological Hygiene, *The Biology of Human Starvation* (Minneapolis: University of Minnesota Press, 1950); R. Dirks, 'Famine and Disease', in K. Kiple (ed.), *Cambridge World History of Human Disease* (Cambridge: Cambridge University Press, 1993), 157–63.
24 K. Marx, *Capital: A Critical Analysis of Capitalist Production, trans from the 3rd German Edition by Samuel Moore and Edward Aveling* (New York: International Publishing Co, 1939).
25 *Ibid.*, 366–7, quoting Richardson (1863).
26 *Ibid.*, 365, quoting *Morning Star*.
27 B. W. Richardson, *The Diseases of Modern Life* (New York: Bermingham, 1882); A. Rabinbach, *The Human Motor: Energy, Fatigue, and the Origins of Modernity* (New York: Basic Books, 1990).
28 J. C. Scott, *Weapons of the Weak: Everyday Forms of Peasant Resistance* (New Haven, CT: Yale University Press, 1985).
29 K. Thomas, *Religion and the Decline of Magic* (New York: Scribner's, 1971); R. Porter (ed.), *Patients and Practitioners: Lay Perceptions of Medicine in*

Pre-Industrial Society (Cambridge: Cambridge University Press, 1985); L. M. Beier, *Sufferers and Healers: The Experience of Disease in Seventeenth-Century England* (London: Routledge and Kegan Paul, 1987); R. K. Rittgers, *The Reformation of Suffering Pastoral Theology and Lay Piety in Late Medieval and Early Modern Germany* (Oxford: Oxford University Press, 2012); S. C. Karant-Nunn, *The Reformation of Feeling: Shaping the Religious Emotions in Early Modern Germany* (Oxford: Oxford University Press, 2010).
30 S. Zlotnick, '"The law's a bachelor": Oliver Twist, bastardy, and the New Poor Law', *Victorian Literature and Culture*, 34:1 (2006), 131–46; U. R. Q. Henriques, 'Bastardy and the New Poor Law', *Past & Present*, 37 (1967), 103–29.
31 David Lean et al., *Oliver Twist* (Independent Producers: Criterion Collection, 1948).
32 Here, too, Lean's film is more positive than Dickens in depicting a sympathetic nurse and surgeon. Persons like Agnes may have often had more of a clear sense of what to request and what to expect than Dickens allocates to Agnes (King, 'Negotiating').
33 R. A. Soloway, *Prelates and People: Ecclesiastical Social Thought in England 1783–1852* (London: Routledge and Kegan Paul, 1969); P. Mandler, 'The making of the New Poor Law redivivus', *Past & Present*, 117 (1987), 131–57; P. Mandler, 'Tories and paupers: Christian political economy and the making of the New Poor Law', *Historical Journal*, 33 (1990), 81–101.
34 At least on a regional basis, 'misery' had a specific medical meaning – like 'complaint', it was shorthand for a particular bodily pain (*OED* 'misery', #6).
35 Notably, there is not only no reflexive form, but no verb. If one could once say 'I complain myself', one cannot 'miserate' though, oddly, one can 'co-miserate'.
36 R. Emerson, 'Numbering the Medics', in *Essays on David Hume, Medical Men and the Scottish Enlightenment: Industry, Knowledge and Humanity* (Burlington VT: Ashgate, 2009), 163–224; A. Chitnis, *The Scottish and Early Victorian English Society* (London: Croom Helm, 1986).
37 Jackson, *The Age of Stress*, 41.
38 J. Pringle, *Observations on the Diseases of the Army* (London, 1752); Hamlin, *More than Hot*.
39 H. Marland, *Dangerous Motherhood: Insanity and Childbirth in Victorian Britain* (New York: Palgrave Macmillan, 2004).
40 C. Hamlin, *Public Health and Social Justice in the Age of Chadwick: Britain, 1800–1854* (Cambridge: Cambridge University Press, 1998); C. Hamlin, 'The "necessaries of life" in British political medicine, 1750–1850', *Journal*

of Consumer Policy, 29 (2006), 373–97; C. Hamlin, 'William Pulteney Alison, the Scottish philosophy, and the making of a political medicine', *Journal of the History of Medicine and Allied Sciences*, 61 (2006), 44–86.

41 Royal College of Physicians in Ireland, DC 2/4/2–3, 'Hardwicke Fever Hospital case books', 1840–46 and 1843–45. The actual entries are by anonymous students. Each of the seven handwritings in these books reflects a distinct case-recording approach. On Irish medical charities, see R. D. Cassell, *Medical Charities, Medical Politics: The Irish Dispensary System and the Poor Law, 1836–1872* (Woodbridge: The Royal Historical Society/ The Boydell Press, 1997), 4–15; L. Geary, *Medicine and Charity in Ireland, 1718–1851* (Dublin: University College Dublin Press, 2004); P. Gray, *The Making of the Irish Poor Law, 1815–43* (Manchester/New York: Manchester University Press, 2009).

42 I have explored these issues in 'Public Sphere to Public Health: The Transformation of nuisance', in S. Sturdy (ed.), *Medicine, Health and the Public Sphere in Britain, 1600–2000* (London: Routledge, 2002), 190–204; C. Hamlin, *Sanitary Reform in the Provinces*, vol. 2 of M. Allen-Emerson, *Sanitary Reform in Victorian Britain*, 5 vols (London: Pickering and Chatto, 2012); 'Nuisances and community in mid-Victorian England: the attractions of inspection', *Social History*, 38 (2013), 346–79. See also T. Crook, 'Sanitary inspection and the public sphere in late Victorian and Edwardian Britain: a case study in liberal governance', *Social History*, 32:4 (2007), 369–93; T. Crook, *Governing Systems: Modernity and the Making of Public Health in England, 1830–1910* (Berkeley: University of California Press, 2016).

43 *OED* 'annoy', ## 4a, 5.

44 Elias, *History of Manners*; M. Douglas, *Purity and Danger: An Analysis of the Concepts of Pollution and Taboo* (London: Routledge and Kegan Paul, 1966); M. Douglas, 'Environments at Risk', in B. Barnes and D. Edge (eds), *Science in Context* (Cambridge, MA: MIT Press, 1982), 260–75.

45 Bassetlaw Museum, East Retford, 2004. 3260, 3526; 'Worksop Inspectors' Notebooks'. Mellars was succeeded in June 1876 by Sampson White. My general views draw from both. On Mellars see www.genuki.org.uk/big/eng/NTT/Worksop/worksop_PLU. Accessed 22 August 2016.

46 Page numbers from D. H. Lawrence, *Lady Chatterley's Lover* (New York: Grove Press, 1962).

47 Worksop Heritage Trail, 'Worksop History, Part 4: 19th and 20th Century Worksop', www.worksopheritagetrail.org.uk/index.asp?page=history. See also W. Lee, 'Worksop Public Health Inspection, 1850', www.worksopheritagetrail.org.uk/resources/worksop_public_health_inspection_1851.pdf. Both accessed 29 March 2017.

48 'Worksop Inspectors' Notebooks', 7 August 1871, 4; 18 October 1875, 3; 18 September, 1876, 3; 30 October, 1876, 5.
49 'Worksop Inspectors' Notebooks', 17 April 1871, 6; 15 May 1871, 5.
50 'Worksop Inspectors' Notebooks', 29 May 1871, 3; 7 August 1871, 6; 4 September 1871, 2, 7; 2 October 1871, 1.
51 'Worksop Inspectors Notebooks', 7 August 1871, 2; 3 September 1871, 3; 26 June 1876, 1; 18 September 1876, 2; 13 November 1876, 1; 5 February 1877, 3.
52 'Worksop Inspectors Notebooks', 7 August 1876, 5; 15 May 1871, 5.
53 'Worksop Inspectors Notebooks', 21 August 1871, 4; 2 October 1871, 5; 30 October 1871, 2; 28 June 1875, 1; 1 November 1875, 1.
54 'Worksop Inspectors Notebooks', 2004.3258, 1 May 1882, 5; 15 May 1882, 7; 25 September 1882, 6; Lawrence, *Lady Chatterley*, 207.
55 Worksop Inspectors Notebooks', 7 August 1871, 5.
56 A. M. McBriar, *An Edwardian Mixed Doubles: The Bosanquets versus the Webbs: A Study in British Social Policy 1890–1929* (Oxford: Clarendon, 1987); B. Webb, *My Apprenticeship* (New York: AMS Press, 1977).
57 www.euro.who.int/en/health-topics/environment-and-health/urban-health/activities/healthy-cities/who-european-healthy-cities-network. Accessed 2 April 2017.
58 S. L. Smith, *Sick and Tired of Being Sick and Tired: Black Women's Health Activism in America, 1890–1950* (Philadelphia: University of Pennsylvania Press, 1995). J. C. Riley's *Sick, Not Dead: The Health of British Workingmen during the Mortality Decline* (Baltimore, MD: Johns Hopkins University Press, 1997) similarly reminds us of the unhelpful fixation of many historians on mortality as the foundation of medical signification.
59 For populations, an exception is skeletal evidence. See C. B. Ruff, E. Garofalo, and M. A. Holmes, 'Interpreting skeletal growth in the past from a functional and physiological perspective', *American Journal of Physical Anthropology*, 150:1 (January 1, 2013), 29–37, https://doi.org/10.1002/ajpa.22120. For a very different approach, see R. Wilkinson and M. Marmot, *Social Determinants of Health*, 2nd edn (Oxford: Oxford University Press, 2006).
60 C. Kent, 'Victorian social history: post-Thompson, post-Foucault, post-modern', *Victorian Studies*, 40:1 (1996), 97–133; R. Cooter, '"Framing" the End of the Social History of Medicine', in J. H. Warner and F. Huisman (eds), *Locating Medical History* (Baltimore, MD: Johns Hopkins University Press, 2004), 309–37.
61 Cooter, '"Framing"'.
62 E. P. Thompson, 'Moral Economy Reviewed', in *Customs in Common* (New York: New Press, 1991), 259–305.

63 J. Vernon, *Hunger: A Modern History* (Cambridge MA: Harvard University Press, 2007).
64 N. Götz, '"Moral economy": its conceptual history and analytical prospects', *Journal of Global Ethics*, 11 (2015), 147–62, https://doi.org/10.1080/17449626.2015.1054556.
65 This is well developed in D. Porter, *Health, Civilization and the State* (London: Routledge, 1999). See also my *Public Health and Social Justice in the Age of Chadwick: Britain, 1800–1854* (Cambridge: Cambridge University Press, 1998). For an example of how this might be done, see J. Livingston, *Debility and the Moral Imagination in Botswana* (Bloomington: Indiana University Press, 2005). See also R. Levins and C. Lopez, 'Toward an ecosocial view of health', *International Journal of Health Services*, 29 (1999), 261–93.

Bibliography

'A comparative statistical study of cancer mortality. V. General summary (concluded), *British Medical Journal*, 1:2211 (1903).
'A physician', 'Fatigue', *Quiver*, 429 (1908), 1012.
Abernethy, J. *Surgical Observations on Tumours* (London: Longman, Hurst, Rees, Orme, and Brown, Paternoster Row, 1811).
Adair, J. *Essays on Fashionable Diseases* [...] (London: Bateman, n.d.).
Adams, J. 'Mental fatigue', *The Practical Teacher*, 22 (April 1902).
Aisenberg, A. R. *Contagion: Disease, Government, and the 'Social Question' in Nineteenth-Century France* (Stanford, CA: Stanford University Press, 1999).
Alavi, S. *Islam and Healing: Loss and Recovery of an Indo-Muslim Medical Tradition, 1600–1900* (Basingstoke: Palgrave Macmillan, 2008).
Albisetti, J. C. *Secondary School Reform in Imperial Germany* (Princeton, NJ: Princeton University Press, 1983).
Allbutt, T. C. 'Nervous diseases and modern life', *Contemporary Review*, 67 (February 1895).
Allott, K. *Jules Verne* (London: Cresset Press, 1940).
Alston, P. L. *Education and the State in Tsarist Russia* (Stanford, CA: Stanford University Press, 1969).
Alter, J. S. (ed.). *Asian Medicine and Globalization (Encounters in Asia)* (Philadelphia: University of Pennsylvania Press, 2005).
American Medical Association, 'The propaganda for reform', *Journal of the American Medical Association* (10 November 1917).
Amery, J. *The Life of Joseph Chamberlain* (London: Macmillan & Co., 1951).
Armstrong, T. 'Two types of shock in modernity', *Critical Quarterly*, 42 (2000), 61–73.
Armstrong, T. *The Power of Neurodiversity: Unleashing the Advantages of Your Differently Wired Brain* (Cambridge, MA: DeCapo Books, 2010).
Arnold, D. *Colonizing the Body: State Medicine and Epidemic Disease in Nineteenth-Century India* (Berkeley: University of California Press, 1993).
Arnold, D. *Everyday Technology: Machines and the Making of India's Modernity* (Chicago: University of Chicago Press, 2013).

Arnold-Forster, A. 'Mapmaking and mapthinking: cancer as a problem of place in nineteenth-century England', *Social History of Medicine*, 32:1 (2019).
Aronowitz, R. A. *Unnatural History: Breast Cancer and American Society* (Cambridge: Cambridge University Press, 2007).
Arps, L. *Auf sicheren Pfeilern: Deutsche Versicherungswirtschaft vor 1914* (Göttingen: Vandenhoeck & Ruprecht, 1965).
Asperger, H. '"Autistic Psychopathy" in Childhood' [1944], in Uta Frith (ed.), *Autism and Asperger Syndrome* (Cambridge: Cambridge University Press, 1991), 37–92.
Asperger, H. 'Die "Autischen Psychopathen" im Kindesalter' [1944], *Archiv für Psychiatrie und Nervenkrankheiten*, 117 (1994), 76–136.
Attewell, G. N. A. *Refiguring Unani Tibb: Plural Healing in Late Colonial India* (New Delhi: Orient Longman, 2007).
Australasian Medical Association, 'Public Health', *The Australasian Medical Gazette* (20 August 1897).
Baczko, B. *Ending the Terror: The French Revolution after Robespierre* (Cambridge: Cambridge University Press, 1994 [1989]).
Bakhtin, M. *Rabelais and his World* (Cambridge, MA: MIT Press, 1968).
Barlow, T. 'Buying in: Advertising and the Sexy Modern Girl Icon in Shanghai in the 1920s and 1930s', in A. E. Weinbaum et al. (eds), *The Modern Girl around the World: Consumption, Modernity, and Globalization* (Durham, NC/London: Duke University Press, 2008), 288–319.
Barnert, E. *Der eingebildete Dritte: Eine Argumentationsfigur im Zivilrecht* (Tübingen: Mohr Siebeck, 2008).
Barnes, D. S. *The Great Stink of Paris and the Nineteenth-Century Struggle Against Filth and Germs* (Baltimore, MD: Johns Hopkins University Press, 2006).
Baron-Cohen, S. 'Two new theories of autism: hyper-systemising and assortative mating', *Archives of Disease in Childhood*, 91 (2006), 2–5.
Bashford, E. F. 'An address entitled are the problems of cancer insoluble?', *British Medical Journal*, 2:2345 (1905).
Bataille, G. *Visions of Excess: Selected Writings, 1927–1939*, trans. Allan Stoekl (Minnesota: University of Minnesota Press, 1985).
Baumann, U. *Vom Recht auf den eigenen Tod* (Weimar: Verl. Hermann Böhlaus Nachf., 2001).
Bayertz, K. (ed.). *Verantwortung: Prinzip oder Problem?* (Darmstadt: Wissenschaftliche Buchgesellschaft, 1995).
Bean, P. and J. Melville, *Lost Children of the Empire* (London: Unwin Hyman, 1989).
Bear, L. G. 'Miscegenations of modernity: constructing European respectability and race in the Indian railway colony, 1857–1931', *Women's History Review*, 3:4 (1994), 531–48.

Beard, G. M. 'Neurasthenia, or nervous exhaustion', *The Boston Medical and Surgical Journal*, 80:13 (29 April 1869).
Beard, G. M. *American Nervousness: Its Causes and Consequences* (New York: G. P. Putnam's, 1881).
Beatty, H. *Nervous Disease in Late Eighteenth-Century Britain: The Reality of a Fashionable Disorder* (London: Pickering and Chatto, 2012).
Beddoes, G. *Habit and Health: A Book of Golden Hints for Middle Age* (London: Swan, Sonnenschein & Co, 1890).
Beier, L. M. *Sufferers and Healers: The Experience of Disease in Seventeenth-Century England* (London: Routledge and Kegan Paul, 1987).
Bell, C. *Surgical Observations; Being a Quarterly Report of Cases in Surgery; Treated in the Middlesex Hospital, in the Cancer Establishment, and in Private Practice* (London: Longman, Hurst, Rees, Orme, and Brown, Paternoster Row, 1816).
Benzaquén, A. *Encounters with Wild Children: Temptation and Disappointment in the Study of Human Nature* (Montreal: McGill-Queen's University Press, 2006).
de Berdt Hovell, D. *On Some Conditions of Neurasthenia* (London: J. & A. Churchill, 1886).
Berger, R. *Ayurveda Made Modern: Political Histories of Indigenous Medicine in North India, 1900–1955* (Basingstoke: Palgrave Macmillan, 2013).
Bergère, M.-C. *Shanghai: China's Gateway to Modernity* (Stanford, CA: Stanford University Press, 2009).
Berman, M. *All That is Solid Melts into Air: The Experience of Modernity* (London: Verso, 1983).
Bettleheim, B. *The Empty Fortress: Infantile Autism and the Birth of the Self* (New York/London: Free Press, 1967).
Binet, A. and V. Henri. *La Fatigue intellectuelle* (Paris: C. Reinwald, 1898).
Bittel, C. 'Woman, know thyself: producing and using phrenological knowledge in 19th-century America', *Centaurus*, 55 (2013), 104–30.
Bivins, R. *Alternative Medicine? A History* (Oxford/New York: Oxford University Press, 2007).
Blake, R. *Religion in the British Navy 1815–1879* (Woodbridge: Boydell Press, 2014).
Blaser, M. *Missing Microbes: How Killing Bacteria Creates Modern Plagues* (London: Oneworld, 2015).
Bleiler, E. F. *Science Fiction: The Early Years* (Kent, OH: Kent State University Press, 1990).
Blevins, S. M. and M. S. Bronze, 'Robert Koch and the "golden age" of bacteriology', *International Journal of Infectious Diseases*, 14 (2010), 744–51.
le Bon, G. *The Crowd. A Study of the Popular Mind* (London: Penguin, 1977).

Bonea, A., M. Dickson, S. Shuttleworth, and J. Wallis. *Anxious Times: Medicine and Modernity in Nineteenth-Century Britain* (Pittsburgh, PA: University of Pittsburgh Press, 2019).
Borsay, A. *Disability and Social Policy in Britain since 1750* (Basingstoke: Palgrave Macmillan, 2005).
Borsay, A. and P. Dale, *Disabled Children: Contested Caring, 1850–1979* (London: Pickering and Chatto, 2012).
Boucher, E. *Empire's Children: Child Emigration, Welfare, and the Decline of the British World, 1869–1967* (Cambridge: Cambridge University Press, 2014).
Boxtröm, A. *Jemförande befolknings-statistik: med särskildt afseende å förhållandena I Finland* (Helsingfors: G. W. Edlund, 1891).
Brancaccio, M. '"The fatal tendency of civilized society": Enrico Morselli's suicide, moral statistics, and positivism in Italy', *Journal of Social History*, 46:3 (2013), 700–15.
Brinton, C. *The Shaping of Modern Thought* (Englewood Cliffs, NJ: Prentice-Hall, 1963).
Brookes, L. 'The hygiene hypothesis – redefine, rename, or just clean it up?', *Medscape*, 6 April 2015, www.medscape.com/viewarticle/842500. Accessed 9 August 2017.
Brown, J. W. and M. Lal, 'An inquiry into the relation between social status and cancer mortality', *Journal of Hygiene*, 14:2 (1914), 186–200.
Brown, M. 'Medicine, reform, and the "end" of charity in early nineteenth-century England', *English Historical Review* 124:511 (2009), 1353–88.
Brown, N. *Life against Death: The Psychoanalytic Meaning of History* (Middletown, CT: Wesleyan University Press, 1985).
Brush, S. G. *The Temperature of History: Phases of Science and Culture in the Nineteenth Century* (New York: Burt Franklin & Co., 1978).
Burnet, E. *The Campaign Against Microbes*, trans. E. E. Austen (London: J. Bale & Sons and Danielsson Ltd, 1909).
Bynum, W. *The History of Medicine: A Very Short Introduction* (Oxford: Oxford University Press, 2008).
Cabanis, P. J. G. *Rapports du physique et du moral de l'homme* (Paris: J. B. Baillière, 1844 [1798]).
Caird, M. 'The evolution of compassion', *Westminster Review*, 145 (1896), 643.
Campbell, B. 'The making of "American": race and nation in neurasthenic discourse', *History of Psychiatry*, 18:2 (2007), 131–56.
Campbell, H. *Nervous Exhaustion and the Diseases Induced by It, with Observations on the Origin and Nature of Nerve Force* (London: Longmans, Green, Reader, and Dyer, 1873).
Campbell, H. *The Anatomy of Nervousness and Nervous Exhaustion* (London: Henry Renshaw, 1886).

'Cancer Deaths Increasing: Porter Says the Malady is Assuming Menacing Proportions', *New York Times* (5 November 1907).
'Cancer in the colonies', *British Medical Journal*, 1:2362 (1906).
'Cancer Increasing at an Alarming Rate', *Vogue* (15 April 1909).
Carpenter, W. B. 'On the voluntary and instinctive actions of living beings', *Edinburgh Medical and Surgical Journal*, 48 (1837), 22–44.
Carpenter, W. B. *Principles of Human Physiology* (London: John Churchill, 1842).
Carpenter, W. B. *Principles of Mental Physiology* (London: Henry S. King & Co., 1874).
Cassell, R. D. *Medical Charities, Medical Politics: The Irish Dispensary System and the Poor Law, 1836–1872* (Woodbridge: Royal Historical Society/ Boydell Press, 1997).
Cawelti, J. G. *Apostles of the Self-Made Man* (Chicago: University of Chicago Press, 1989).
Chakrabarty, D. *Provincializing Europe: Postcolonial Thought and Historical Difference* (Princeton, NJ: Princeton University Press, 2009).
Chamberlain, H. S. *Foundations of the Nineteenth Century*, trans. John Lees (New York: John Lane, 1913).
Chamberlin, J. E. and S. L. Gilman. *Degeneration: The Dark Side of Progress* (New York: Columbia University Press, 1985).
Channing, W. *Self-Culture: An Address Introductory to the Franklin Lectures* (Boston: Dutton and Wentworth, 1838).
Chappey, J. L. *La Société des observateurs de l'homme (1799–1804). Des anthropologues au temps de Bonaparte* (Paris: Société des Études Robespierristes, 2002).
Chappey, J. L. *Sauvagerie et civilisation. Une histoire politique de Victor de l'Aveyron* (Paris: Fayard, 2017).
Chappey, J. L., C. Christen, and I. Mouiller (eds). *Joseph-Marie de Gérando. Connaître et réformer la société* (Rennes: Presses Universitaires de Rennes, 2014).
Chatterjee, P. *Our Modernity* (Rotterdam/Dakar: Sephis/Codesria, 1997).
Chelebourg, C. *Jules Verne. L'Oeil et le ventre* (Paris: Minard, 1999).
Chen, T. S. and P. S. Y. Chen, 'Intestinal autointoxication: a medical leitmotif', *Journal of Clinical Gastroenterology*, 11 (1989), 434–41.
Cheng, M. 'Kids with ADHD have some brain regions that are smaller than normal, new study finds', *TIME Health* (15 February 2017) http://time.com/4670266/adhd-children-brains-study-normal/. Accessed 16 February 2017.
Chevrel, Y. 'Questions de méthodes et d'idéologies chez Verne et Zola. *Les Cinq cents millions de la Bégum* et *Travail*', in F. Raymond (ed.), *Jules*

Verne 2. *L'Ecriture vernienne* (Paris: Lettres Modernes, 1978), vol. 2, 69–96.
Chitnis, A. *The Scottish and Early Victorian English Society* (London: Croom Helm, 1986).
Christie, A. *The Mysterious Affair at Styles* (New York: John Lane, 1920).
Cochran, S. 'Transnational Origins of Advertising in Early Twentieth-Century China', in S. Cochran (ed.), *Inventing Nanjing Road* (Ithaca, NY: Cornell University Press, 1999).
Coffin, J. 'Credit, consumption, and images of women's desires: selling the sewing machine in late nineteenth-century France', *French Historical Studies*, 18 (1994), 749–83.
Cohen, W. A. 'Introduction: Locating Filth', in Cohen and Johnson (eds), *Filth*, pp. vii–xxxvii.
Cohen, W. A. and R. Johnson (eds), *Filth: Dirt, Disgust, and Modern Life* (London: University of Minnesota Press, 2005).
Colbert, C. *A Measure of Perfection: Phrenology and the Fine Arts in America* (Chapel Hill: University of North Carolina Press, 1998).
Collin, P. 'Ehrengerichtliche Rechtssprechung im Kaiserreich und der Weimarer Republik. Mulitnormativität in einer mononormativen Rechtsordnung?', *Rechtsgeschichte/Legal History*, 25 (2017), 138–50.
Combe, G. *The Constitution of Man Considered in Relation to External Objects*, 6th edn (Edinburgh: Maclachlan and Stewart, 1851).
Combe, G. *A System of Phrenology* (Boston: B. B. Mussey & Co., 1851).
Conan Doyle, A. *The Sign of Four* (London: Spencer Blackett, 1890).
Condorcet, M. J. *Esquisse d'un tableau historique des progrès de l'esprit humain. Ouvrage posthume de Condorcet* (Paris: Agasse, 1795).
Constant, B. *Des effets de la terreur* (s.l., 1797).
'Cool Things – Pink Pills for Pale People', Kansas Historical Society, n.d., www.kshs.org/kansapedia/pink-pills-for-pale-people/10240. Accessed 28 November 2016.
Cooter, R. *The Cultural Meaning of Popular Science: Phrenology and the Organization of Consent in Nineteenth-Century Britain* (Cambridge: Cambridge University Press, 1984).
Cooter, R. '"Framing" the End of the Social History of Medicine', in J. H. Warner and F. Huisman (eds), *Locating Medical History* (Baltimore, MD: Johns Hopkins University Press, 2004), 309–37.
Cooter, R. 'Medicine and Modernity', in Mark Jackson (ed.), *The Oxford Handbook of the History of Medicine* (Oxford: Oxford University Press, 2015), 100–16.
Corbin, A. *The Foul and the Fragrant: Odour and the Social Imagination* (London: Papermac, 1996).

Cox, P. *Bad Girls in Britain: Gender, Justice and Welfare, 1900–1950* (Basingstoke: Palgrave Macmillan, 2013).
Coze, L. and V. Feltz, 'Physiologie pathologique', *Gazette Médicale de Strasbourg*, 26:61 (1866), 115–208.
Crabtree, A. '"Automatism" and the emergence of dynamic psychiatry', *Journal of the History of the Behavioural Sciences*, 39:1 (2003), 51–70.
Crane, J. '"The bones tell a story the child is too young or too frightened to tell": the battered child syndrome in post-war Britain and America', *Social History of Medicine*, 28:4 (2015), 767–88.
Creighton, C. 'Address in pathology', *British Medical Journal*, 2:1179 (1883).
Crompton, F. *Workhouse Children* (Stroud: Sutton, 1997).
Crook, T. 'Sanitary inspection and the public sphere in late Victorian and Edwardian Britain: a case study in liberal governance', *Social History*, 32:4 (2007), 369–93.
Crook, T. *Governing Systems: Modernity and the Making of Public Health in England, 1830–1910* (Berkeley: University of California Press, 2016).
Crow, C. 'Pills for the Ills of China', in *Four Hundred Million Customers* (New York/London: 1937).
Cullen, J. *The American Dream: A Short History of an Idea that Shaped a Nation* (Oxford: Oxford University Press, 2003).
Cunningham, H. *Children of the Poor: Representations of Childhood since the Seventeenth Century* (London: Blackwell, 1991).
Cunningham, H. *The Invention of Childhood* (London: BBC Books, 2006).
Dana, C. L. 'The partial passing of neurasthenia', *Boston Medical and Surgical Journal*, 150:13 (1904), 339–44.
David, P. *Epître à l'abbé Sicard, sur les mots avec lesquels on nous a gouverné pendant la Révolution* (Paris: Chez les Marchands de Nouveautés, 1801).
Davies, J. D. *Phrenology Fad and Science: A 19th-Century American Crusade* (New Haven, CT: Yale University Press, 1955).
Davin, A. 'Imperialism and motherhood', *History Workshop Journal*, 5 (1978), 9–65.
Davin, A. *Growing up Poor: Home, School and Street in London, 1870–1914* (London: Rivers Oram, 1995).
De Castro, E. V. 'Cosmological deixis and Amerindian perspectivism', *Journal of the Royal Anthropological Institute*, 4:3 (1998), 469–88.
'Death of Commodore Goodenough and two seamen of H. M. S. Pearl at Santa Cruz', *Sydney Morning Herald* (3 September 1875).
Deichert, H. *Geschichte des Medizinalwesens im Gebiet des ehemaligen Königreichs Hannover* (Hanover and Leipzig: Hahn, 1908).
Denman, T. *Observations on the Cure of Cancer* (London: J. Johnson and Co., 1810).

Destutt de Tracy, A. L. C. *Quels sont les moyens de fonder la morale chez un peuple* (Paris: Agasse, 1798).
Diamond, M. *Emigration and Empire: The Life of Maria S. Rye* (New York: Routledge, 2016).
Dirks, R. 'Famine and Disease', in K. Kiple (ed.), *Cambridge World History of Human Disease* (Cambridge: Cambridge University Press, 1993), 157–63.
Douglas, J. *The Social Meaning of Suicide* (Princeton, NJ: Princeton University Press, 1967).
Douglas, M. *Purity and Danger* (Routledge: London, 1966).
Douglas, M. 'Environments at Risk', in B. Barnes and D. Edge (eds), *Science in Context* (Cambridge, MA: MIT Press, 1982), 260–75.
Dowbiggin, I. *Inheriting Madness: Professionalization and Psychiatric Knowledge in Nineteenth-Century France* (Berkeley: University of California Press, 1991).
Dowse, T. S. *On Brain and Nerve Exhaustion: 'Neurasthenia', Its Nature and Curative Treatment* (London: Ballière, Tindall, and Cox, 1880).
Dubos, R. *Louis Pasteur: Free Lance of Science* (New York: DaCapo, 1960).
Dumas, O. et al. (eds). *Correspondance inédite de Jules Verne et de Pierre-Jules Hetzel*, 3 vols. (Geneva: Slatkine, 1999–2003).
Dunn, H. P. 'An inquiry into the causes of the increase of cancer', *British Medical Journal*, 1:1163 (1883).
Dunn, H. P. 'An inquiry into the causes of the increase of cancer (continued)', *British Medical Journal*, 1:1164 (1883).
Dunn, H. P. 'English experience with cancer', *The Popular Science Monthly* (March 1885).
Durbach, N. *Bodily Matters: The Anti-Vaccination Movement in England, 1853–1907* (Durham, NC/London: Duke University Press, 2007).
Durham, A. E. 'The physiology of sleep', *Guy's Hospital Reports*, 3rd series, 6 (1860).
Durkheim, E. *Suicide: A Study in Sociology* (London: Routledge & Kegan Paul, 1970).
Eckart, W. U. and R. Jütte (eds). *Das europäische Gesundheitssystem. Gemeinsamkeiten und Unterschiede in historischer Perspektive* (Stuttgart: Franz Steiner Verlag, 1994).
Eisenstadt, S. N. 'Multiple modernities', *Daedalus* 129:1 (Winter, 2000), 1–29.
Eisenstadt, S. N. (ed.). *Multiple Modernities, Daedalus*, 129:1 (Winter, 2000).
Elias, N. *The History of Manners* (New York: Pantheon Books, 1982).
Elinder, E. 'How international can European advertising be?' *Journal of Marketing*, 29 (1965), 7–11.
Elkeles, B. *Der moralische Diskurs über das medizinische Menschenexperiment im 19. Jahrhundert* (Stuttgart: Fischer, 1996).

Emerson, R. 'Numbering the Medics', in *Essays on David Hume, Medical Men and the Scottish Enlightenment: Industry, Knowledge and Humanity* (Burlington VT: Ashgate, 2009), 163–224.

Emsley, C. *Crime, Police, and Penal Policy: European Experiences 1750–1940* (Oxford: Oxford University Press, 2007).

Englander, D. *Poverty and Poor Law Reform in Nineteenth-Century Britain, 1834–1914, from Chadwick to Booth* (Florence: Taylor and Francis, 2013).

Epstein, J. E. 'Writing the unspeakable: Fanny Burney's mastectomy and the fictive body', *Representations*, 16 (1986), 131–66.

Esquirol, J. É. D. *Des passions considérées comme causes, symptômes et moyens curatifs de l'aliénation mentale* (Paris: Didot jeune, 1805).

Esquirol, J. É. D. 'De la folie', in J. É. D. Esquirol, *Des maladies mentales considées maladies mentales considcal, hygiies menet médico-légal* (Paris: Baillière 1838 [1816]).

Evans, A. B. *Jules Verne Rediscovered: Didacticism and the Scientific Novel* (New York: Greenwood Press, 1988).

Ewald, F. *Der Vorsorgestaat* (Frankfurt am Main: Suhrkamp, 1993).

Ewen, S., and E. Ewen, *Typecasting: On the Arts & Sciences of Human Inequality* (New York: Seven Stories Press, 2006).

Eyler, J. M. 'The Conceptual Origins of William Farr's Epidemiology: Numerical Methods and Social Thought in the 1830s', in A. M. Lilienfeld (ed.), *Times, Places, and Persons* (Baltimore, MD: Johns Hopkins University Press, 1980), 1–27.

Faber, K. *Nosography in Modern Internal Medicine* (New York: Paul Hoeber, 1922).

Fabian, J. *Time and the Other: How Anthropology Makes its Object* (New York: Columbia University Press, 2014).

Farquharson, R. 'On overwork', *Lancet*, 107 (1 January 1876).

Ferrier, D. 'Introductory lecture on life and vital energy considered in relation to physiology and medicine', *British Medical Journal*, 2:512 (22 October 1870).

Fielden, K. 'Samuel Smiles and self-help', *Victorian Studies*, 12:2 (1968), 155–76.

Fine, E. 'Women Physicians and Medical Sects in Nineteenth-Century Chicago', in E. S. More, E. Fee, and M. Parry (eds), *Women Physicians and the Cultures of Medicine* (Baltimore, MD: Johns Hopkins University Press, 2009), 245–73.

Finger, S. *Minds Behind the Brain: A History of the Pioneers and their Discoveries* (New York: Oxford University Press, 2000).

Finnane, A. (ed.). *Changing Clothes in China: Fashion, History, Nation* (New York: Columbia University Press, 2008).

Finnane, A. 'The Fashion Industry in Shanghai', in A. Finnane (ed.), *Changing Clothes in China: Fashion, History, Nation* (New York: Columbia University Press, 2008), 101–38.
Flammarion, C. *Uranie* (Paris: Librairie Spirite Francophone, 2011).
Folger Fowler, L. *Familiar Lessons on Physiology and Phrenology: Designed for the Use of Children and Youth in Schools and Families* (New York: Fowler and Wells, 1847).
Fonssagrives, J.-B. *La Maison. Étude d'hygiène et de bien-être* (Montpellier: de Gras, 1871).
Forbes, L. 'Notes on Fiji', *Lancet*, 107:2732 (1876).
Forde, K. (ed.). *Dirt: The Filthy Reality of Everyday Life* (London: Profile Books, 2011).
Formigari, L. 'Les Idéologues. Philosophie du langage et hégémonie bourgeoise', in W. Busse and J. Trabant (eds), *Les Idéologues. Sémiotique, théories et politiques linguistiques pendant la Révolution française* (Amsterdam: John Benjamins, 1986)
Foster, M. 'Weariness', *The Nineteenth Century*, 34 (September 1893).
Foucault, M. *The Order of Things: An Archaeology of the Human Sciences* (New York: Pantheon, 1970).
Foucault, M. *The Birth of the Clinic: An Archaeology of Medical Perception* (New York: Pantheon, 1973).
Foucault, M. *Discipline and Punish: The Birth of the Prison* (New York: Random House, 1975).
Foucault, M. *Surveiller et punir. Naissance de la prison* (Paris: Gallimard, 1975).
Foucault, M. *Power/Knowledge: Selected Interviews and Other Writings, 1972–1977* (New York: Random House, 1980).
Foucault, M. *Madness and Civilization* (London: Routledge, 2009 [1961]).
Fowler, O. S. 'The phrenological facts', *American Phrenological Journal* 5:1 (January 1843), 29–30.
Fowler, O. S. *Education and Self-Improvement, Founded on Physiology and Phrenology*, 2nd edn (New York: O. S. & L. N. Fowler, 1844).
Fowler, O. S. *The Octagon House: A Home for All* (New York: Dover Publications, 1973 [1848]).
Fowler, O. S. *Self-Culture and the Perfection of Character* (New York: Fowler and Wells, 1853 [1847]).
Fox, D. *Power and Illness: The Failure and Future of American Health Policy* (Berkeley: University of California Press, 1993).
Freeland, N. 'The Dustbins of History: Waste Management in Late-Victorian Utopias', in Cohen and Johnson (eds), *Filth*, 225–49.
Freud, S. 'Character and Anal Erotism' [1908], in A. Richards (ed.), *On Sexuality: Three Essays on the Theory of Sexuality and Other Works* (London: Penguin, 1977), 205–15.

Freud, S. *Civilization and its Discontents* [1930], trans. J. Strachey (New York: Norton, 1961).
Frevert, U. *Krankheit als politisches Problem 1770–1880. Soziale Unterschichten in Preußen zwischen medizinischer Polizei und staatlicher Sozialversicherung* (Göttingen: Vandenhoeck und Ruprecht, 1984).
Fritzsche, P. *Stranded in the Present: Modern Time and the Melancholy of History* (Cambridge MA: Harvard University Press, 2004).
Froude, J. A. 'England's war', *Fraser's Magazine*, 3 (February 1871).
Frühstück, S. 'Male anxieties: nerve force, nation, and the power of sexual knowledge', *Journal of the Royal Asiatic Society*, 15 (2005), 71–88.
Gabriel, A. *Die staatliche Organisation des Deutschen Ärztestandes* (Berlin, 1920).
Galton, F. *Inquiries into Human Faculty and its Development* (London: Macmillan & Co., 1883).
Galton, F. 'Remarks on replies by teachers to questions respecting mental fatigue', *Journal of the Anthropological Institute*, 18 (1889), 157–68.
Galton, F. *Essays on Eugenics* (London: The Eugenics Education Society, 1909).
Ganim, R. and J. Persels (eds). *Fecal Matters in Early Modern Literature and Art: Studies in Scatology* (Aldershot: Ashgate, 2004).
Gant, F. J. *The Science and Practice of Surgery* (London: J. & A. Churchill, 1871).
Gauchet, M. 'De Pinel à Freud', in G. Swain (ed.), *Le Sujet de la folie. Naissance de la psychiatrie* (Paris: Calmann-Lévy, 1997), 7–57.
Geary, L. *Medicine and Charity in Ireland, 1718–1851* (Dublin: University College Dublin Press, 2004).
Gebhardt, H. 'Siveellisyystilastot ja ihmistahdon vapaus', *Valvoja*, 21 (1891).
Gelbart, N. 'The French Revolution as medical event: the journalistic gaze', *History of European Ideas*, 10:4 (1989), 417–27.
Gérando, J. M. *Des signes et de l'art de penser considérés dans leur rapports mutuels*, 4 vols (Paris: Chez Goujon, 1800).
Giessen, O. 'Cancer in domestic animals', *Journal of Comparative Pathology and Therapeutics*, 18 (1905), 278–9.
Gijswijt-Hofstra, M. and R. Porter (eds). *Cultures of Neurasthenia from Beard to the First World War* (Amsterdam: Rodopi, 2001).
Gilbert, P. *The Citizen's Body: Desire, Health, and the Social in Victorian England* (Columbus: Ohio State University Press, 2007).
Gilbert, P. *Cholera and Nation: Doctoring the Social Body in Victorian England* (Albany: State University of New York Press, 2008).
Gillespie, R. 'Industrial fatigue and the discipline of physiology', in J. C. Wood and M. C. Wood (eds), *George Elton Mayo: Critical Evaluations in Business Management* (London: Routledge, 2004), 429–57.

Gineste, T. *Victor de l'Aveyron. Dernier enfant sauvage, premier enfant fou* (Paris: Hachette Littératures, 2004 [1981]).
Glosser, S. 'Milk for Health, Milk for Profit: Shanghai's Chinese Dairy Industry under Japanese Occupation', in S. Cochran (ed.), *Inventing Nanjing Road: Commercial Culture in Shanghai, 1900–1945* (Ithaca, NY: Cornell University Press, 1999), 207–33.
Go, S. *Hong Kong Apothecary: A Visual History of Chinese Medicine Packaging* (New York: Princeton Architectural Press, 2003).
de Gobineau, A. 'The Inequality of Human Races', in R. Bernasconi and T. L. Lott (eds), *The Idea of Race* (Indianapolis: Hackett Publishing Company, 2000), 45–53.
Göckenjan, G. *Kurieren und Staat machen. Gesundheit und Medizin in der bürgerlichen Welt* (Frankfurt am Main: Suhrkamp, 1985).
Goddard, N. 'Nineteenth-century recycling: the Victorians and the agricultural utilisation of sewage', *History Today*, 31 (June 1981), 32–6.
Goering, L. 'Russian nervousness: neurasthenia and national identity in nineteenth-century Russia', *Medical History*, 47:1 (2003), 23–46.
Goldstein, J. *Console and Classify: The French Psychiatric Profession in the Nineteenth Century* (New York: Cambridge University Press, 1987).
Goldstein, J. *The Post-Revolutionary Self: Politics and Psyche in France, 1750–1850* (Cambridge, MA: Harvard University Press, 2005).
Goschler, C. *Rudolf Virchow. Mediziner – Anthropologe – Politiker*, 2nd edn (Köln/Weimar/Wien: Böhlau, 2009).
Gosling, F. *Before Freud: Neurasthenia and the American Medical Community* (Chicago: University of Illinois Press, 1987).
Götz, N. '"Moral economy": its conceptual history and analytical prospects', *Journal of Global Ethics*, 11 (2015), 147–62, https://doi.org/10.1080/17449626.2015.1054556. Accessed 6 February 2019.
Gourevitch, M. 'La Psychiatrie sous l'empire', *Histoire des sciences medicales*, 23:1 (1989), 27–32.
Gowers, W. R. *Epilepsy and Other Chronic Convulsive Diseases* (London: J. & A. Churchill, 1881).
Gowers, W. R. 'Fatigue', *The Quarterly Review*, 200 (October 1904).
Gray, P. *The Making of the Irish Poor Law, 1815–43* (Manchester/New York: Manchester University Press, 2009).
Greenblatt, S. 'Filthy rites', *Daedalus*, 111:3 (Summer 1982), 1–16.
Greenslade, W. *Degeneration, Culture, and the Novel, 1880–1940* (Cambridge: Cambridge University Press, 2010).
Greg, W. R. 'Life at High Pressure', *Contemporary Review* (December 1874), 623–38.
Guerrini, A. *Obesity and Depression in the Enlightenment: The Life and Times of George Cheyne* (Norman: University of Oklahoma Press, 2000).

Hacking, I. *The Taming of Chance* (Cambridge: Cambridge University Press, 1990).
Haig, A. *Diet and Food* (London: J. & A. Churchill, 1898).
Hamilton, C. I. 'Naval hagiography and the Victorian hero', *Historical Journal*, 23:2 (1980), 381–98.
Hamlin, C. *Public Health and Social Justice in the Age of Chadwick: Britain, 1800–1854* (Cambridge: Cambridge University Press, 1998).
Hamlin, C. 'Public Sphere to Public Health: The Transformation of Nuisance', in S. Sturdy (ed.), *Medicine, Health and the Public Sphere in Britain, 1600–2000* (London: Routledge, 2002), 190–204.
Hamlin, C. 'The "necessaries of life" in British political medicine, 1750–1850', *Journal of Consumer Policy*, 29 (2006), 373–97.
Hamlin, C. 'William Pulteney Alison, the Scottish philosophy, and the making of a political medicine', *Journal of the History of Medicine and Allied Sciences*, 61 (2006), 44–86.
Hamlin, C. *Sanitary Reform in the Provinces*, vol. 2 of M. Allen-Emerson, *Sanitary Reform in Victorian Britain*, 5 vols (London: Pickering and Chatto, 2012).
Hamlin, C. 'Nuisances and community in mid-Victorian England: the attractions of inspection', *Social History*, 38 (2013), 346–79.
Hamlin, C. *More than Hot: A Short History of Fever*, Johns Hopkins Biographies of Disease (Baltimore, MD: Johns Hopkins University Press, 2014).
Hampton, C. 'The Feast's Beginning: *News from Nowhere* and the Utopian Tradition', in S. Coleman and P. O'Sullivan (eds), *William Morris & News from Nowhere: A Vision for our Time* (Bideford: Green Books, 1990), 43–55.
Harrison, J. F. C. 'The Victorian gospel of success', *Victorian Studies*, 1:2 (1957), 155–64.
Harrison, M. 'Scurvy on sea and land: political economy and natural history, c. 1780–c. 1850', *Journal for Maritime Research*, 15 (2013), 7–25.
Haughton, S. *On the Natural Constants of the Healthy Urine of Man, and a Theory of Work Founded Thereon* (Dublin: Trinity College Dublin Press, 1860).
Hausman, J. G. 'Siddhars, Alchemy and the Abyss of Tradition: "Traditional" Tamil Medical Knowledge in "Modern" Practice' (PhD dissertation, University of Michigan, 1996).
Hehir, P. *The Medical Profession in India* (London: H. Frowde and Hodder & Stoughton, 1923).
Helvétius, C. A. *De l'homme, de ses facultés intellectuelles et de son éducation* (London: Société typographique, 1773).
Hendrick, H. *Child Welfare in England, 1872–1989* (London: Routledge, 1994).
Hennen, J. *Principles of Military Surgery* (Edinburgh: Archibald Constable and Co., 1820).

Henniker, B. P. 'Deaths from several zymotic and other causes, and inquest cases, in the divisions, counties, and districts of England', *Forty-Second Annual Report of the Registrar-General* (1879), 186–97.

Henriques, U. R. Q. 'Bastardy and the New Poor Law', *Past & Present*, 37 (1967), 103–29.

Herman, A. *The Idea of Decline in Western History* (New York: Free Press, 1997).

Heron, D. *On the Relation of Fertility in Man to Social Status etc.* (London: Dulau and Co., 1906).

Herrnstadt, M. 'Verwaltung des Selbst – Epistemologie des Staates. Joseph-Marie de Gérando, die Wissenschaft vom Menschen & der 18. Brumaire des Jahres VIII' (PhD dissertation, Frankfurt am Main, 2017).

Higgs, E. 'The Annual Report of the Registrar-General, 1839–1920: A Textual History', in E. Magnello and A. Hardy (eds), *The Road to Medical Statistics* (Leiden: Brill, 2002), 55–76.

Higgs, E. 'Registrar General's Reports for England and Wales, 1838–1858', *Online Historical Population Reports* http://histpop.org/. Accessed 13 October 2016.

Hill-Climo, W. 'Cancer in Ireland: an economic question', *Empire Review*, 6:34 (November 1903).

Hilton, B. *The Age of Atonement: The Influence of Evangelicism on Social and Economic Thought, 1795–1865* (Oxford: Clarendon Press, 1988).

Holmes, T. *A System of Surgery: Theoretical and Practical* (London: Longmans, Green, and Co., 1870).

Homan, P. G., B. Hudson, and R. C. Rowe. *Popular Medicines: An Illustrated History* (London/Chicago: Pharmaceutical Press, 2008).

Home, E. *Observations on Cancer: Connected with Histories of the Disease* (London: W. Bulmer and Co., 1805).

Hooff, A. *From Autothanasia to Suicide: Self-Killing in Classical Antiquity* (London: Routledge, 1990).

Howard, J. *The Plan Adopted by the Governors of the Middlesex-Hospital for the Relief of Persons Afflicted with Cancer: With Notes and Observations* (London: H. L. Galabin, 1792).

Howard Okie, A. *Ruoff's Repertory of Homoeopathic Medicine, Nosologically Arranged* (Philadelphia: J. Dobson, Kay & Brothers, & H. Hooker, 1844).

Hudemann-Simon, C. *Die Eroberung der Gesundheit 1750–1900* (Frankfurt am Main: Fischer-Taschenbuch-Verlag, 2000).

Huerkamp, C. *Aufstieg der Ärzte im 19. Jahrhundert. Vom gelehrten Stand zum professionellen Experten. Das Beispiel Preußens* (Göttingen: Vandenhoeck & Ruprecht, 1985).

Humphries, J. *Childhood and Child Labour in the British Industrial Revolution* (Cambridge: Cambridge University Press, 2010).

Huntley, H. A. *Thermo Dynamical Phenomena, or the Origin and Physical Doctrine of 'Life'* (Madras: Foster & Co., 1875).
Hurren, E. *Protesting about Pauperism* (Woodbridge: Boydell and Brewer, 2007).
Hutchinson, W. 'The cancer problem: or, treason in the republic of the body', *Contemporary Review* (July 1899), 105–17.
Huxley, T. H. *Lessons in Elementary Physiology* (London: Macmillan & Co., 1866).
Huxley, T. H. 'On the physical basis of life', *Fortnightly Review*, 5 (February 1869), 136–7.
Huxley, T. H. *Collected Essays* (London: Macmillan & Co., 1904).
Inglis, D. *A Sociological History of Excretory Experience* (Lewiston: Edwin Mellen Press, 2000).
Itard, J. *Trait, J. Edwin Mellen Press, 20et de l'audition* (Paris: Chez Méquignon-Marvis, 1821).
Itard, J. M. G. 'Second rapport fait au Ministre de l'intérieur sur les nouveaux développements et l'état actuel du sauvage de l'Aveyron', in J. M. G. Itard, *Rapports et mémoires sur le sauvage de l'Aveyron, l'idiotie et la surdi-mutité* (Paris: Progrès Médical, 1894 [1806]).
Jackson, L. *Child Sexual Abuse in Victorian England* (London: Routledge, 2000).
Jackson, M. *The Age of Stress: Science and the Search for Stability* (Oxford: Oxford University Press, 2013).
Jacyna, L. S. *Medicine and Modernism: A Biography of Sir Henry Head* (London: Pickering and Chatto, 2008).
Jacyna, L. S. *Medicine and Modernism: A Biography of Henry Head* (London: Routledge, 2015).
Jainchill, A. *Reimagining Politics after the Terror* (Ithaca, NY: Cornell University Press, 2008).
Jenkins, B. 'Phrenology, heredity and progress in George Combe's *Constitution of Man*', *British Journal for the History of Science*, 48:3 (September 2015), 455–73.
Jenner, M. S. R. 'Civilization and Deodorization? Smell in Early Modern English Culture', in P. Burke, B. Harrison, and P. Slack (eds), *Civil Histories: Essays Presented to Sir Keith Thomas* (Oxford: Oxford University Press, 2000), 127–44.
Jewson, N. D. 'The disappearance of the sick-man from medical cosmology, 1770–1870', *Sociology*, 10 (1976), 225–44.
Jones, H. B. *Lectures on Some of the Applications of Chemistry and Mechanics to Pathology and Therapeutics* (London: John Churchill & Sons, 1867).
Jones, H. B. *Croonian Lectures on Matter and Force* (London: John Churchill & Sons, 1868).

Jürgens, O. *Die Beschränkung der strafrechtlichen Haftung für ärztliche Behandlungsfehler* (Frankfurt am Main: Lang, 2005).
Kalisch, M. *Die Kunstfehler der Ärzte* (Leipzig: Veit und Comp., 1860).
Kanner, A. M. and S. C. Schachter, *Psychiatric Controversies in Epilepsy* (Amsterdam: Elsevier/Academic Press, 2008).
Karant-Nunn, S. C. *The Reformation of Feeling: Shaping the Religious Emotions in Early Modern Germany* (Oxford: Oxford University Press, 2010).
Karimi, P., E. Kamali, et al., 'Environmental factors influencing the risk of autism', *Journal of Research in the Medical Sciences* 22:27 (16 February 2017), doi 10.4103/1735-1995.200272.
Katzenmeier, C. *Arzthaftung* (Tübingen: Mohr-Siebeck, 2002).
Kelvin, N. 'The Erotic in *News from Nowhere* and *The Well at the World's End*', in C. Silver and J. R. Dunlap (eds), *Studies in the Late Romances of William Morris* (New York: William Morris Society, 1976), 97–114.
Kent, C. 'Victorian social history: post-Thompson, post-Foucault, postmodern', *Victorian Studies*, 40:1 (1996), 97–133.
Kerr, I. J. *Engines of Change: The Railroads that made India* (Westport, CA: Greenwood Publishing Group, 2007).
Killen, A. *Berlin Electropolis: Shock, Nerves, and German Modernity* (Berkeley: University of California Press, 2006).
King, G. and A. Newsholme, 'On the alleged increase of cancer', *Proceedings of the Royal Society of London*, 54 (1893), 209–42.
King, S. *Poverty and Welfare in England 1700–1850: A Regional Perspective* (Manchester: Manchester University Press, 2000).
King, S. '"Stop this overwhelming torment of destiny": negotiating financial aid at times of sickness under the English Old Poor Law, 1800–1840. Author Abstract)', *Bulletin of the History of Medicine*, 79:2 (22 June 2005), 228–60, https://doi.org/10.1353/bhm.2005.0072.
King, S. 'Regional patterns in the experiences and treatment of the sick poor, 1800–40: rights, obligations and duties in the rhetoric of paupers', *Family & Community History*, 10:1 (1 May 2007), 61–75, https://doi.org/10.1179/175138107x185256.
King, S. 'Negotiating the law of poor relief in England, 1800–1840', *History*, 96:324 (2011), 410–35, https://doi.org/10.1111/j.1468-229X.2011.00527.x.
King, S. 'Constructing the disabled child in England, 1800–1860', *Family and Community History*, 18:2 (2015), 104–21.
Kirby, P. *Child Workers and Industrial Health in Britain 1780–1850* (Woodbridge: The Boydell Press, 2013).
Kivivuori, J. *Discovery of Hidden Crime* (Oxford: Oxford University Press, 2011).
Kleinman, A. *The Illness Narratives: Suffering, Healing, and the Human Condition* (New York: Basic Books, 1988).

Kleinman, A. *Social Origins of Distress and Disease: Depression, Neurasthenia, and Pain in Modern China* (New Haven, CT: Yale University Press, 1990).
Klement, J. H. *Verantwortung. Funktion und Legitimation eines Begriffs im Öffentlichen Recht* (Tübingen: Mohr Siebeck, 2006).
Klemettilä, H. *Keskiajan julmuus* (Jyväskylä: Atena Kustannus, 2008).
Klinge, M. *Keisarin Suomi* (Espoo: Schildts Miktor, 1997).
Klinge, S. and L. Schlicht, Differenz Automat. Ein Ausschnitt aus der Geschichte des Menschen: Taubstummenforschung (um 1800) und Kybernetik (1946–1953), in M. C. Gruber, J. Bung, and S. Ziemann (eds), *Autonome Automaten. Künstliche Körper und artifizielle Agenten in der technisierten Gesellschaft* (Berlin: trafo, 2014), 103–34.
Kolnai, A. *On Disgust* (Chicago: Open Court, 2004).
Kolshus, T. and E. Hovdhaugen, 'Reassessing the death of Bishop John Coleridge Patteson', *Journal of Pacific History*, 45:3 (2010), 331–55.
König, F. F. 'Geschichte und Begriff des Kunstfehlers', *Zeitschrift für die gesamte gerichtliche Medizin*, 20 (1933), 161–72.
Kontler, L. 'Mankind and its histories: William Robertson, Georg Forster and a late eighteenth-century German debate', *Intellectual History Review*, 23:3 (2013), 411–29.
Kowalski, R. M. *Complaining, Teasing, and Other Annoying Behaviors* (New Haven, CT: Yale University Press, 2003).
Krähe, J. *Die Diskussion um den ärztlichen Kunstfehler in der Medizin des neunzehnten Jahrhunderts. Zur Geschichte eines umstrittenen Begriffes* (Frankfurt am Main: Peter Lang, 1982).
Kühner, A. *Die Kunstfehler der Ärzte vor dem Forum der Juristen* (Frankfurt am Main: Knauer, 1886).
Kühner, A. *Der ärztliche Stand und dessen besondere Gefahren. Supplement zu der Abhandlung über 'Die Kunstfehler der Aerzte' nebst einer Casuistik* (Frankfurt am Main: Knauer, 1889).
Kumar, K. '*News from Nowhere*: the renewal of utopia', *History of Political Thought*, 14 (1993), 133–43.
Kuriyama, S. 'Between Mind and Eye: Japanese Anatomy in the Eighteenth Century', in C. Leslie and A. Young (eds), *Paths to Asian Medical Knowledge* (Berkeley: University of California Press, 1992), 21–43.
Kushner, H. *Self-Destruction in the Promised Land: A Psychocultural Biology of American Suicide* (New Brunswick: Rutgers University Press, 1989).
Kushner, H. 'Suicide, gender, and the fear of modernity in nineteenth-century medical and social thought', *Journal of Social History*, 26:3 (1993), 461–90.
Kushner, H. 'Suicide, Gender and the Fear of Modernity', in J. Weaver and D. Wright (eds), *Histories of Suicide* (Toronto: University of Toronto Press, 2009), 19–52.

La Berge, A. E. *Mission and Method: The Early Nineteenth-Century French Public Health Movement* (Cambridge: Cambridge University Press, 1992).
Lahiri Choudhury, D. K. *Telegraphic Imperialism: Crisis and Panic in the Indian Empire, c. 1830–1920* (Basingstoke: Palgrave Macmillan, 2010).
Laing, E. J. *Selling Happiness: Calendar Posters and Visual Culture in Early Twentieth-Century Shanghai* (Honolulu: University of Hawai'i Press, 2004).
Landouzy, H. *Trait de l'hysterie* (Paris: J. B. & G. Balliere, 1846).
Lankester, E. R. *Degeneration: A Chapter in Darwinism* (London: Macmillan and Co., 1880).
Laporte, D. *History of Shit* (Cambridge, MA: The MIT Press, 2002).
Laprade, V. *L'Éducation homicide. Plaidoyer pour l'enfance* (Paris: Didier, 1868).
Latour, B. *The Pasteurization of France* (Cambridge: Cambridge University Press, 1988).
Lawler, C. *Consumption and Literature: The Making of the Romantic Disease* (Basingstoke: Palgrave Macmillan, 2006).
Lawrence, C. 'Disciplining Disease: Scurvy, the Navy, and Imperial Expansion, 1750–1825', in D. P. Miller and P. H. Reill (eds), *Visions of Empire* (Cambridge: Cambridge University Press, 1996), 80–106.
Lawrence, D. H. *Lady Chatterley's Lover* (New York: Grove Press, 1962).
Lears, J. *Rebirth of a Nation: The Making of Modern America, 1877–1920* (New York: Harper Collins, 2009).
Lederer, D. 'Sociology's "One Law": moral statistics, modernity, religion, and German nationalism in the suicide studies of Adolf Wagner and Alexander von Oettingen', *Journal of Social History*, 46:3 (2013), 688–9.
Ledger, S. and S. McCracken (eds), *Cultural Politics at the Fin de Siècle* (Cambridge: Cambridge University Press, 1990).
Ledger, S. and R. Luckhurst (eds), *The Fin de Siècle: A Reader in Cultural History, c. 1880–1900* (Oxford: Oxford University Press, 2000).
Leuf, E. 'Low morals at a high latitude? Suicide in nineteenth-century Scandinavia', *Journal of Social History*, 46:3 (2013), 1–16.
Levene, A. *The Childhood of the Poor: Welfare in Eighteenth-Century London* (Basingstoke: Palgrave Macmillan e-book, 2012).
Levins, R. and C. Lopez, 'Toward an Ecosocial view of health', *International Journal of Health Services*, 29 (1999), 261–93.
Levitt, T. 'The globalization of markets', *Harvard Business Review*, 83:3 (1983), 92–102.
Lewis, R. J. Sr. *Hawley's Condensed Chemical Dictionary*, 15th edn (Chichester: Wiley, 2007).
Lezay-Marnésia, A. *Des causes de la Révolution et de ses résultats* (Paris: Imprimerie du Journal d'économie publique, 1797).

Liang, S. Y. *Mapping Modernity in Shanghai: Space, Gender, and Visual Culture in the Sojourner's City, 1853–98* (London: Routledge, 2010).
Linker, B. 'On the borderland of medical and disability history', *Bulletin of the History of Medicine*, 87:4 (2013), 540–59.
Livingston, J. *Debility and the Moral Imagination in Botswana* (Bloomington: Indiana University Press, 2005).
Loeb, L. 'Doctors and patent medicines in modern Britain: professionalism and consumerism', *Albion: A Quarterly Journal Concerned with British Studies*, 33:3 (Autumn, 2001), 404–25.
Lovejoy, E. P. *Women Doctors of the World* (New York: Macmillan Company, 1957).
Löwy, I. '"Because of their praiseworthy modesty, they consult too late": regimes of hope and cancer of the womb, 1800–1910', *Bulletin of the History of Medicine*, 85 (2001), 356–83.
Luther, G. *Suomen tilastotoimen historia vuoteen 1970* (Helsinki: WSOY, 1993).
'Lydia Folger Fowler' (obituary), *Englishwoman's Review of Social and Industrial Questions* (15 February 1879), 82–3.
McBriar, A. M. *An Edwardian Mixed Doubles: The Bosanquets versus the Webbs: A Study in British Social Policy 1890–1929* (Oxford: Clarendon, 1987).
MacCabe, F. 'On mental strain and overwork', *Journal of Mental Science*, 21:95 (1 October 1875), 388–402.
McDougall, W. 'Fatigue', in *Report of the British Association for the Advancement of Science 1908* (London: John Murray, 1909).
McGinn, C. *The Meaning of Disgust* (Oxford: Oxford University Press, 2011).
MacGregor, W. 'Some problems of tropical medicine', *Lancet*, 2:13 (1900).
McIvor, A. 'Employers, the government, and industrial fatigue in Britain, 1890–1918', *British Journal of Industrial Medicine* 44:11 (1987), 724–32.
McIvor, A. 'Manual work, technology, and industrial health, 1918–39', *Medical History*, 31 (1987), 160–89.
Macleod, 'Annual Report of the Royal Naval Lunatic Asylum at Great Yarmouth', in A. Egerton (ed.), *Statistical Report of the Health of the Navy for the Year 1875* (House of Commons, 1876).
Maehle, A.-H. 'Professional ethics and discipline: the Prussian medical courts of honour, 1899–1920', *Medizinhistorisches Journal*, 34 (1999), 309–38.
Maehle, A.-H. *Doctors, Honour, and the Law: Medical Ethics in Imperial Germany* (Basingstoke: Palgrave Macmillan, 2009).
Mandler, P. 'The making of the New Poor Law redivivus', *Past & Present*, 117 (1987), 131–57.
Mandler, P. 'Tories and paupers: Christian political economy and the making of the New Poor Law', *Historical Journal*, 33 (1990), 81–101.

Margerison, K. 'P. L. Roederer: political thought and practice during the French Revolution', *Transactions of the American Philosophical Society*, 73:1 (1983), 1–166.
Marland, H. *Dangerous Motherhood: Insanity and Childbirth in Victorian Britain* (New York: Palgrave Macmillan, 2004).
Marsh, I. *Suicide: Foucault, History and Truth* (Cambridge: Cambridge University Press, 2010).
Marsh, J. 'Concerning Love: *News from Nowhere* and Gender', in S. Coleman and P. O'Sullivan (eds), *William Morris & News from Nowhere: A Vision for our Time* (Bideford: Green Books, 1990), 107–27.
Martinelli, A. *Global Modernization: Rethinking the Project of Modernity* (London: SAGE, 2005).
Marx, K. *Capital: A Critical Analysis of Capitalist Production, trans from the 3rd German Edition by Samuel Moore and Edward Aveling* (New York: International Publishing Co, 1939).
'The Massacre at Santa Cruz', *Sydney Mail and New South Wales Advertiser* (28 August 1875).
Mathews, W. 'Civilization and suicide', *The North American Review*, 152:413 (1891).
Mathias, M. 'Recycling excrement in Flaubert and Zola', *Forum for Modern Language Studies* 54:2 (2017), 224–43.
Mathisen, A. '"So that they may be useful to themselves and the community": charting childhood disability in an eighteenth-century institution', *The Journal of the History of Childhood and Youth*, 8:2 (2015), 191–210.
Matus, J. *Shock, Memory and the Unconscious in Victorian Fiction* (Cambridge: Cambridge University Press, 2009).
Maudsley, H. 'Sex in mind and in education', *Fortnightly Review*, 15 (April 1874).
Medina, J. *Brain Rules for Baby: How to Raise a Smart and Happy Child from Zero to Five* (Seattle, WA: Pear Press, 2014).
Mediratta, S. 'Beauty and the breast: the poetics of physical absence and narrative presence in Frances Burney's mastectomy letter (1811)', *Women: A Cultural Review*, 19:2 (2008), 188–207.
Menninghaus, W. *Disgust: The Theory and History of a Strong Sensation*, trans. H. Eiland and J. Golb (New York: State University of New York Press, 2003).
Merchant, C. *Autonomous Nature: Problems of Prediction and Control from Ancient Times to the Scientific Revolution* (Abingdon: Routledge, 2006).
Messer, A. B. 'An Enquiry into the Reputed Poisonous Nature of the Arrows of the South Sea Islanders', in A. Egerton (ed.), *Statistical Report of the Health of the Navy for the Year 1875* (House of Commons, 1876), 149–63.

Messer, A. B. 'Continuation of an Enquiry into the Reputed Poisonous Nature of the Arrows of the South Sea Islanders', in A. Egerton (ed.), *Statistical Report of the Health of the Navy for the Year 1876* (House of Commons, 1877), 184–98.

Messer, A. B. 'On "An inquiry into the reputed poisonous nature of the arrows of the South Sea Islanders"', *Journal of the Anthropological Institute of Great Britain and Ireland*, 7 (1878), 209–11.

Meulenbeld, G. J. *The Madhavanidana and its Chief Commentary* (Leiden: Brill, 1974).

Meulenbeld, G. J. *The History of Indian Medical Literature* (Groningen: Egbert Forsten, 1999).

Micale, M. S. *The Mind of Modernism: Medicine, Psychology, and the Cultural Arts in Europe and America, 1880–1940* (Stanford, CA: Stanford University Press, 2004).

Micale, M. S. 'Two Cultures Revisited: The Case of the Fin de Siècle', in R. Bivins and J. V. Pickstone (eds), *Medicine, Madness and Social History: Essays in Honour of Roy Porter* (Basingstoke: Palgrave Macmillan, 2007), 210–23.

Micale, M. S. *Hysterical Man: The Hidden History of Male Nervous Illness* (Cambridge, MA: Harvard University Press, 2008).

Micale, M. S. and P. Lerner (eds). *Traumatic Pasts: History, Psychiatry and Trauma in the Modern Age, 1870–1930* (Cambridge: Cambridge University Press, 2001).

Miles, M. 'Proselytizing for profit and consuming self-help: Fowlers and Wells phrenological and water-cure publications', *New York History Review* (2016) http://nyhrarticles.blogspot.com/2016/08/proselytizing-for-profit-and-consuming.html. Accessed 2 November 2017.

Milner Fothergill, J. 'Work and overwork', *Good Words*, 23 (December 1882).

Minerva, N. *Jules Verne aux confins de l'utopie* (Paris: L'Harmattan, 2001).

Minois, G. *History of Suicide: Voluntary Death in Western Culture* (Baltimore, MD: Johns Hopkins University Press, 1999).

Mittler, B. *A Newspaper for China?* (Cambridge, MA: Harvard University Asia Center, 2004).

Möhle, J. *Die Haftpflichtversicherung im Heilwesen. Eine Studie über die versicherungsrechtliche Deckung medizinischer Haftpflichtschäden* (Frankfurt am Main: Lang, 1992).

Mohun, A. *Risk: Negotiating Safety in American Society* (Baltimore, MD: Johns Hopkins University Press, 2013).

Morantz-Sanchez, R. *Sympathy and Science: Women Physicians in American Medicine* (Oxford: Oxford University Press, 1985).

More, E. S. *Restoring the Balance: Women Physicians and the Profession of Medicine, 1850–1995* (Cambridge, MA: Harvard University Press, 1999).

Morris, W. *News from Nowhere* (Oxford: Oxford University Press, 2009).

Morse, M. S. 'Facing a bumpy history; the much-maligned theory of phrenology gets a tip of the hat from modern neuroscience', *The Smithsonian Magazine* (October 1997), www.smithsonianmag.com/history/facing-a-bumpy-history-144497373/. Accessed 28 March 2017.
Morselli, E. *Suicide: An Essay on Comparative Moral Statistics* (New York: D. Appleton, 1882).
Mortimer Granville, J. *Nerve-Vibration and Excitation as Agents in the Treatment of Functional Disorder and Organic Disease* (London: J. & A. Churchill, 1883).
Moscucci, O. 'Gender and cancer in Britain, 1860–1910', *American Journal of Public Health*, 95:8 (2005), 1312–21.
Moscucci, O. *Gender and Cancer in England, 1860–1948* (Basingstoke: Palgrave Macmillan, 2016).
Moses, J. *The First Modern Risk: Workplace Accidents and the Origins of European Social States* (Cambridge: Cambridge University Press, 2018).
'Mr. Braxton Hicks on Nostrums', *The Chemist and Druggist*, 60 (March 1902), 330.
Mukharji, P. B. *Nationalizing the Body: The Medical Market, Print and Daktari Medicine* (London: Anthem Press, 2009).
Mukharji, P. B. *Doctoring Traditions: Ayurveda, Small Technologies, and Braided Sciences* (Chicago: University of Chicago Press, 2016).
Mukherjee, S. *The Emperor of All Maladies: A Biography of Cancer* (Scribner: New York, 2011).
Murard, L. and P. Zylberman (eds). *L'Hygiène dans la république: la santé publique en France, ou l'utopie contrariée (1870–1918)* (Paris: Fayard, 1996).
Murdoch, L. *Imagined Orphans: Poor Families, Child Welfare, and Contested Citizenship in London* (New Brunswick: Rutgers University Press, 2006).
Murray, A. *Suicide in the Middle Ages* (Oxford: Oxford University Press, 1999).
Murswiek, D. *Die staatliche Verantwortung für die Risiken der Technik. Verfassungsrechtliche Grundlagen und immissionsschutzrechtliche Ausformung* (Berlin: Duncker & Humblot, 1985).
Myllykangas, M. *Rappeutuminen, tiedostamaton vai yhteiskunta? Lääketieteellinen itsemurhatutkimus Suomessa vuoteen 1985 [Degeneration, unconscious, or society? Medical suicide research in Finland until 1985, doctoral thesis]* (Oulu: Universitatis Ouluensis, B 120, 2014).
Myllykangas, M. 'The History of Suicide Prevention in Finland, 1860s–2010s', in D. Kritsotaki, V. Long, and M. Smith (eds), *Preventing Mental Illness: Past, Present, Future* (London: Palgrave Macmillan, 2019), 151–70.
Myllykangas, M. 'The social engineering of suicide: psychiatric epidemiology and suicide research in Finland in the 1960s and 1970s', *Medizinhistorisches Journal*, 54:2 (2019), 145–68.

Myrtle, A. S. 'Neurasthenia – true and false', *Provincial Medical Journal*, 8:86 (1 February 1889).
Ne'eman, A. 'The Future (and the Past) of Autism Advocacy, or Why the ASA's Magazine, *The Advocate*, Wouldn't Publish This Piece', [2010], in J. Bascom (ed.), *Loud Hands: Autistic People, Speaking* (Washington: The Autistic Press, 2012).
Noakes, R. 'Natural Causes? Spiritualism, Science, and the Supernatural in Mid-Victorian Britain', in N. Brown, C. Burdett, and P. Thurschwell (eds), *The Victorian Supernatural* (Cambridge: Cambridge University Press, 2004), 23–43.
Nordau, M. *Degeneration* (London: William Heinemann, 1896 [1892]).
Nye, R. *Crime, Madness and Politics in Modern France: The Medical Concept of National Decline* (Princeton, NJ: Princeton University Press, 1984).
Oakley, C. 'Vital Forms: Bodily Energy in Medicine and Culture, 1870–1925' (PhD dissertation, University of York, 2016).
'Obituary', *British Medical Journal*, 2:3073 (1919).
O'Connor, E. *Raw Material: Producing Pathology in Victorian Culture* (London/Durham, NC: Duke University Press, 2000).
Oesterlen, O. A. 'Kunstfehler der Ärzte und Wundärzte', in J. Maschka (ed.), *Handbuch der gerichtlichen Medizin*, vol. 3 (Tübingen: Verlag der H. Laupp'schen Buchhandlung, 1882), 589–647.
Ogorek, R. *Untersuchungen zur Entwicklung der Gefährdungshaftung im 19. Jahrhundert* (Köln and Wien: Böhlau, 1975).
Omran, A. 'The epidemiological transition: a theory of the epidemiology of population change', *The Milbank Quarterly*, 83:4 (1971), 731–57.
'On the law of fatigue in the work done by men or animals', *Nature*, 22 (10 June 1880).
Oppenheim, J. *'Shattered Nerves': Doctors, Patients, and Depression in Victorian England* (Oxford: Oxford University Press, 1991).
Otis, L. *Membranes: Metaphors of Invasion in Nineteenth-Century Literature, Science, and Politics* (Baltimore, MD/London: Johns Hopkins University Press, 1999).
Otis, L. *Networking: Communicating with Bodies and Machines in the Nineteenth Century* (Ann Arbor: University of Michigan Press, 2001).
Otis, L. 'The metaphoric circuit: organic and technological communication in the nineteenth century', *Journal of the History of Ideas*, 63:1 (2002), 105–28.
Ozouf, M. 'La Révolution française et l'idée de l'homme nouveau', in C. Lucas (ed.), *The Political Culture of the French Revolution* (Oxford: Pergamon, 1988), 213–32.
Paget, J. 'Notes for a clinical lecture on dissection poisons', *Lancet*, 97 (3 June 1871).

Palmer, J. F. (ed.). *The Works of John Hunter, F.R.S.* (London: Longman, Rees, Orme, Brown, Green, & Longman, 1835).
Parker, R. *Away from Home: A History of Childcare* (Ilford: Barnardo's, 1990).
Parr, J. *Labouring Children: British Immigrant Apprentices to Canada, 1869–1924* (London: Croom Helm, 1980).
Parrinder, P. 'News from Nowhere, The Time Machine, and the break-up of classical realism', *Science Fiction Studies*, 3:3 (November 1976), 265–74.
Payne, J. F. 'The Goulstonian Lectures on the origin and relations of new growths', *British Medical Journal*, 1:688 (1874).
Pearson, J. *Practical Observations on Cancerous Complaints: With an Account of Some Diseases Which Have Been Confounded with the Cancer* (London: J. Johnson, 1792).
Petit, M. A. *Essai sur la médecine du cœur* (Lyon: Chez Garnier/Chez Reymann, 1806).
'Phrenology in England', Center for the History of Medicine (Harvard University, 2015). https://collections.countway.harvard.edu/onview/exhibits/show/talking-heads/phrenology-in-england. Accessed 13 July 2017.
Pick, D. *Faces of Degeneration: A European Disorder c. 1848–c. 1918* (Cambridge: Cambridge University Press, 1989).
Pietikäinen, P. *Neurosis and Modernity: The Age of Nervousness in Sweden* (Leiden: Brill, 2007).
Pietikäinen, P. *Madness: A History* (London: Routledge, 2015).
Pietsch, R. 'Hearts of oak and jolly tars? Heroism and insanity in the Georgian navy', *Journal for Maritime Research*, 15:1 (2013), 69–82.
Pike, D. *Subterranean Cities: The World beneath Paris and London, 1800–1945* (Ithaca, NY: Cornell University Press, 2005).
Poe, C. H. *Where Half the World is Waking Up* (Garden City, NY: Doubleday, 1912).
'Poisoned Arrows', *Tribune* (28 April 1877).
'Poisoned Arrows and Their Antidotes', *Australian Town and Country Journal* (21 April 1877).
Poore, G. V. 'On fatigue', *Lancet*, 106 (31 July 1875).
Poore, G. V. 'Exhaustion', in R. Quain (ed.), *A Dictionary of Medicine: Including General Pathology, General Therapeutics, Hygiene, and the Diseases Peculiar to Women and Children* (London: Longmans, Green, & Co, 1882).
Poovey, M. *Making a Social Body: British Cultural Formation, 1830–1864* (Chicago: University of Chicago Press, 1995).
Pordié, L. (ed.). *Tibetan Medicine in the Contemporary World: Global Politics of Medical Knowledge and Practice* (New York: Routledge, 2008).
Porter, D. *Health, Civilization and the State* (London: Routledge, 1999).
Porter, R. (ed.). *Patients and Practitioners: Lay Perceptions of Medicine in Pre-Industrial Society* (Cambridge: Cambridge University Press, 1985).

Porter, R. *The Greatest Benefit to Mankind: A Medical History of Humanity from Antiquity to the Present* (Fontana Press: London, 1999).
Porter, R. 'Nervousness, Eighteenth and Nineteenth Century Style: From Luxury to Labour', in M. Gijswijt-Hofstra and R. Porter (eds), *Cultures of Neurasthenia* (Amsterdam: Rodopi, 2001), 31–49.
Porter, T. *The Rise of Statistical Thinking 1820–1900* (Princeton, NJ: Princeton University Press, 1986).
Prebel, J. 'Head bumps to brain scans: a visual rhetorical history of scientific surveillant looking', *Enculturation* (21 August 2015), http://enculturation.net/head-bumps-to-brain-scans. Accessed 30 January 2017.
Pringle, J. *Observations on the Diseases of the Army* (London, 1752).
Püster, D. *Entwicklungen der Arzthaftpflichtversicherung* (Berlin: Springer, 2013).
Putzke, S. *Die Strafbarkeit der Abtreibung in der Kaiserzeit und in der Weimarer Zeit. Eine Analyse der Reformdiskussion und der Straftatbestände in den Reformentwürfen (1908–1931)* (Berlin: Berliner Wissenschafts-Verlag, 2003).
Quaiser, N. 'Politics, Culture and Colonialism: Unani's Debate with Doctory', in B. Pati and M. Harrison (eds), *Health, Medicine and Empire: Perspectives on Colonial India* (Hyderabad: Orient Longman, 2001), 317–55.
Quartararo, A. *Deaf Identity and Social Images in Nineteenth-Century France* (Washington: Gallaudet University Press, 2008).
R. I. S. (ed.). *The Christian Hero of Santa Cruz* (London: S. W. Partridge & Co., 1876).
Rabi, B. *Ärztliche Ethik – eine Frage der Ehre? Die Prozesse und Urteile der ärztlichen Ehrengerichtshöfe in Preußen und Sachsen 1918–1933* (Frankfurt am Main: Lang, 2002).
Rabinbach, A. 'The Body Without Fatigue: A Nineteenth-Century Utopia', in S. Drescher, D. Sabean, and A. Sharlin (eds), *Political Symbolism in Modern Europe: Essays in Honor of George L. Mosse* (New Brunswick: Transaction Books, 1982), 42–62.
Rabinbach, A. *The Human Motor: Energy, Fatigue, and the Origins of Modernity* (New York: Basic Books, 1990).
Radkau, J. 'The Neurasthenic Experience in Imperial Germany: Expeditions into Patient Records and Side-Looks upon General History', in M. Gijswijt-Hofstra and R. Porter (eds), *Cultures of Neurasthenia from Beard to the First World War* (Amsterdam: Rodopi, 2001), 199–217.
Rankin, G. 'Fatigue dyspepsia', *British Medical Journal*, 1:2842 (19 June 1915).
Rasila, V. *Torpparikysymyksen ratkaisuvaihe* (Helsinki: Suomen Historiallinen Seura, 1970).
Ray, B. 'Abataranika' [Inaugural Preface], *Chikitshak*, 1:1 (1296 BE).
Ray, B. 'Sharir Kriya Bigyan', *Chikitshak*, 1:1 (1296 BE).

Ray, B. 'Vayu Pitta Kapha', *Chikitshak*, 1:1 (1296 BE).
Ray, B. 'Rasayan Bigyan', *Chikitshak*, 1:2 (1296 BE).
Ray, B. 'Sharir Kriya Bigyan', *Chikitshak*, 1:2 (1296 BE).
Ray, B. 'Rasayan Bigyan', *Chikitshak*, 1:3 (1296 BE).
Ray, B. 'Vayu Pitta Kapha', *Chikitshak*, 1:3 (1296 BE).
Ray, B. 'Sharir Kriya Bigyan', *Chikitshak*, 1:4 (1296 BE).
Ray, B. 'Vayu Pitta Kapha', *Chikitshak*, 1:4 (1296 BE).
Ray, B. 'Ayurbbed Baigyanik?', *Chikitshak*, 3:3 (1306 BE).
Ray, B. *Podyo Ayurbbed-Shikkha* (Calcutta: Leela Printing Works, 1315 BE).
Ray, B. *Srishti-Sthiti-Pralay-Tattwa* (Calcutta: India Press, 1911).
Read, I. 'A triumphant decline? Tetanus among slaves and freeborn in Brazil', *História, ciências, saúde – Manguinhos*, 19:1 (2012), 107–32.
Reid, D. *Paris Sewers and Sewermen: Realities and Representations* (Cambridge, MA: Harvard University Press, 1991).
Renner, W. 'The spread of cancer among the descendants of the liberated Africans or Creoles of Sierra Leone', *British Medical Journal*, 2:2592 (1910).
Report on the Progress and Condition of the Royal Gardens at Kew (London: George E. Eyre and William Spottiswoode, 1879).
Riant, A. *Le Surménage intellectuel et les exercices physiques* (Paris: J. B. Baillère, 1889).
Richardson, B. W. *Diseases of Modern Life* (London: Macmillan, 1876).
Riese, W. *The Conception of Disease: Its History, Its Versions, and Its Nature* (New York: Philosophical Library, 1953).
Riley, J. C. *Sick, Not Dead: The Health of British Workingmen during the Mortality Decline* (Baltimore, MD: Johns Hopkins University Press, 1997).
Rimke, H. and A. Hunt, 'From sinners to degenerates: the medicalization of morality in the 19th century', *History of the Human Sciences*, 15:1 (2002), 59–88.
Rittgers, R. K. *The Reformation of Suffering Pastoral Theology and Lay Piety in Late Medieval and Early Modern Germany* (Oxford: Oxford University Press, 2012).
Rivers, W. H. R. *The Influence of Alcohol and Other Drugs on Fatigue* (London: Edward Arnold, 1908).
Roederer, P. L. *De la philosophie moderne et de la part qu'elle a eue a la Révolution française* (Paris: Imprimerie de Journal de Paris, 1799).
Roederer, P. L. *L'Esprit de la Révolution de 1789* (Paris: Chez les principaux libraires, 1831).
Roemer, K. M. 'Paradise Transformed: Varieties of Nineteenth-Century Utopias', in G. Claeys (ed.), *The Cambridge Companion to Utopian Literature* (Cambridge: Cambridge University Press, 2010), 79–106.

Rook, G. A. W. '99th Dahlem Conference on infection, inflammation and chronic inflammatory disorders: Darwinian medicine and the "hygiene" or "old friends" hypothesis', *Clinical and Experimental Immunology*, 160 (2010), 70–9.

Rosen, G. 'Social stress and mental disease from the eighteenth century to the present: some origins of social psychiatry', *Millibank Memorial Fund Quarterly*, 37:1 (1959), 5–32.

Rosenberg, C. E. 'The place of George M. Beard in nineteenth-century psychiatry', *Bulletin of the History of Medicine*, 36 (January 1962), 245–59.

Rosenberg, C. E. 'Catechisms of health: the body in the prebellum classroom', *Bulletin of the History of Medicine*, 69 (Summer 1995), 175–97.

Rosenberg, C. E. 'Pathologies of progress: the idea of civilization as risk', *Bulletin of the History of Medicine*, 72:4 (1998), 714–30.

Rosenberg, C. E. 'The tyranny of diagnosis: specific entities and individual experience', *The Millbank Quarterly*, 80 (2002), 237–60.

Rosenberg, C. E. 'Contested boundaries: psychiatry, disease, and diagnosis', *Perspectives in Biology and Medicine*, 49:3 (2006), 407–24, https://doi.org/10.1353/pbm.2006.0046.

Rosenberg, C. E. 'Epilogue: airs, waters, places. A status report', *Bulletin of the History of Medicine*, 86:4 (2012), 661–70.

Rosenfeld, S. *A Revolution in Language: The Problems of Signs in Late Eighteenth-Century France* (Stanford, CA: Stanford University Press, 2001).

Rosenfeld, S. 'The political uses of sign language: the case of the French Revolution', *Sign Language Studies*, 6:1 (2005), 1–37.

Rousseau, J.-J. *Émile, or on Education*, trans. Allan Bloom (New York: Basic Books, 1979).

Rousseau, J.-J. *Emile*, trans. Barbara Foxley (London: Everyman's Library, 1992).

Rozin, P. et al. 'Disgust', in L. Feldman Barrett, M. Lewis, and J. M. Haviland-Jones (eds), *Handbook of Emotions* (New York/London: Guildford Press, 2000), 637–53.

Ruff, C. B., E. Garofalo, and M. A. Holmes. 'Interpreting skeletal growth in the past from a functional and physiological perspective', *American Journal of Physical Anthropology*, 150:1 (January 1, 2013), 29–37, https://doi.org/10.1002/ajpa.22120.

Ruggiero, K. *Modernity in the Flesh: Medicine, Law, and Society in Turn-of-the-Century Argentina* (Stanford, CA: Stanford University Press, 2004).

Ruoff, A. J. F. *Repertorium für die homöopathische Praxis* (Stuttgart: Hallberger'sche Verlagshandlung, 1837).

Russell, A. F. and P. S. Twentyman-Jones, 'Dr Williams Medicine Co. vs. Alexander', *Cases Decided in the Supreme Court of the Cape of Good Hope During the Year 1905*, vol. 22 (Cape Town: J. C. Juta & Co., 1907).

Russett, C. *Sexual Science: The Victorian Construction of Womanhood* (Cambridge, MA: Harvard University Press, 1989).
Rütten, T. 'Early Modern Medicine', in M. Jackson (ed.), *The Oxford Handbook of the History of Medicine* (Oxford: Oxford University Press, 2011), 60–81.
Sachsenmaier, D., S. N. Eisenstadt, and J. Riedel (eds). *Reflections on Multiple Modernities: European, Chinese, and Other Interpretations* (Leiden: Brill, 2002).
Saelan, T. *Om sjelfmordet I Finland I statistiskt och rättsmedicinskt afseende* (Helsingfors: J. C. Frenckell & Son, 1864).
Saler, M. '"Clap if you believe in Sherlock Holmes": mass culture and the re-enchantment of modernity, c. 1890–c. 1940', *The Historical Journal*, 46:3 (2003), 599–622.
Saler, M. (ed.). *The Fin-de-Siècle World* (London: Routledge, 2015).
Salisbury, L. and A. Shail (eds). *Neurology and Modernity: A Cultural History of Nervous Systems, 1800–1950* (Basingstoke: Palgrave Macmillan, 2010).
Samson, J. *Imperial Benevolence: Making British Authority in the Pacific Islands* (Hawaii: University of Hawai'i Press, 1998).
Samson, J. 'Hero, fool or martyr? The many deaths of Commodore Goodenough', *Journal for Maritime Research*, 10:1 (2008), 1–22.
Sappol, M. *Body Modern: Fritz Kahn, Scientific Illustration, and the Homuncular Subject* (Minneapolis: University of Minnesota Press, 2017).
Savarese, R. 'From neurodiversity to neurocosmopolitanism: beyond mere acceptance and inclusion', in A. Perry and C. Herrera (eds), *Ethics and Neurodiversity* (Newcastle upon Tyne: Cambridge Scholars Publishing, 2013), 191–205.
Schacht, J. O. *Dissertatio medica inauguralis de terrore ejusque effectis in corpus humanum* [...] (Utrecht: Alexander van Megen, 1733).
Scheidemantel, F. C. G. *Die Leidenschaften als Heilmittel betrachtet* (Hildburghausen: Johann Gottfried Hanisch, 1787).
Schivelbusch, W. *The Railway Journey: The Industrialization of Time and Space in the 19th Century* (Berkeley: University of California Press, 1986).
Schoenberg, B. 'A program for the conquest of cancer: 1802', *Journal of the History of Medicine and Allied Sciences*, 30:1 (1975), 3–22.
Scott, J. C. *Weapons of the Weak: Everyday Forms of Peasant Resistance* (New Haven, CT: Yale University Press, 1985).
Scott, J. W. 'The evidence of experience', *Critical Inquiry*, 17 (1991), 773–97.
Schulman, P. 'Jules Verne's *Very* Far West: America as testing ground in *Les 500 millions de la Bégum*', *Dalhousie French Studies*, 76 (Autumn 2006), 63–71.
Schuster, D. *Neurasthenic Nation: America's Search for Health, Happiness, and Comfort, 1869–1920* (New Brunswick: Rutgers University Press, 2011).

Scull, A. *Madness in Civilization: A Cultural History of Insanity from the Bible to Freud, from the Madhouse to Modern Medicine* (Princeton, NJ: Princeton University Press, 2015).

Searle, G. R. *Eugenics and Politics in Britain, 1900–1914* (Leyden: Noordhoff International Publishing, 1976).

Seeger, P. and P. Dubois Jacobs, 'Pink Pills for Pale People', in *Pete Seeger's Storytelling Book* (San Diego/New York/London: Harcourt, 2000),

Sekula, A. 'The body and the archive', *October* 39 (Winter 1986), 3–64.

Sengoopta, C. "A Mess of Incoherent Symptoms"? Neurasthenia in British Medical Discourse, 1860–1920', in M. Gijswijt-Hofstra and R. Porter (eds), *Cultures of Neurasthenia from Beard to the First World War* (Amsterdam: Rodopi, 2001), 97–116.

Seymour, C. C. B. *Self-Made Men* (New York: Harper and Brothers, 1858).

Shakespeare, T. *Disability Rights and Wrongs* (London: Routledge, 2006).

Shapin, S. and S. Schaffer. *Leviathan and the Air Pump: Hobbes, Boyle and the Experimental Life* (Princeton, NJ: Princeton University Press, 2011).

Sharma, S. *Caraka-Samhita: Mul o Bonganubad* (Calcutta: Bhaisajya Steam Machine Jantra, 1904).

Sheffer, E. *Asperger's Children: The Origins of Autism in Nazi Vienna* (New York/London: W. W. Norton & Company, 2018).

Shuttleworth, S. *The Mind of the Child: Child Development in Literature, Science, and Medicine, 1840–1900* (Oxford: Oxford University Press, 2010).

Sicard, R. A. *Cours d'instruction d'un sourd-muet de naissance, pour servir a l'éducation des sourds-muets* (Paris: Le Cere, 1799/1800).

Sicard, R. A. 'Relation adressée par M. Abbé Sicard, Instituteur des sourds et muets, à un de ses amis, sur les dangers qu'il a courus les 2 et 3 septembre 1792', in P. J. B. Buchez and P. C. Roux (eds), *Histoire parlementaire de la Révolution française* (Paris: Paulin, vol. 18, 1835 [1797]), 72–103.

Siegel, D. J. and T. Payne Bryson, *The Whole-Brain Child: Twelve Revolutionary Strategies to Nurture Your Child's Developing Mind* (New York: Bantam Books, 2011).

Sieyès, E.-J. 'Qu'est-ce que le tiers-état?' (s.l., 1789).

Signe Morrison, S. *Excrement in the Late Middle Ages* (New York: Palgrave Macmillan, 2008).

Silberman, S. *Neurotribes: The Legacy of Autism and the Future of Neurodiversity* (New York: Avery, 2015).

Simmons, D. 'Waste not, want not: excrement and economy in nineteenth-century France', *Representations*, 96 (Autumn 2006), 73–98.

Simpson, D. 'For Science, Friendship or Personal Gain? Alexander Collie and the Origins of Naval Ethnography at Haslar Hospital Museum', in G. Sculthorpe and M. Nugent (eds), *Yurlmun: Mokare Mia Boodja* (Albany: Western Australian Museum, 2016).

Simpson, D. 'Medical collecting on the frontiers of natural history: the rise and fall of Haslar Hospital Museum (1827–1855)', *Journal of the History of Collections*, 30:2 (2018), 253–67.
Sipe, D. *Text, Image, and the Problem with Perfection in Nineteenth-Century France: Utopia and its Afterlives* (Burlington, VT: Ashgate, 2013).
Sivaramakrishnan, K. *Old Potions, New Bottles: Recasting Indigenous Medicine in Colonial Punjab (1850–1945)* (New Delhi: Orient Longman, 2006).
Skinner, A. and N. Thomas, '"A pest to society": the Charity Organisation Society's domiciliary assessments into the circumstances of poor families and children', *Children & Society*, doi 10.111/chso.12237.
Skinner, C. *Women Physicians and Professional Ethos in Nineteenth-Century America* (Carbondale, IL: Southern Illinois University Press, 2014).
Smith, F. M. and D. Wujastyk (eds), *Modern and Global Ayurveda: Pluralism and Paradigms* (Buffalo: SUNY Press, 2008).
Smith, P. J. *Between Two Stools: Scatology and its Representations in English Literature, Chaucer to Swift* (Manchester: Manchester University Press, 2012).
Smith, R. *Medical Discipline: The Professional Conduct Jurisdiction of the General Medical Council, 1858–1990* (Oxford: Clarendon Press, 1994).
Smith, R. *Between Mind and Nature: A History of Psychology* (London: Reaktion Books, 2013).
Smith, S. L. *Sick and Tired of Being Sick and Tired: Black Women's Health Activism in America, 1890–1950* (Philadelphia: University of Pennsylvania Press, 1995).
Smith, V. *Clean: A History of Personal Hygiene and Purity* (Oxford: Oxford University Press, 2007).
Snellman, J. V. 'Om Finsk Statistik', in *J. V. Snellman Samlade Arbeten IV 1844–1845* (Helsingfors: Statsrådets Kansli, 1994).
Soares, C. 'Neither Waif nor Stray: Home, Family and Belonging in the Victorian Children's Institution, 1881–1914' (PhD dissertation, University of Manchester, 2014).
Soloway, R. A. *Prelates and People: Ecclesiastical Social Thought in England 1783–1852* (London: Routledge and Kegan Paul, 1969).
Sontag, S. *Illness as Metaphor and AIDS and its Metaphors* (London: Penguin, 1991 [1968]).
Southam, G. 'The nature and treatment of cancer: being the address in surgery', *British Medical Journal*, 1:53 (1858).
Spencer, H. *First Principles* (London: Williams & Norgate, 1862).
Stanley Jevons, W. 'On the natural laws of muscular exertion', *Nature*, 2 (30 June 1870).
Stanley-Wilde, F. G. *Sleeplessness: Its Treatment by Homoeopathy, Hydropathy, and Other Accessory Means* (London: E. Gould & Son, 1879).

Starling, E. H. *Elements of Human Physiology* (London: J. & A. Churchill, 1892).

'Statue to Captain Cook, at Randwick', *The Sydney Morning Herald* (28 October 1874).

Staum, M. 'The Class of Moral and Political Sciences, 1795–1803', *French Historical Studies*, 11:3 (1980), 371–97.

Stewart, J. '"The dangerous age of childhood": child guidance and the "normal" child in Great Britain, 1920–1950', *Paedagogica Historica*, 47:6 (2011), 785–803.

Stern, M. *Heads and Headlines: The Phrenological Fowlers* (Norman: University of Oklahoma Press, 1971).

Stocking, G. *Victorian Anthropology* (London: Simon and Schuster, 1991).

Stockton, W. *Playing Dirty: Sexuality and Waste in Early Modern Comedy* (Minneapolis/London: University of Minnesota Press, 2011).

Stoddart, W. H. B. 'A theory of the toxic and exhaustion psychoses', *Journal of Mental Science*, 56:234 (July 1910).

Stolberg, M. 'Metaphors and images of cancer in early modern Europe', *Bulletin of the History of Medicine*, 88:1 (2014), 48–74.

Strachan, D. P. 'Hay fever, hygiene, and household size', *British Medical Journal*, 299 (1989), 1259–60.

Strasser, S. *Waste and Want: A Social History of Trash* (New York: Metropolitan Books, 1999).

Strauss, J. *Human Remains: Medicine, Death and Desire in Nineteenth-Century Paris* (New York: Fordham University Press, 2012).

Stroud, J. *Thirteen Penny Stamps: The Story of the Church of England Children's Society (Waifs and Strays) from 1881 to the 1970s* (London: Hodder and Stoughton, 1971).

Sullivan, H. I. 'Dirt theory and material ecocriticism', *Interdisciplinary Studies in Literature and Environment*, 19:3 (Summer 2012), 515–31.

Sullivan-Fowler, M. 'Doubtful theories, drastic therapies: autointoxication and faddism in the late nineteenth and early twentieth centuries', *Journal of the History of Medicine and Allied Sciences*, 50 (July 1995), 364–90.

Summers, A. '"The constitution violated": the female body and the female subject in the campaigns of Josephine Butler', *History Workshop Journal*, 48 (1999), 1–15.

'Superstitions of Seamen', *Leisure Hour*, 44 (28 October 1852), 692–4.

Swain, S., and M. Hillel, *Child, Nation, Race and Empire: Child Rescue Discourse, England, Canada and Australia, 1850–1915* (Manchester: Manchester University Press, 2010).

Symonds, J. A. 'A comparison of Elizabethan with Victorian poetry', *Fortnightly Review*, 45 (January 1889), 60.

Szreter, S. *Fertility, Class and Gender in Britain, 1860–1940* (Cambridge: Cambridge University Press, 1996).
Tableau des opérations de l'Assemblée nationale d'après le Journal de Paris, 2 vols (Lausanne: Chez Hignou & Comp., 1789).
Talleyrand-Périgord, C. M. *Rapport sur l'instruction publique fait au nom du Comité de constitution a l'assemblée nationale* (Paris: Baudouin/Du Pont, 1791).
Tallien, J. L. 'Speech before the *Comité de salut public*', *Moniteur* (Tridi, 13 fructidor an II = 30 August 1794, no. 343), 613.
Tarnas, R. *The Passion of the Western Mind: Understanding the Ideas that have Shaped our World View* (London: Pimlico, 1996).
Taylor, S. J. 'Insanity, philanthropy and emigration: dealing with insane children in late-nineteenth-century north-West England', *History of Psychiatry*, 25:2 (2014), 224–36.
Taylor, S. J. 'Poverty, emigration and family: experiencing childhood poverty in late-nineteenth-century Manchester', *Family and Community History*, 18:2 (2015), 89–103.
Taylor, S. J. *Child Insanity in England, 1845–1907* (Basingstoke: Palgrave Macmillan, 2016).
Teich, M., and R. Porter (eds). *Fin de Siècle and its Legacy* (Cambridge: Cambridge University Press, 1990).
Temkin, O. 'Metaphors of Human Biology', in R. C. Stauffer (ed.), *Science and Civilisation* (Madison: University of Wisconsin Press, 1949), 178–82.
Tharps, L. L. *Same Family, Different Colors: Confronting Colorism in America's Diverse Families* (Boston: Beacon Press, 2016).
Thomas, K. *Religion and the Decline of Magic* (New York: Scribner's, 1971).
Thompson, E. P. 'The moral economy of the English crowd in the eighteenth century', *Past & Present*, 50 (February 1971), 76–136.
Thompson, E. P. *Customs in Common* (New York: New Press, 1991).
Thomson, W. 'On the age of the sun's heat', *Macmillan's Magazine*, 5 (1862), 388–9.
Thomson, W. *Mathematical and Physical Papers* (Cambridge: Cambridge University Press, 1882).
Thraikill, J. F. 'Railway Spine, Nervous Excess and the Forensic Self', in Laura Salisbury and Andrew Shail (eds), *Neurology and Modernity: A Cultural History of Nervous Systems, 1800–1950* (Basingstoke: Palgrave Macmillan, 2010), 96–112.
Tobin, A. 'Brains of Those with Autism are Not Shaped Differently, Study Shows', *Times of Israel* (5 November 2014) www.timesofisrael.com/brains-of-those-with-autism-are-not-shaped-differently-study-shows/. Accessed 30 January 2017.

Tomes, N. *The Gospel of Germs: Men, Women, and the Microbe in American Life* (Cambridge, MA: Harvard University Press, 1998).
Tomlinson, S. *Head Masters: Phrenology, Secular Education, and Nineteenth-Century Social Thought* (Tuscaloosa: University of Alabama Press, 2005).
Traill, H. D. *Number Twenty: Fables and Fantasies* (London: Henry & Co., 1892).
Trautmann, T. R. *Aryans and British India* (New Delhi: Yoda Press, 2004).
Tresch, J. *The Romantic Machine: Utopian Science and Technology after Napoleon* (Chicago: University of Chicago Press, 2012).
Tresch, J. 'Cosmologies Materialized: History of Science and History of Ideas', in Darrin M. McMahon and Samuel Moyn (eds), *Rethinking Modern European Intellectual History* (New York: Oxford University Press, 2014), 153–72.
Trimble, M. R. *Post-Traumatic Neuroses: From Railway Spine to Whiplash* (Chichester: John Riley, 1981).
Triolo, V. A. 'The institution for investigating the nature and cure of cancer: a study of four excerpts', *Medical History*, 13:1 (1969), 11–28.
Trotter, D. *The Uses of Phobia: Essays on Literature and Film* (Oxford: Wiley Blackwell, 2010).
Trotter, T. *A View of the Nervous Temperament* (Newcastle: Edward Walker, 1807).
Trower, S. *Senses of Vibration: A History of the Pleasure and Pain of Sound* (London: Continuum, 2012).
Tsai, W. *Reading* Shenbao: *Nationalism, Consumerism and Individuality in China, 1919–37* (London: Palgrave Macmillan, 2010).
Turmel, A. *A Historical Sociology of Childhood* (Cambridge: Cambridge University Press 2008).
Turner, D. M. 'Impaired children in eighteenth-century England', *Social History of Medicine* 30:4 (2017), 788–806.
Turpeinen, O. *Nälkä vai tauti tappoi? Kauhunvuodet 1866–1868* (Helsinki: Suomen historiallinen seura, 1986).
United States Pharmacopeial Convention, *Food Chemicals Codex*, 7th edn (Rockville, MD: United States Pharmacopeial Convention, 2010).
University of Minnesota: Laboratory of Physiological Hygiene, *The Biology of Human Starvation* (Minneapolis: University of Minnesota Press, 1950).
Unwin, T. *Jules Verne: Journeys in Writing* (Liverpool: Liverpool University Press, 2005).
Urwin, C. 'Constructing Motherhood: The Persuasion of Normal Development', in C. Steedman, C. Urwin, and V. Walkerdine (eds), *Language, Gender and Childhood* (London: Routledge, 1985), 164–202.
Verne, J. *Les Cinq cents millions de la Bégum* (Lyon: Editions Drôles de, 2013).

Vernon, J. *Hunger: A Modern History* (Cambridge MA: Harvard University Press, 2007).
Vertinsky, P. A. *The Eternally Wounded Woman: Women, Doctors, and Exercise in the Late Nineteenth Century* (Manchester: Manchester University Press, 1990).
Vidal, F. 'Brainhood, anthropological figure of modernity', *History of the Human Sciences*, 22:1 (2009), 5–36.
Vigarello, G. *Concepts of Cleanliness: Changing Attitudes in France since the Middle Ages*, trans. J. Birrel (Cambridge: Cambridge University Press, 1988).
Virchow, R. 'Kunstfehler der Aerzte', in R. Virchow, *Gesammelte Abhandlunge aus dem Gebiet der Öffentlichen Medizin*, vol. 2 (Berlin, 1879), 514–22.
Vuorinen, H. *Tautinen historia* (Tampere: Vastapaino, 2002).
'W. T. Hanson Co. v. Collier et. Al', *The New York Supplement: Containing the Decisions of the Supreme and Lower Courts of Record of New York State. June 3–July 15, 1907*, vol. 104 (St Paul, MN: West Publishing Co., 1907), 792.
Wagar, W. W. (ed.). *The Idea of Progress Since the Renaissance* (New York: John Wiley, 1964).
Wahnich, S. *Les Émotions, la Révolution française et le present. Exercices pratiques de conscience historique* (Paris: CNRS Éd., 2009).
Wahrmann, D. *The Making of the Modern Self: Identity and Culture in Eighteenth-Century England* (New Haven, CT: Yale University Press, 2004).
Waite, F. 'Lydia Folger Fowler', *Annals of Medical History*, n.s. 4 (1932), p. 293.
Wakefield, A., S. Murch, A. Anthony, et al., 'Ileal-lymphoid-nodular hyperplasia, non-specific colitis, and pervasive developmental disorder in children', *Lancet*, 351 (1998), 637–41.
Walker, N. 'Throw Away the Master's Tools: Liberating Ourselves from the Pathology Paradigm', in J. Bascom (ed.), *Loud Hands: Autistic People, Speaking* (Washington: The Autistic Press, 2012), 225–37.
Wallerstein, I. 'Citizens all? Citizens some! The making of the citizen', *Comparative Studies in Society and History*, 45:4 (2003), 650–79.
Walshe, W. H. *The Anatomy, Physiology, Pathology and Treatment of Cancer* (Boston: William D. Ticknor & Company, 1854).
Watt, J. (ed.). *From Sin to Insanity: Suicide in Early Modern Europe* (Ithaca, NY: Cornell University Press, 2004).
Wear, A. 'Place, health, and disease: the *air, water, places* tradition in early modern England and North America', *Journal of Medieval and Early Modern Studies*, 38:3 (2008), 443–65.
Weaver, J. *A Sadly Troubled History: The Meanings of Suicide in the Modern Age* (Montreal: McGill-Queen's University Press, 2009).

Webb, B. *My Apprenticeship* (New York: AMS Press, 1977).
Wehle, W. 'Kunst und Subjektivität. Von der Geburt ästhetischer Anthropologie aus dem Leiden an Modernität – Nodier, Chateaubriand', in R. Fetz, R. Hagenbüchle, and P. Schulz (eds), *Geschichte und Vorgeschichte der modernen Subjektivität* (Berlin/New York: De Gruyter 1998), vol. 2, 901–41.
Weidner, T. *Die unpolitische Profession. Deutsche Mediziner im langen 19. Jahrhundert* (Frankfurt am Main: Campus, 2012).
Weiss, R. S. *Recipes for Immortality: Healing, Religion, and Community in South India* (Oxford: Oxford University Press, 2009).
Westcott, W. *Suicide: Its History, Literature, Jurisprudence, Causation, and Prevention* (London: H. K. Lewis, 1885).
Westerlund, F. W. *Bidrag till kännedom af Finlands natur och folk* (Helsingfors: Finska Vetenskaps-Societeten, 1900).
'Wheaton Graduate Becomes Doctor', http://wheatoncollege.edu/college-history/1850s/wheaton-graduate-doctor/. Accessed 25 March 2017.
Whitbourne, S. K. 'MRI's: the new phrenology?' *Psychology Today* (21 February 2011), https://psychologytoday.com/blog/fulfillment-any-age/201102/mris-the-new-phrenology?#. Accessed 30 January 2017.
Whorton, J. C. *Inner Hygiene: Constipation and the Pursuit of Health in Modern Society* (Oxford: Oxford University Press, 2000).
Wilde, O. *The Picture of Dorian Gray* (London: Penguin Classics, 2003 [1891]).
Wilkinson, R. and M. Marmot. *Social Determinants of Health*, 2nd edn (Oxford: Oxford University Press, 2006).
Wilks, S. 'On overwork', *Lancet*, 105 (26 June 1875).
Willan, R. *Reports on the Diseases in London* (London: H. L. Galabin, 1801).
Williams, E. *The Physical and the Moral: Anthropology, Physiology, and Philosophical Medicine in France, 1750–1850* (Cambridge: Cambridge University Press, 1994).
Williams, R. *Keywords: A Vocabulary of Culture and Society* (Oxford: Oxford University Press, 1976).
Williams, W. R. 'Cancer in the lower animals', *British Medical Journal*, 2:2021 (1899).
Williams, W. R. 'Cancer in Egypt and the causation of cancer', *British Medical Journal*, 2:2177 (1902).
Wokler, R. 'From the moral and political sciences to the sciences of society by way of the French Revolution', *Annual Review of Law and Ethics*, 8 (2000), 33–45.
World Health Organisation. *Traditional Medicine Strategy: 2014–2023* (Geneva: WHO Press, 2013).
World Health Organisation. Mission Statement. Appendix 1. http://healthydocuments.org/appendices/doc49.html. Accessed 14 March 2017.

Wright, D. 'Familial Care of "Idiot" Children in Victorian England', in P. Horden and R. Smith (eds), *The Locus of Care: Families, Communities, Institutions and the Provision of Welfare since Antiquity* (London: Routledge, 1997), 176–97.
Wright, D. *Mental Disability in Victorian England: The Earlswood Asylum, 1847–1901* (Oxford: Clarendon 2001).
Wujastyk, D. (ed.). *The Roots of Ayurveda: Selections from Sanskrit Medical Writings* (New Delhi: Penguin Books, 2003).
Wujastyk, D. 'Interpreting the image of the human body in premodern India', *International Journal of Hindu Studies*, 13:2 (2009), 189–228.
van Wyhe, J. *Phrenology and the Origins of Victorian Scientific Naturalism* (Aldershot, Ashgate, 2004).
Wyllie, I. G. *The Self-Made Man in America* (New York: Free Press, 1966).
Yeazell, R. B. 'Introduction', in R. B. Yeazell (ed.), *Sex, Politics, and Science in the Nineteenth-Century Novel* (Baltimore, MD: Johns Hopkins University Press, 1986).
Yoon, S. *Die Gefährdungshaftung für moderne Techniken. Zugleich eine Stellungnahme zum neuen Schadensersatzrecht* (Frankfurt am Main: Lang, 2002).
Young, R. M. *Mind, Brain, and Adaptation in the Nineteenth Century* (London: Oxford University Press, 1970).
Yousef, N. *Isolated Cases: The Anxieties of Autonomy in Enlightenment Philosophy and Romantic Literature* (Ithaca, NY: Cornell University Press, 2004).
Zenderland, L. *Measuring Minds: Henry Herbert Goddard and the Origins of American Intelligence Testing* (Cambridge: Cambridge University Press, 2001).
Zimmermann, F. *The Jungle and the Aroma of Meats: An Ecological Theme in Hindu Medicine* (Delhi: Motilal Banarsidass, 1999).
Zinneker, J. 'What Does the Future Hold? Youth and Sociocultural Change in the FRG', in L. Chisholm, P. Büchner, H. H. Krüger, and P. Brown (eds), *Childhood, Youth and Social Change: A Comparative Perspective* (Basingstoke: Falmer Press, 1990), 17–32.
Zlotnick, '"The law's a bachelor": Oliver Twist, bastardy, and the New Poor Law', *Victorian Literature and Culture*, 34:1 (2006), 131–46.

Index

Page references for figures are given in *italics*; for tables in the format 206t; and for notes in the format 265n.4.

abnormality 81–2, 90–1
accidents 57, 71, 92, 316
accountability 56–8, 69–72
advertisements 17–18, 247–65
   in China 254–64, 259, 261–4, 262
   Chinese language 257–64, 259, 262
   English language 251, 257, 261
   testimonials 257–8
Africa 178–9, 253
agency 46–7, 319
alternative medicine *see* Ayurveda; phrenology; 'traditional' medicine
America *see* United States of America
amputation 89
anatomy 222, 232–3
anthrax 136
antisepsis 61
anti-vaccination movements 108, 116

Asia 179, 220, 237, 275
   China 248–9, 254–65, 259, 262, 265n.4
   India 237–8, 241, 253
Asperger, Hans 113–14, 123n.94
asylums 278–9
Australia 270–1
Austria 70
authoritarianism 32–4, 46–7
autism 113–14, 115–18
Ayurveda 217–42
   versus biomedicine 222–3, 232–3
   and the body 227–35
   decline of 221–2
   doshas (elements) 226–33
      kapha (fluid) 228–9, 230, 231
      pitta (heat) 228–9, 230, 231, 232–3
      vayu (force) 228–9, 230, 231
   modernity of 219–20, 222–3
   physiograms 234–5, *234, 235*
   physiology 227–35
   prakriti (nature) 224–5

Index

and religion 230, 231
scientificity 224–7
six objects of 226–7
Snayubik Man 231–5
snayus (threads) 229, 231–2
Susruta Samhita 232–3

bacteriology 131, 133, 136, 271
Bangladesh 220
Beard, George Miller 1–3, 158–9, 209
biomedicine 108, 217–18, 222–3, 232–3
Blackwell, Elizabeth 110
blood poisoning 279, 280
body
   Ayurvedic 227–35
   baseness of 136–7
   economy of 161–2
   embodiment 19, 321
   escape from 138
   and fatigue 157–9, 163–6
   metaphors of 163–4, 183, 187
   and modernity 7, 17, 22n.25, 144
   natural rhythms 160
   optimisation of 163–6
   reticulated 227–32
   as thermodynamic engine 154, 157, 163–4
   see also anatomy; disability/impairment; physiology
brain 105–7, 116, 233, 234
British Empire 89, 186–7, 237, 241, 270–1
   see also imperialism
British Phrenological Society 103

Cabanis, Pierre-Jean-Georges 35, 42
cancer 173–88
   civilisation, disease of 177–82
   and degeneration theories 181–4

   as 'epidemic' 176–9, 184–5
   health, disease of 185–7
   metaphors of 182–5
   modernity, consequence of 173–4, 187–8
   mortality rates 176–7
   and race 178–82
   treatment of 175–6
Cannon, Walter 302–3
capitalism 100, 104, 105, 118, 161, 304–5, 314
Carpenter, William 282–3, 284
cellular pathology 183
charity 78–9, 81–8, 89–93
childbirth 65–6, 306–7
childhood 80, 84–5
children
   in advertisements 260, *262*, 263
   autistic 113
   criminal 81
   disabled/impaired 78, 80–3, 86–90, 91–2
   disease in 89–90, 92
   girls 83–4
   health of 79–80
   medical information for 112–13
   normality/abnormality of 81–2, 90–1
   orphans 84–5, 89
   'rescue'/removal of 79, 80, 86–7, 89–94
   sexual abuse of 86
   'wild' 39–42
   work of 84, 87
children's homes 83, 86, 90
China 248–9, 254–65, *259*, *262*, 265n.4
cholera 79, 139
Christianity 270–1, 274, 275, 287
cities 129–30, 131–2, 133–5, 138, 141
   see also urbanisation

civilisation 2, 6–7, 42, 146n.18, 160–3
  diseases of 177–82, 186
  fatigue, cause of 4–5, 21n.16, 160–3
  and mental illness 201–3, 278
  progress of 18–19, 274, 275
class, social 89, 102, 162, 207, 313–15, 317, 319
  middle class 87, 97n.52, 100, 102, 114, 162
  and phrenology 100–1, 114
  and stress 303–4
  working class 85–6, 100–1, 102, 167–8
cleanliness *see* hygiene
colonialism *see* British Empire; imperialism
Combe, George 102, 105
communications technology 7, 228, 229, 237
complaint 299–301, 307–8, 321
Conan Doyle, Arthur, *The Sign of Four* 272
Condillac, Etienne Bonnot de 31
Constant, Benjamin 34
control, social 45–6
Cooter, Roger 9, 217–18
cosmology 220–1, 238–41
Creole peoples 181–2
crime 81, 84, 134, 141
Cullen, William 309
culpability 84, 310, 311

deaf-muteness 36–8
death 61, 134, 137, 142, 176–7, 188, 196–7, 273
  see also suicide
debility 309–10
decadence 153–4

degeneration theories 12, 13, 15–16, 79, 139, 179–80, 212n.25
  and cancer 181–4
  and fatigue 155–6, 158–9
  and suicide 199–200
deservingness 89–93
despotism 32–3, 34
Destutt de Tracy, Antoine Louis Claude 31–2, 33–4
determinism 181, 198, 202, 207–8
diagnosis 222, 271–2, 273–4, 281–6
Dickens, Charles, *Oliver Twist* 306–9, 320
dirt 127–33, 135, 136, 139, 144–5, 312–18
  see also excrement; hygiene
disability/impairment 36–8, 117
  in children 78, 80–3, 86–90, 91–2
discrimination 89–93, 105, 114, 138
  racism 2, 102, 114, 138–9, 237
disease
  anthrax 136
  in children 89–90, 92
  cholera 79, 139
  of civilisation 177–82, 186
  debility 309–10
  eradication of 134, 137–8, 139–40, 141
  excrement-borne 79, 127–9, 130–2, 139
  gangrene 61
  of modernity 115, 158–9, 173–4, 187–8, 209–10
  moral 27–8, 29
  and mortality rates 176–7
  and progress 6–7
  scurvy 282
  sepsis 61
  syphilis 61
  tetanus 269–70, 271–3, 281–6

theories of 131, 132–4, 136, 138–9, 174
  tuberculosis 177–8
  of women 47n.4
  see also cancer
disgust 128, 136–7, 142–3
doctors
  expertise of 46, 61–2
  'failures' of 62
  and liability insurance 70–1
  licensing 63, 64–5, 67, 70, 110, 221
  litigation 59–60, 63
  misconduct 57
  power of 44
  status of 61–2
  women 109–13
  see also medicine
Dowse, Thomas Stretch 4–5, 159
Dr. Williams' Pink Pills 247–64, 265n.10, 267n.34
  advertisements 250, 251, 252, 254–64, 259, 262
  formula 251–2, 252t
  marketing 250–1, 255–6
  testimonials 257–8
  yuefenpai (poster advert) 261–4, 262
drugs 17–18
Dunn, Hugh P. 185, 186
Durkheim, Émile, *Le Suicide* 16, 198, 203
dystopias 131–2, 134

education
  of deaf-mute pupils 36–9
  of disabled/impaired pupils 89–90
  medical 221, 275–7
  'natural' 37–9
  and shock 40–1
  systems 4, 84

  and urbanisation 11–12
  of 'wild' children 39–42
efficiency 164–8
ego 41, 47
Eisenstadt, Shmuel N. 6, 219
electricity 228, 229, 237–8
embodiment 19, 321
emotion 43–7, 135, 138, 143
energy 14, 154, 156–9, 161
enlightenment 34, 35, 36, 42
entitlements 298–9, 310
entropy 157–9
environmental health *see* nuisances inspectors; public health
epidemics 176–9, 184–5
Esquirol, Jean-Étienne 43–4, 197, 203
eugenics 102, 114, 117, 123n.94, 166
evolution, theories of 12, 13, 15–16, 199–200, 202
excrement
  and disease 79, 127–9, 130–2, 139
  eradication of 135, 137
  sewerage 140–1, 315, 317
  symbolism of 141–2
  value of 140, 151n.112
exhaustion *see* fatigue; neurasthenia
experimentation 223–4, 238, 281, 284–5

faeces *see* excrement
families 83, 85–8, 92–3
famine 204–5
Farr, William 176
fatigue 153–68
  and the body 157–60, 163–6
  civilisation, consequence of 4–5, 21n.16, 160–3
  and class 162
  and degeneration 155–6, 158–9
  eradication of 163–6

metaphors of 14, 161
as 'natural' limit 159–60
overwork 158, 302–3, 304–5
pathology of 154, 158–9, 309–10
psychological 165–6
and thermodynamics 156–9
fear 32–4, 37, 39, 283, 309–10
feminism 111–12, 114
Fiji 275
filth *see* dirt; excrement
fin-de-siècle period 153–68
in Britain 155, 162–3, 167–8
decadence 153–4
optimism 163–8
Finland 194, 196–8, 204–8, 206t, 211n.13
Flammarion, Camille, *Uranie* 129, 135–9, 143
food 136–7, 204–5, 297–8, 320
Fowler, Edward Payson 109
Fowler, Lorenzo (L. N.) 100–1, 103–5, *106*, *107*, 109–10, 118
Fowler, Lydia Folger 103–5, 109–13
Fowler, Orson (O. S.) 99–101, 103, 105–7, *106*, *107*, 108–9
Fowler Ormsbee Breakspear, Almira 109
Fowler Phrenological Institute (London) 103
Fowler Wells, Charlotte 103
France 4, 27, 129–30
Institution nationale des sourds-muets 36–42
public hygiene 130–1, 140–1
Society of the Observers of Man 35–6, 39–40
see also French Revolution
free will 198, 202, 207–8
French Revolution 27–47
Consulate 36–44
and moral shock 45–7
post-Terror period 31–5
September Massacres (1792) 37
Terror 39, 43, 45
Thermidorian Convention 32–4

Gall, Franz Joseph 99–100, 101–2
Galton, Francis 114, 166
gangrene 61
Gebhardt, Hannes 208
gender 29, 83–4, 284, 285
General Medical Council (UK) 69–70
General Registry Office (GRO, UK) 176, 184–5
genetics 92, 102, 116, 139
Gérando, Joseph Marie de 41–2
germ theory 131, 132–3, 136, 138–9
Germany 4, 56, 59–60
Hanover 63–5, 66–7
legislation 58–9, 62–4, 67–8, 71
medicine, regulation of 62–4, 67–8, 70
Prussia 59–60, 65–7, 68
Goldfinch, Henry 285
Goodenough, James Graham 269–71, 273–5, 285–6
Goodman, Geoffrey 279
Grandville, J. J., *Un autre monde* 135
Great Britain *see* United Kingdom (UK)
Greg, W. R. 5

Hang Zhiying 262, 263
Hanover 63–5, 66–7
health 79–80, 116–17, 139, 185–7, 298–9
as moral economy 297–301, 307–9
national 5, 185–7
reform 111–12, 130
see also public health

heat 228, 229, 232–3
heredity 92, 102, 116, 139
Heron, David 185–6
historiography 142, 318–20
Horn, Ernst 59–60
hospitals 59–60, 61, 275–6, 278–9, 310–11
human sciences 35–6, 45
humanity 41–2, 45–6
hunger 136–7, 297–8, 320
Hutchinson, Woods 173, 174, 186
hygiene 127–31, 282
   and civilisation 127, 129, 146n.18
   and morality 136–7, 140–2
   public 130–1, 140–1, 316, 317
   sewerage 140–1, 315, 317
   utopian 131–5, 139–44
   see also dirt; excrement
hypochondria 304
hysteria 7, 59, 202, 279, 282, 284
hysterical tetanus 269–75, 281–6

illness *see* disease
impairment *see* disability/impairment
imperialism 138–9, 253–4
   and cancer 178–9, 181–2, 184, 186–7
   and Christianity 270–1, 287
   and civilisational progress 18–19, 274, 275
   and technology 237–8, 241–2
India 237–8, 241, 253
industrialisation 16, 57, 205–6, 313–14
insanity *see* mental illness
Institution nationale des sourds-muets 36–42
insurance 57, 58, 70–1
interiority 28, 30, 42

Ireland 310–11
Itard, Jean Marc Gaspard 40–1, 42

Koch, Robert 131
Kohlrausch, Heinrich 59–60
Kolnai, Aurel 142
König, Friedrich Franz 56

laboratory medicine 100, 108
labour *see* work
Lawrence, D. H., *Lady Chatterley's Lover* 313–15
legislation
   child welfare 79–80, 84
   medical negligence 58–9, 63, 67–9
   medical research 60–1
   and morality 33–4
   Poor Laws (UK) 79, 84–5, 87–8, 306–7, 308–9
Lezay-Marnésia, Adrien 34
liability 57, 58, 71
litigation 57, 58–60, 63
Locke, John 84–5

MacGregor, Sir William 181–2
Marx, Karl 304
materiality 136–8, 154, 225
Mathews, William 203
medical negligence 56–72
   definitions of 57–8, 58–9
   and innovation 60–1
   investigations 62, 64–7
   legislation 58–9, 63, 67–9
   litigation 58–60, 63
   and status of doctors 61–2
medicine
   and accountability 56–8, 69–72
   biomedicine 108, 217–18, 222–3, 232–3
   Chinese 255–6

diagnosis 222, 271–2, 273–4, 281–6
'eclectic' 109–10
education 221, 275–7
laboratory 100, 108
and modernity 9, 18–19, 101, 218–20
naval 272–7, 282
psychiatry 197–8, 200, 202–3
psychology 165–6, 282–4
quackery 17–18, 250–1
regulation 61–2, 62–4, 67–70, 108
see also Ayurveda; doctors; drugs; hospitals; 'traditional' medicine
Mellars, Henry 313, 315–19
mental illness 29, 42, 92–3, 197–8, 282–3, 287
and civilisation 202–3, 278
hysteria 7, 59, 202, 279, 282, 284
hysterical tetanus 269–75, 281–6
neurasthenia 1–3, 7–8, 158–9, 161–2
psychiatry 197–8, 200, 202–3
of sailors 275–9
stress 4–5, 28, 299, 301–6, 321
treatment of 29, 32, 43–4, 49n.19, 59
Messer, Adam Brunton 269–85
education 275–7
'hysterical tetanus', diagnosis of 269–75, 281–6
poison, investigation of 279–81
rationalism of 274–5
metaphors 14–15, 161–2, 182–5
in Ayurveda 235–41
of the body 163–4, 183, 187
of fatigue 14, 161
modern 4, 17, 235–8
technological 4, 229, 235–8, 239–40

metaphysics 37, 38
miasma theory 131, 132–3
microbes 131, 132, 136
middle class *see* class, middle class
mind, theories of 30, 31, 41–2, 233
missionaries 270–1, 274, 277–8
modernity/modernities
and the body 7, 17, 22n.25, 144
Chinese 249, 254–5
and cultural hybridity 263–4
definitions of 5–6, 21n.20
and dirt 144–5
diseases of 1–3, 115, 158–9, 173–4, 187–8, 209–10
imperial 240–2
metaphors of 17, 235–8
multiple 218–19, 240–2, 264–5
versus nature 159–60
subjectivity 28–30
and suicide 16, 194–7, 200–1, 209–10
and 'traditional' medicine 219–20, 222–3
Moi (ego) 41, 47
moral economy 297–301, 307–9, 319–21
moral shock 29–32, 43–7
morality 27–9, 33–4, 136–7, 140–2, 282
Morris, William, *News from Nowhere* 129, 139–44
Morselli, Enrico 15–16, 201–3, 207
mortality rates 61, 134, 176–7, 196–7
muteness 36–8

nations 5, 42, 183–4, 185–7
natural selection 15–16, 199–200, 202
nature 37–9, 159–60, 224–5
negligence *see* medical negligence
Neisser, Albert 61

Index

nervous system 20n.2, 161, 231, *234*, *236*, 281, 282–3
neurasthenia 1–3, 7–8, 158–9, 161–2
neurodiversity movement 116–18
neurological conditions 101, 115–18
newspapers 251, 253–4, 256–8, 259
Nordau, Max, *Degeneration* 13
normality 81–2, 90–1
nuisances 312–13
nuisances inspectors 312, 315–19

objectivity 302, 321
Oettingen, Alexander von 203, 207–8
orphans 84–5, 89
overwork 299, 302–3, 304–5

pain 137, 279, 296, 300, 305, 310–11
Papua New Guinea (British New Guinea) 182
parents/parenting 83, 85–8, 92–3
passion 43–7, 135, 138, 143
past time 141, 142
Pasteur, Louis 131, 133
patent medicines *see* Dr. Williams' Pink Pills
pathology
  cellular 183
  of civilisation 201–3
  definitions of 80–1
  of difference 90–3
  of fatigue 154, 158–9, 309–10
  of neurodiversity 114
  see also disease
Pearl, HMS 269–70, 275
Petit, Antoine 27–8, 47n.4
philanthropy 78–9, 81–8, 89–93
Phrenological Depot (New York) 103, 110
Phrenological Journal 103
Phrenologist, The (journal) 103

phrenology 99–118, *106*, *107*
  development of 99–102
  and eugenics 102, 114, 117
  and neurodiversity 113–18
  'practical' 100–1, 102, 104–7
  scientificity 107–8
  for self-improvement 100–1, 102, 104–7
physiognomy 123n.94
physiograms 231–2, *234*, *235*, *236*
physiology 112, 164–5, 222–3, 231
  Ayurvedic 227–32, 233–5
Pinel, Philippe 29, 32, 40, 45
poison 251–2, 269, 271–3, 276, 277, 279–81, 287
Poor Laws (UK) 79, 84–5, 87–8, 306–7, 308–9
Poor Law Crusade 80
Poore, George 158, 161
poverty 85, 186, 304, 306–11
pregnancy 306–7, 308–9
prejudice *see* discrimination
progress
  civilisational 18–19, 274, 275
  'dark side' 13, 34
  of enlightenment 34, 35, 42
  and imperialism 18–19, 274, 275
  metaphors of 4
  and rationality 283
  of reason 32–3, 274
  and risk 6–7
  see also degeneration theories
Prussia 59–60, 65–7, 68
psychiatry 197–8, 200, 202–3
psychology 165–6, 282–4
public health 299
  information 103, 115–16
  inspections 312–18
  reform 130–1, 140–1
  sanitation 140–1, 315–17

quackery 17–18, 250–1

race 2, 178–82, 267n.34, 278
racism 2, 102, 114, 138–9, 237
railway 5, 161, 228, 229, 237
rationality 32–3, 36, 49n.19, 274
Ray, Binodbihari 220–3, 224–9
  Ayurvedic physiology 227–35
  Chikitshak ('Physician') 221, 223, 225–6
  cosmological works 220–1, 238–41
  metaphors, use of 235–41
  Podyo Ayurbbed Siksha ('Medical Educational Verses') 220, 227–8
reform
  health 111–12, 130
  public health 130–1, 140–1
  social 104, 108–13, 317–18
religion
  and Ayurveda 230, 231
  Christianity 103, 107, 270–1, 274, 275, 287
  missionaries 270–1, 274, 277–8
  and phrenology 107
Renner, W. 181–2
research
  experimentation 223–4, 238, 281, 284–5
  laboratory medicine 100, 108
  legislation for 60–1
  mental illness 275–6
  suicide 201–3
responsibility 57, 84, 85
rest 160
revolution *see* French Revolution
rhythms, natural 160–1
Richardson, Benjamin Ward 8, 132, 305
rights 298–9, 310

risk 6–7, 57–8, 61–2, 69–72
Roederer, Pierre Louis 38–9
Rousseau, Jean-Jacques 11, 78, 80, 85
Royal Naval Hospital Haslar (UK) 275–6
Royal Navy (UK) 276–7
Rudolf, Edward 82, 86, 87
rural communities 204

Saelan, Thiodolf 197–8, 199, 201
sanitary inspectors 312, 313, 315–19
sanitation 140–1, 315–17
Santa Cruz Islands 269–70, 277, 278–80
scurvy 282
self-help 12, 100–1, 102, 103, 104–7
selfhood *see* subjectivity
Sengupta, Gopalchandra 235
Sengupta, Nagendranath 234
septicaemia 280
sewerage 140–1, 315, 317
sex/sexuality 138, 140, 143–4
sexual abuse/violence 86, 93
sexually transmitted disease 61
Seyle, Hans 302–3, 304
Shanghai 248, 264–5, 265n.4
shock 27–8, 40–1, 47
  moral 29–32, 43–7
  therapeutic 29, 32, 43–4
Sicard, Roch Ambroise 36–9, 40
Sierra Leone 181–2
sign language 36–7
slavery 138, 182
Smiles, Samuel, *Self-Help* 12
Snellman, Johan Wilhelm 196–7
Society of the Observers of Man 35–6, 39–40
Sontag, Susan, *Illness as Metaphor* 14–15
South Africa 253
South America 253–4

Index 373

South Pacific 269–70, 272, 274–80, 287
Spurzheim, Johann Gaspar 102
statistical analysis 196–7, 201, 211n.13
stress 4–5, 28, 299, 301–6, 321
strychnine 272, 280
subjectivity 46–7, 233, 302, 319, 321
  and education 40–1
  embodied 19, 321
  and fatigue 165–6
  interiority 28, 30, 42
  modern 28–30
suffering, expression of 296, 305, 307–8, 321
suicide 15–16, 194–210, 206t
  civilisation, consequence of 201–3
  as crime or sin 195–6
  and degeneration 199–200
  determinist model of 198, 202, 207–8
  medical model of 197–8, 213n.42
  modernity, consequence of 16, 194–5, 196–7, 200–1, 209–10
  research 201–3
  social model of 198–9, 204–5, 206–7
  universality of 208–10
  and urbanisation 16, 204, 213n.49
superstition 277–80, 283, 287
surgeons/surgery 61, 65–6
syphilis 61

Tallien, Jean-Lambert 33
taxonomy 105, 114, 117
technology
  communications 7, 228, 229, 237
  and imperialism 237–8, 241–2
  metaphors 4, 229, 235–8, 239–40

telegraph 7, 228, 229, 237
terror 32–3, 34, 37, 39
tetanus 269–70, 271–3, 281–6
thermodynamics 154, 156–9, 163–4
Thiele, Louise 59–60
Thompson, E. P. 297–8, 320
toilets 315, 317
'traditional' medicine 16–17, 217–20, 222–3, 255–6
  see also Ayurveda
Traill, Henry Duff 153–4
transport 5, 7, 22n.26, 161, 228, 229, 237
Trotter, Thomas 276
tuberculosis 177–8
tyranny 32–3, 34

United Kingdom (UK)
  cancer 'epidemic' 176–9
  fatigue, anxiety about 155
  fin-de-siècle period 183–4
  General Registry Office (GRO, UK) 176, 184–5
  London 103, 129–30, 141
  medicine, regulation of 69–70
  phrenology in 102, 104, 108, 110
  Poor Laws 79, 84–5, 87–8, 306–7, 308–9
  public hygiene 130–1, 140–1
  Royal Naval Hospital Haslar 275–6
  Royal Navy 276–7
  Waifs and Strays Society 78, 81–7, 89–93
United States of America (USA) 1–3, 102, 103, 107–8, 141, 252
upper class 102
urbanisation 11–12, 129–31, 204, 213n.49
  see also cities

utopias 131–45
　hygienic 131–2, 139–45
　and sex/sexuality 138, 140, 143–4

vaccination 108, 116
Verne, Jules, *Les Cinq cents millions de la Bégum* 129, 131–5, 138, 139, 143
Victor (the 'wild boy') 39–42
Virchow, Rudolph 60–1

Wagner, Adolph 203, 207–8
Waifs and Strays Society (UK) 78, 81–7, 89–93
water 32, 131, 316, 317
welfare state 57, 71
Wells, Samuel 103, 105
Westcott, William Wynn 203
Westerlund, Fredrik Wilhelm 16, 194, 195, 201, 203, 204–9
Westernisation 249, 254–5, 263
'wild' children 39–42

Wilde, Oscar, *The Picture of Dorian Gray* 167
Williams, W. Roger 182
women
　in advertisements 248–9, 260–4, 262
　and disease 47n.4
　doctors 109–13
　girls 83–4
　medical care of 111–12
　and mental illness 29
　philanthropic 79
　poor 306–11
　and technology 7
work 21n.16, 138, 154, 164, 165, 167–8
　of children 84, 87
　overwork 158, 302–3, 304–5
workhouses 90–1, 93, 306, 309, 320
working class *see* class, working class

Zhiying, Hang 262, 263